Neurological Physiotherapy

A problem-solving approach

For Churchill Livingstone:

Editorial Director (Health Professions): Mary Law
Project Development Manager: Dinah Thom
Project Manager: Derek Robertson
Design Direction: George Ajayi

Neurological Physiotherapy

A problem-solving approach

Edited by

Susan Edwards FCSP
Consultant in Neurological Physiotherapy,
London, UK

SECOND EDITION

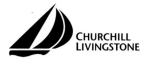

CHURCHILL LIVINGSTONE

EDINBURGH LONDON NEW YORK OXFORD PHILADELPHIA ST LOUIS SYDNEY TORONTO 2002

CHURCHILL LIVINGSTONE
An imprint of Elsevier Science Limited

First edition 1996
Second edition 2002
Reprinted 2002, 2003

ISBN 0 443 06440 7

British Library Cataloguing in Publication Data
A catalogue record for this book is available from the British Library

Library of Congress Cataloging in Publication Data
A catalog record for this book is available from the Library of Congress

Note
Medical knowledge is constantly changing. As new information becomes available, changes in treatment, procedures, equipment and the use of drugs become necessary. The editor, contributors and the publishers have taken care to ensure that the information given in this text is accurate and up to date. However, readers are strongly advised to confirm that the information, especially with regard to drug usage, complies with the latest legislation and standards of practice.

 ELSEVIER SCIENCE your source for books, journals and multimedia in the health sciences

www.elsevierhealth.com

The publisher's policy is to use paper manufactured from sustainable forests

Printed in China
N/03

Contents

Contributors

Philippa Carter MCSP
Superintendent Physiotherapist,
King's College Hospital, London, UK

Paul T. Charlton DipOrthotics DipOTC
Senior Orthotist specialising in Neurology,
J.C. Peacock & Son Ltd, Orthotic Services,
Newcastle upon Tyne

Susan Edwards FCSP
Consultant in Neurological Physiotherapy,
London, UK

Jennifer A. Freeman PhD BAppSc MCSP
Research Fellow, Institute of Neurology,
London, UK; Lecturer, University of Plymouth,
Plymouth, UK

Dawn Wendy Langdon MA MPhil PhD
CClinPsychol AFBS
Department of Psychology, Royal Holloway,
University of London, Egham, UK

Margaret J. Mayston PhD MSc BAppSc MCSP
Director, The Bobath Centre for Children with
Cerebral Palsy and Adults with Neurological
Disability; Lecturer, Department of Physiology,
University College London, London, UK

Cecily Partridge PhD BA(Hons) FCSP
Reader in Physiotherapy,
Centre for Health Services Studies,
The University of Kent, Canterbury, UK

Pauline M. Pope MSc BA FCSP
Consultant in Disability Therapy,
Mary Marlborough Centre,
Nuffield Orthopaedic Centre NHS Trust,
Oxford, UK

Alan J. Thompson MD FRCP FRCPI
Garfield Weston Professor of Clinical
Neurology and Neurorehabilitation,
Institute of Neurology, London, UK

Preface

This book aims to provide both undergraduate and qualified therapists with an improved understanding of problems commonly encountered in their work with people with neurological disability. It is a daunting process, particularly in the light of the ever-increasing availability of knowledge and information related to the control of human movement.

It must be emphasised that the perspective of this book is clinical and arises from clinical experience. This approach to management is based on using the analysis of movement as a means to evaluate disability resulting from a wide variety of neurological conditions. The need for evidence-based practice is recognised and, wherever possible, references are given to support the text. However, I have not been constrained by lack of publications in making assertions about treatment approaches. There is a continuing challenge to substantiate the constructive and functional changes demonstrated by patients treated in this manner.

There are many people who have provided invaluable support and assistance to me in compiling this second edition. Jon Marsden, senior physiotherapist at the Human Movement and Balance Unit, Queen's Square, London provided a constant supply of articles and books that enabled me to produce the first edition. For this second edition, in spite of his PhD commitments, he again found time to provide constructive comment and must take full credit for the revised section on ataxia in Chapter 5.

Numerous colleagues have read and critically appraised many of the chapters, for which I am most grateful. I hesitate to name them all for fear of inadvertently omitting one from such a large number of individuals. My thanks also go to the other authors in this book: Margaret Mayston for 'setting the scene'; Jenny Freeman for her chapter on assessment and outcome measures; Dawn Langdon and Pauline Pope for updating their previous contributions; Alan Thompson for his chapter on drug management; and Cecily Partridge for proposing 'the way forward'.

I would like to acknowledge the therapy staff in the Directorate of Neurorehabilitation and Therapy Services at the National Hospital for their continued support, despite the fact that I no longer work there, and for taking part in the original, and some of the new, photographic sessions. I also wish to thank George Kaim, head of the Audio-visual Department at the National Hospital who was responsible for many of the original photographs which, some readers may note, are unchanged from the first edition and David Waldman for the new photographs in the splinting section.

And finally my thanks to family and friends who, in spite of questioning my reasoning for embarking on a second edition, have continued to provide invaluable support and appropriate distraction. The regular bridge and sports events have gone some way to preserving some degree of sanity in an otherwise frenzied 2 years of my life.

Susan Edwards

Introduction

Susan Edwards

The purpose of this book is to describe aspects of posture and movement and difficulties which may arise as a result of neurological damage. The emphasis is on the analysis of the abnormal pathology which prevails and determining appropriate treatment interventions.

The ability to solve problems has been described as an integral part of physiotherapy practice (Newman Henry 1985). 'Problem solving' is a term often used in the management and treatment of patients with a variety of disabilities and particularly for those with neurological dysfunction. Patients with neurological disability may present with complex and extensive movement disorders in addition to cognitive and sensory impairments. Analysing these deficits and determining the most appropriate course of treatment is the aim of all staff working in this field.

Problem solving may be considered in the context of both the physiotherapist identifying the patient's problems and adopting an appropriate treatment approach and the patient himself learning to contend with the movement deficit through compensatory strategies. Much has been written with respect to the former, the terms 'clinical reasoning' and 'problem solving' often being used synonymously (Higgs 1992). The concept of the patient being a problem solver is perhaps less well recognised.

The physiotherapist as a problem solver is dependent upon an accurate and extensive knowledge of movement, taking into consideration all aspects of the impairment which may contribute to the movement deficit. The patient, unable to function in the same way as before the onset of his neurological deficit, must determine the most efficient way to contend with his disability. Function is the ultimate goal for both parties but the means by which this is attained raises several issues.

The current clinical environment requires that the therapist makes judgements that weigh the advantages and disadvantages of each intervention (Shewchuk & Francis 1988). While quality of movement is imperative for optimal function, it must be recognised that, for the majority of patients with neurological disability, restoration of normal movement is often an unattainable goal. There must be a balance between re-education of more normal movement patterns and acceptance, and indeed promotion, of necessary and desirable compensation. Patients, therefore, must be involved in the decision-making process. 'In essence, they have a PhD in their own uniqueness that is very powerful in solving complex problems' (Weed & Zimny 1989).

REFERENCES

Higgs J 1992 Developing clinical reasoning competencies. Physiotherapy 78: 575–581

Newman Henry J 1985 Identifying problems in clinical problem solving. Perceptions and interventions with nonproblem-solving behaviors. Physical Therapy 65(7): 1071–1074

Shewchuk R M, Francis K T 1988 Principles of clinical decision making – an introduction to decision analysis. Physical Therapy 68(3): 357–359

Weed L L, Zimny N J 1989 The problem-orientated system, problem knowledge coupling and clinical decision making. Physical Therapy 69(7): 565–568

1

Problem solving in neurological physiotherapy – setting the scene

Margaret J. Mayston

HISTORY

A therapist using a problem-solving approach to the management of neurological patients prior to the 1940s may have asked: How can I train the person to use their unaffected body parts to compensate for the affected parts, and how can I prevent deformity? The result was a strong emphasis on orthopaedic intervention with various types of splints, strengthening exercises and surgical intervention. However, in the 1940s several other ideas emerged, the most popular being the Bobath approach. Bobath (1985) with others, such as Peto (Forrai 1999), Kabat & Knott (1954), Voss (1967) and Rood (1954), pioneered the neurological approach to these disorders, recognising that patients with neurological impairment, in particular stroke patients, had potential for functional recovery of their affected body parts. For the child with a neurodevelopmental disorder, the approach was based on the idea that each child's development could be guided by the therapist, to maximise their potential for functional independence and minimise contractures and deformities. While the Bobath approach is one of the most used and accepted in the UK, little has been written about it in recent years, and there is no robust evidence for its efficacy (Davidson & Waters 2000).

In the last few years there has been a further progression in the neurorehabilitation field, with increasing interest in different models of central nervous system (CNS) function, skill acquisition and training. For example, for some therapists, the emphasis for retraining of the neurologically

3

impaired person now is on the biomechanical requirements of a task (Carr & Shepherd 1998), accepting that the patient has to compensate for their damaged nervous system. Carr and Shepherd are to be applauded for their well-researched approach; however, it should be recognised that their actual ideas for management largely arose from the work of Bobath. The emphasis on patient participation and practice is helpful for the cognitively and physically able person, but it is unclear how the approach can be used with people who have significant neurological impairments.

It must be realised that the nervous and musculoskeletal systems cannot be separated; they interact with each other to meet the demands of both the internal and external environment. Thus it is important to approach the person with movement disorder with a balanced view of the neural control of movement, the biomechanical requirements for a task and the limitations of CNS damage on both of these systems.

In order to use a problem-solving approach for the treatment of people with neurological disability, it is necessary to have an understanding of the control of movement, the result of damage to different areas of the CNS, neuroplasticity and ways to promote skill learning.

CONTROL OF MOVEMENT

There are many models of motor control. Some examples are neurophysiological, systems/distributed model, neurobehavioural, engineering model, information processing and biomechanical. All have value, but individually do not provide the therapist with complete information on which to base their practice. Therefore an understanding of different approaches is helpful for the therapist working in the neurorehabilitation field. The most relevant of these are discussed below.

Neurophysiological/information processing

It is recognised that there is an interaction between central and peripheral components of the CNS (see Dietz 1992 for a review). Dietz (1992) points out that neuronal mechanisms are a part of biomechanical strategies but are themselves constrained by biomechanics. This view is supported by Martenuik et al (1987) who make the following comment: 'While there are biomechanical factors which constrain movement control processes, there are also brain mechanisms which are potentially complementary to the biomechanical factors that take part in the planning and control processes. We cannot neglect one at the expense of the other ...'. What then do we need to know about the neurophysiological control of movement?

Early ideas suggested that the CNS controlled movement primarily by reacting to sensory input (Foster 1985, Sherrington 1906). Roland et al (1980) demonstrated the presence of brain activity when simply imagining a movement by studying changes in regional cerebral blood flow. This work alongside other studies of CNS activity during function (Deecke et al 1969, Shibasaki & Nagae 1984, Kristeva et al 1994) has demonstrated activity of the brain before a movement begins, and has shown that the nervous system is largely proactive and not simply reactive, in response to sensory feedback. Central (feedforward) mechanisms are based on innate and ongoing experiences of the individual and can take place in the absence of any kind of sensory feedback. Keele (1968) suggested that the CNS organises a general plan in advance of the task to be executed, referred to as the motor programme, on the basis of prior experience. Schmidt (1991) has taken up this idea of programme-based motor control, describing the comparative nature of how the brain organises the preparation and execution of movements. Much debate has taken place about the role of the motor programme and sensory feedback from the periphery in motor control (Morris et al 1994). However, it is clear that both central and peripheral factors are important in the efficient execution of motor tasks.

Central programming requires the integration of many neural structures, both supraspinal and in the periphery, to produce the required output to achieve the task goal. It is helpful to consider

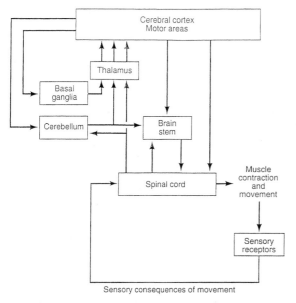

Figure 1.1   Knowledge of how different parts of the CNS connected to each other can be helpful in understanding the control of movement. (From Kandel et al 1991, p. 539.)

the wiring-type diagram which gives an idea of how different parts of the CNS interact (Fig. 1.1), but this gives little insight into the contribution of different systems to the control of movement. The advent of imaging techniques such as positron emission tomography (PET) and functional magnetic resonance imaging (fMRI) have enabled a window into the CNS to provide greater insight into how tasks are organised. For example, a recent PET study by Jueptner & Weiller (1998) shows that the cerebellum is mostly concerned with processing of sensory information during an ongoing task whereas the basal ganglia are more concerned with organisation of well-learned tasks. Neurophysiologists suggest that the CNS organises the required neural activity to perform a task on the basis of past experience, but, if prior knowledge is lacking, feedback systems will play a greater role. These of necessity take longer to effect a response. Information needs to be transmitted from the periphery to supraspinal structures for processing and the result sent via efferent pathways to the spinal cord and muscles acted on.

Feedback systems are therefore less efficient and inadequate to effect fast action.

For example, take the task of drinking from a cup. There are several stages in this process. First, there needs to be a stimulus generated, either internally or externally; for example, thirst or a social situation. On the basis of past experience, the CNS organises the required strategy to achieve the goal. Perceptual aspects such as the weight, shape and texture of the cup are essential in order for the correct grip and load forces to be computed by the CNS. Spatial concepts are important for the grading and timing of postural adjustments and the actual limb movements required to take the cup to the mouth. Oral and swallowing musculature need to be coordinated with breathing in order to have the drink without choking. A decision also needs to be made when sufficient liquid has been ingested.

Although sensory information is not necessary for tasks to occur, it is important for the fine-tuning and learning of any motor/postural task. Studies on the 'deafferented man' (neuropathy of the large-diameter pathways), have shown that tasks previously experienced by the individual can be performed in the same way, but the need for repetition results in a deterioration in the performance of the task, and an inability to learn new skills (Rothwell et al 1982). This is clearly demonstrated by the inability of the 'deafferented man' to drive a new car because the gears were organised differently from the car he had driven previously (Rothwell, personal communication). This highlights the importance of the perception and processing of sensory information not only for learning but also for the efficient execution of a required task. This is important when considering training neurologically impaired patients who may have difficulties of sensory perception or sensory processing.

It seems that the CNS operates in a task- or goal-directed way, an idea embraced by therapists using a motor learning approach (Carr & Shepherd 1998). Studies using transcranial magnetic stimulation (TMS) have shown that a muscle can be activated the same amount in two tasks, e.g. power and pincer grip, but that the task is organised in a different way by the cortex;

i.e. depending on the complexity of the task, or the prior experience of the task, the CNS will select only the necessary information for its execution (Datta et al 1989, Flament et al 1993, Harrison et al 1994). These experiments have shown that the cortex plays a lesser role in simple well-practised movements such as power grip.

Cross-correlation analysis is a useful technique to study the interactions between muscles and to learn more of the neural organisation of their activity. This computer-driven analysis programme analyses the times of occurrence of motor-unit spikes and determines the probability of two motoneurones firing at or around the same time more than expected by chance alone. This technique developed by Moore et al (1970) in their study of the simple CNS of the slug (aplysia), has been successfully applied to the study of respiratory muscles and the control of human muscle activity (Sears & Stagg 1976, Bremner et al 1991, Mayston et al 1997, Farmer et al 1998). Figure 1.2 indicates the three possible

probability histograms that can be computed. The histogram in Figure 1.2a has a short duration peak around time zero, indicating that the motoneurone pools which innervate this muscle pair receive shared synaptic input either due to branched synaptic inputs or from branched common presynaptic inputs. Figure 1.2c shows a flat histogram. From this it can be inferred that the probability of firing of motoneurone A & B is always the same and if the two motoneurones do fire simultaneously such activity occurs purely by chance alone. Figure 1.2b shows a histogram with a short duration central trough, indicating shared synaptic inputs which in this case are reciprocal, i.e. excitatory to one and inhibitory to the other. In this way the reciprocal innervation circuit described by Sherrington (1906) can easily be demonstrated using simple surface electromyographic (EMG) recordings and the appropriate computer-generated software. Using this simple technique applied to surface EMG recordings, changes in motor-unit synchronisation fol-

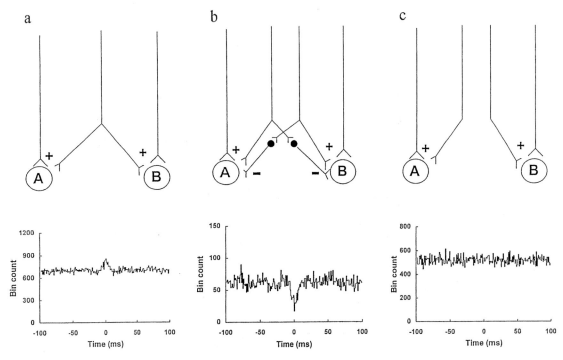

Figure 1.2 Cross-correlation analysis provides a way of examining the synaptic inputs to motoneurone pools which innervate muscle pairs.

lowing stroke have been demonstrated (Farmer et al 1993, Nadler et al 1999a). Similarly, a lack of reciprocal inhibition between antagonistic muscle pairs in healthy children younger than 5 years of age has been demonstrated and found to persist in children with spastic cerebral palsy (Mayston et al 1996, Gibbs et al 1999).

Early ideas underlying the Bobath concept emphasised the importance of reciprocal innervation circuits in the control of antagonistic muscle pairs and thus smooth coordination of movement (Bobath 1990). Bobath (1990) suggested that one of the problems for the patient with increased tone was excessive co-contraction which resulted in stiffness and slow, difficult movements for function. However, reports of abnormal co-contraction in adults with spasticity provide conflicting evidence for the presence of such co-contraction following stroke with muscle changes seemingly the primary problem in the inability to produce adequate force in the agonist, rather than antagonist restraint (Bourbonnais & Van den Noven 1989, Davies et al 1996). In contrast, for children with hypertonic

cerebral palsy, abnormal co-contraction is more common and is likely to contribute to the limb stiffness and associated difficulties in performing postural and voluntary tasks (Berger et al 1982, Leonard et al 1988, Woollacott & Burtner 1996). It is thought that for ataxia pure reciprocal inhibition without the usual overlap period of co-contraction at the reversal of movement direction results in jerky uncoordinated movement (Bobath (1997) course notes).

It is important to understand reciprocal innervation in order to appreciate how a disturbance of this mechanism may contribute to the movement problems encountered by the neurologically impaired client. Reciprocal inhibition is brought about by the reciprocal innervation circuit described by Sherrington (1906). This is shown in the simple diagrammatic representation in Figure 1.3a (Mayston 1996). It is important to note that the inhibitory interneurone which produces the inhibition of activity in the antagonistic muscle is facilitated by descending tracts, in particular the corticospinal tract. The efficiency of this reciprocal inhibition circuit

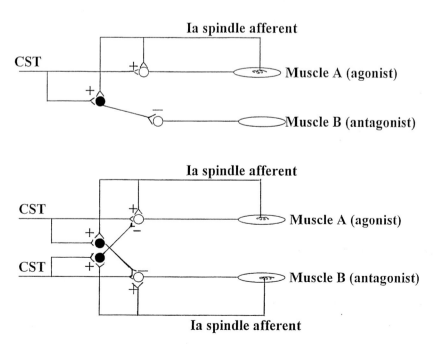

Figure 1.3 The Ia inhibitory interneurone receives input from spinal and supraspinal sources: muscle afferent (spinal) and the corticospinal tract (supraspinal).

increases with maturation of the nervous system and can be altered as a result of a cortical lesion. Reciprocal inhibition allows for the reciprocal activity of agonist and antagonist as required. For example, biceps activity is required to bend the elbow, usually occurring with the triceps relaxed (i.e. reciprocal inhibition). However, in order to produce smooth changes in the direction of the movement, the triceps co-contracts for a short time and then becomes the prime mover and the biceps is reciprocally inhibited. To explain the interaction between the agonist and antagonist when both are actively contracting, Sherrington introduced the term double reciprocal innervation, to explain how the circuits from each muscle will act simultaneously (Sherrington 1906). This is probably why Bobath (1990) emphasised the need for the healthy individual to have all degrees of reciprocal innervation in order to have well coordinated muscle activity for function. In retrospect, it is clear that Bobath placed too much emphasis on abnormalities of co-contraction in his explanation of adult neurological dysfunction, although it seems to be significant in children with spastic cerebral palsy. This is most likely because these children retain characteristics of the immature CNS, including co-contraction of the limb muscles (Forssberg 1985, Woollacott & Burtner 1996).

In summary, the neurophysiological model helps us to understand the interactions between various neural mechanisms, both central and peripheral, and indicates in particular the importance of supraspinal mechanisms for the modulation of spinal systems to produce the required control of movement.

Systems/distributed model

A therapist using a systems-based model on which to base therapy intervention helps the neurologically impaired person to problem-solve the achievement of a task goal, rather than to learn movement patterns (Shumway-Cook & Woollacott 1995). The systems approach has its origin in the work of Bernstein (1967), who suggested that an understanding of the characteristics of the system being moved (in this case the human body), and the internal and external forces acting on it, were necessary in order to understand the neural control of movement. He suggested that the control of movements was most likely distributed throughout several cooperative and interactive systems. This has been described as the distributed model of motor control. Bernstein suggested that we have many degrees of freedom: that is, we have many joints which make several types of movement such as flexion, extension and rotation. In order for coordinated movement to occur, muscles are activated together in synergies such as locomotor, postural and respiratory synergies.

To use this approach as a basis for therapy, several assumptions are made (Horak 1992). The major assumption is that movements are organised around a functional goal and achieved by the interaction of multiple systems such as the sensorimotor and the musculoskeletal systems. In addition, this organisation is also determined by environmental aspects, and emphasises the importance of the interaction between the individual and the environment. The model further hypothesises that the role of sensation is important not only for adaptive control of movement but also to the predictive control of movement. Accordingly, for the neurologically impaired person, abnormal motor control results from impairments in one or more of the systems controlling movement and their resultant attempts at achieving functional goals are produced by activity of the remaining systems, which are doing the best they can. It is the therapist's task to improve the efficiency of the person's compensatory strategies to effectively perform functional tasks. While this model may be useful, some difficulty is encountered when the contribution of each system needs to be identified and evaluated.

Engineering model

This is well described by Miall (1995), who explains that the motor system has to solve problems in response to changing sensory inputs, internal goals or errors in performance. He suggests that the motor system needs to select an appropriate action, transform control signals from sensory to motor frameworks, coordinate the selected movement with other ongoing behaviours and postural activity, and then monitor the movement to ensure its accuracy and efficacy.

In this model, the motor command is sent out to the controlled object (Fig. 1.4). In this example, the arm is the controlled object and the intended position of the arm is the reference. If the controller bases its actions on signals which are not affected by plant output (that is the sensory consequences of the action) it is said to be a feedforward controller; however, if comparisons are required – for example, between a reference signal or changing signal due to interactions with the environment – then it is a feedback controller.

This is useful for understanding how the nervous system can be both proactive and reactive, as already described in the neurophysiological model: proactive to produce activity on the basis of past performance and knowledge of outcome; and reactive to ensure that the task is executed as required in the context of the changing internal and external environments. However, there is usually a need for error correction before the command is executed and during the task performance. As Miall (1995) suggests, there are many examples of feedback control in physi-

ology, such as changes in muscle length which are detected by muscle spindles relayed to both spinal and supraspinal neural structures.

Motor systems also use this information in a feedforward way. For example, the motor command is sent to both alpha and gamma systems to ensure co-contraction of the extrafusal and intrafusal muscle fibres to enable the sensitivity of the muscle spindle to respond to unexpected load.

It must be recognised that feedback systems, although necessary for skill learning and updating of motor performance, are slow. It takes a minimum of approximately 50–100 ms for sensory information to be processed by the CNS, which for efficient postural adjustment and fine motor control is a long time.

While this is a useful model, because it assumes that the CNS acts in a linear way, there are some limitations when it is applied to brain lesions or neurophysiological recordings (Miall 1995, Loeb et al 1999).

Biomechanical model

It is possible that an overemphasis on the neural control of movement has led to a neglect of the importance of muscle strength, force production

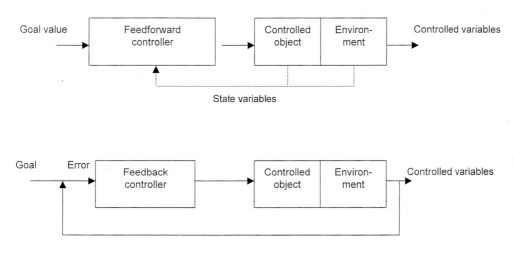

Figure 1.4 Feedforward control in the ideal situation can give perfect performance: i.e. there is no error between the reference signal and the output of the system (upper panel). A feedback system can correct performance by comparing the expected and actual outcome of a movement strategy. (Adapted from Miall 1995.)

and movement velocity. Carr & Shepherd (1998) primarily base their therapy of neurological movement disorder on principles of motor learning and biomechanics, stressing the importance of muscle length, muscle strength and activation of appropriate muscle synergies in a task-specific context. There is good evidence to support this view. Davies et al (1996) showed that a lack of force generation by paretic agonists was the major cause of reduced torque generation in a group of ambulant stroke patients. Biomechanical properties of muscle are also an important aspect of force production and changes in the distribution of muscle fibre types may also contribute to problems of force generation (Edstrom 1970, Dietz et al 1986, Ito et al 1996). It is well known that a muscle will produce optimal force at mid-range where maximal overlap of cross-bridges can occur (Rothwell 1994). Most people with neurological movement disorder demonstrate changes in muscle length which no doubt affects their ability to produce adequate force to achieve an efficient movement strategy. These changes in muscle length also alter joint alignment, which affects the ability to generate sufficient torque and efficient muscle activation patterns. It is possible that the inappropriate co-contraction of agonist and antagonist muscles results from altered biomechanical alignment *in addition* to abnormal neural control of the reciprocal inhibitory circuits between the muscle pair (Woollacott & Burtner 1996). Neurophysiotherapists must therefore consider biomechanical principles in the assessment and management of the neurologically impaired individual.

Hierarchical model

Although this model is considered outdated, it has some value when one considers the effect of the cortex on the control of movement (Lemon 1993). While it is not thought to be useful to think of higher centres controlling lower centres, the cortex is known to exert considerable control over the spinal cord and acts with subcortical areas such as the cerebellum and basal ganglia in the selection, planning and execution of motor commands (Shibasaki et al 1993, Winstein et al 1997). The

cortex though traditionally associated with the control of skilled voluntary movements, has been shown to be active during more automatic activities such as swallowing (Hamdy et al 1998) and locomotion (Schubert et al 1997, Capaday et al 1999). Another departure from the traditional view of motor control is that the spinal cord is capable of producing motor activity without any input from supraspinal centres, just as the cortex can generate commands without feedback from the periphery. This has been well described in the work on central pattern generators (Grillner 1985, Rossignol et al 1988). The central pattern generator is defined as a 'network of neurones … able to produce a repetitive, rhythmic output … that is independent of necessary sensory feedback' (Delcomyn 1980). In this way, the spinal cord via its networks of interneurones and motoneurones, can produce rhythmical, alternating lower limb movements which are the basis of locomotor activity (walking). On the other hand, fractionated finger movements necessary for fine hand control rely on the integrity of the corticospinal tract for their efficiency and are largely under cortical control (Lemon 1993, Olivier et al 1997). It is well known that a lesion affecting the corticospinal tract results in deficits of independent finger movements (Kuypers 1978, Galea & Darian-Smith 1997, Farmer et al 1993).

The view that the cortex has an important influence on control of the spinal cord's organisation of movement is also reflected in reflex studies. Matthews (1991) presents a comprehensive review of the human stretch reflex which consists of a short latency component (M1) and a long latency component (M2). This paper reviews the evidence from studies of latencies of reflex components, lesions and stimulation techniques which show that the simple stretch reflex is more complex than originally proposed by Liddell & Sherrington (1924, as cited in Matthews 1991). Matthews (1991) presents robust evidence for a transcortical route for the transmission of the long latency M2 component.

IMPLICATIONS FOR THE THERAPIST

Successful performance of a sensorimotor task requires the integrated action of the CNS.

Descending commands from the brain interact with spinal neuronal circuits, and incorporate the dynamic properties of muscles and activity of somatosensory receptors (Loeb et al 1999). From the previous discussion it can be concluded that no one model is sufficient for the therapist to apply a problem-solving approach to the management of the neurologically impaired person. The musculoskeletal system is critical to the execution of the motor command, in addition to the various cortical and subcortical areas involved in the organisation of the task. Therapists must understand the nature of the movement disorder to employ effective treatment strategies and to set appropriate goals for those individuals to maximise the potential for functional independence.

Which therapy approach?

It is thought that approximately 88% of therapists in the UK base their intervention on the Bobath concept (Sackley & Lincoln 1996, Davidson & Waters 2000). Although there have been changes to the underlying basis of the concept (Mayston 1992), the lack of relevant literature has resulted in many misconceptions and continuation of outdated ideas, such as an emphasis on reflex activity as a basis of tone and postural activity, a correspondingly misplaced emphasis on the inhibition of spasticity and an overemphasis on the significance of righting and equilibrium reactions. The following discussion attempts to clarify some of the basic ideas underlying the Bobath approach to the management of people with neurological movement disorder.

Normal and abnormal tone

It is clear from the neurophysiological and biomechanical models of motor control that the muscles themselves are important contributors to the concept of tone. The original idea proposed by Sherrington (1906) and adopted by Bobath (1990) that tone is the result of tonic reflex activity is now outdated. Tone comprises both neural and non-neural components (Basmajian et al 1985). Various definitions lead the therapist to

realise that this is the case. Basmajan et al (1985) states 'at rest a muscle has not lost its tone although there is no electrical activity in it'. Ghez (1991) describes tone as 'a slight constant tension of healthy muscles'. The definition by Bernstein (1967) that describes tone as a state of readiness seems a useful explanation. Different individuals can have differing states of readiness, as do patients with movement disorder: for example, the person with hypotonia has a reduced state of readiness, whereas the person with spasticity/hypertonia may be said to have an increased state of readiness. If tone is an important aspect of the control of movement, all factors contributing to it must be taken into account. Tone is not simply produced by tonic reflex activity – viscoelastic properties of muscle are equally important. This has significance for the movement problems of the patient with abnormal tone. It is now known that muscles which are thought to be hypertonic are in fact not usually overactive but cannot generate sufficient electrical activity to exert a force about a joint or to produce a movement (Davies et al 1996).

The controversy regarding the use of the terms 'spasticity' and 'hypertonia' is discussed in Chapter 5, but the therapist must ask this question: Am I managing spasticity, hypertonia or both?

An example of clinical practice may help to clarify the dilemma. Recently a 12-year-old child was referred for physiotherapy because of increasing 'spasticity' for which baclofen (an antispastic agent; see Chapter 7) had not been helpful. This girl presented with increasing stiffness shown by an increased flexion posture of the lower limbs and resistance to extension. Is the increased stiffness due to:

- a lack of power in anti-gravity extensor muscles and associated changes in viscoelastic muscle properties which has resulted in contractures and apparently increased tone over time, or
- is the increased stiffness due to a velocity-dependent increase in hyperreflexia?

After assessment it was clear that the major factor causing increased stiffness was muscle weakness and contracture. Therefore it was not surprising that baclofen had no effect in this case. Careful assessment of what is true spasticity as opposed to weakness, loss of dexterity and contracture (stiffness) is thus essential and may require specific testing, for example using EMG recordings, in order to be accurately determined.

Are inhibitory techniques relevant?

This altered view of tone must influence the way the therapist manages the person with abnormally increased tone. The EMG traces in Figure 1.5a show the activity recorded from the quadriceps and hamstrings of a 10-year-old child during free standing, only possible with some flexion of the hips and knees. When the child is aligned so that the hips and knees are extended, the hamstrings are no longer active and the quadriceps generate larger spike EMG, thus activating larger motor units which results in more dynamic postural activity (Fig. 1.5b). Has this child's hypertonia been 'inhibited', or rather does he now have more appropriate alignment to allow more efficient activation of the quadriceps muscle and hip extensors?

The word 'inhibition' poses many problems. Tone may be influenced (reduced) by elongating and mobilising stiff, tight joints and muscles to enable optimal activation from the required

muscles, but this is not inhibition as understood by physiologists. Inhibition in neurophysiological terms means that synapses are weakened due to reduced transmitter release or that activity in a synapse is dampened down. There are many examples of inhibition in the CNS: for example reciprocal 1a inhibition, lateral inhibition, Renshaw cell inhibition, pre- and post-synaptic inhibition. The term 'inhibition' was introduced by Bobath to explain tone reduction commensurate with the idea that hypertonia was produced by abnormal tonic reflex activity (Bobath 1990). This view can no longer be supported. Bobath therapists achieve tone reduction in various ways: mobilisation of tight joints and muscles, muscle stretch, practice of more normal movements (whole or part practice) and functional tasks.

The changes in explanations of tone and techniques of handling as viewed by paediatric Bobath therapists are summarised in Table 1.1 which shows how the understanding of abnormally increased tone has changed over several decades. Accordingly, the explanation underlying the treatment technique has also changed. It has been suggested that therapists do not so much need to change what they do, but to rethink the explanations for what they do (Gentile, personal communication). Another misleading term related to 'inhibition' is the tech-

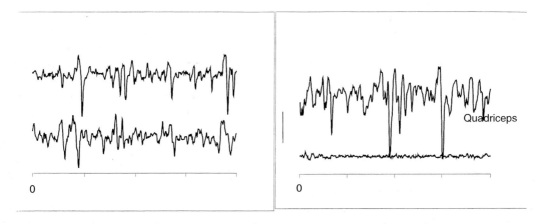

Figure 1.5 The electromyographic (EMG) activity recorded from a 10-year-old child with spastic diplegia standing without support in a typically flexed posture (a) and when held with the hips and knees extended (b). TIP = tone influencing pattern.

Table 1.1 Tone and techniques of handling

Abnormal postural tone	Handling technique	Aim of use of technique	Comment
Released tonic reflexes (1940s)	Reflex inhibiting postures (RIPs)	Inhibition of released tonic reflexes	Static – little or no movements; often opposite to pattern of spasticity
Abnormal tonic (postural) reflex activity (1960s)	Reflex inhibiting patterns (RIPs)	Simultaneous inhibition, facilitation & stimulation	Emphasis on facilitation of postural reactions
Abnormal neural and non-neural aspects of tone (1990 – present)	Tone influencing patterns (TIPs)	'Inhibition', facilitation, stimulation and biomechanical influences	Influence both the control of posture and task performance

nique of specific inhibitory mobilisations (SIMs) introduced by adult Bobath therapists. SIMs apparently stretch tight ligaments and tendons, and are therefore not inhibitory in the physiological sense. The activity of every motoneurone pool depends on the sum of the inhibitory and excitatory inputs at any moment in time. It is by altering sensory feedback due to altered task performance that the CNS, if it has the capacity to adapt, will then provide the neurologically impaired person with the possibility to move more efficiently or to regain lost skills. This neural approach to client management needs to be integrated with a biomechanical approach which takes into account the importance of muscle length, strength and joint alignment.

Postural control

The early work of the Bobaths placed a great emphasis on postural reactions, namely the righting, equilibrium and protective reactions (Bobath & Bobath 1964, 1975). They proposed that postural adjustment took place before, during and after an action, an idea shown by researchers in the postural control field (Massion 1994, Gatev et al 1999).

Unfortunately some users of the Bobath approach are still dominated by an overemphasis on these reactions, and even these are not always clearly understood. Bobath therapy is not facilitation of balance reactions, although this is the perception of some workers (Palmer et al 1988). It is perhaps important to review these reactions before a broader discussion of balance. The righting reactions are a discrete group of reactions which are only seen in the developing infant and in specific animal preparations. In the mature adult these righting reactions cannot be separated from the more complex equilibrium reactions (Bryce 1972). It is therefore incorrect to look for head righting or trunk righting in the mature adult, but rather one should determine whether an individual has the appropriate activity of the head and trunk within the equilibrium response. The equilibrium reactions are either:

- invisible changes in muscle tone which enable the maintenance of the desired posture,
- or, when greater perturbation necessitates visible activity, the response of the body being to extend/elongate the weight-bearing side with flexion of the non-weight-bearing side with some rotation within the body axis. The degree of rotation depends on the direction of the perturbation. When the perturbation is too large or too fast then the protective reactions come in to protect the individual from injury and to assist in restoration of the centre of gravity to lie within the base of support.

In summary, balance in the mature adult is achieved by equilibrium and protective reactions; righting reactions cannot be observed. In the developing infant the various righting reactions can be observed, but early in development become a part of the equilibrium reactions which commence in prone at approximately 3 months of age when the infant can maintain the prone position with head lifting and weight on elbows.

For several years, balance has been viewed in a functional way by the Bobath Centre, London, recognising that the central command for an action includes both the postural and task-related components (Rothwell 1994). Balance reactions are complex responses based on prior experience in addition to the CNS response to unexpected perturbations occurring during task execution (Horak & Nashner 1986). There seems to be much controversy about how balance should be trained in people with neurological movement disorder. Should balance be trained separately or as part of the task goal? For the developing infant the experience of a posture precedes the attainment of postural control in that posture. For example, an infant is propped in sitting to practise using their hands before independent sitting is possible. Thus, for some patients, it could be reasonable to assume that it is necessary to give them the idea of the postural activity required for a task and then to add in the task component. Both components need to be practised simultaneously for the training to be effective. Similarly, testing of sitting balance is not achieved by testing righting and equilibrium reactions, but rather by assessing the person's possibilities to reach in all directions for objects or to carry out activities as in the performance of tasks of daily life. This ability relies not only on sensorimotor activity but also on the perceptual ability of the individual (Massion 1994), which should be considered as part of the postural mechanism to be taken into account during therapy and the goals adjusted accordingly. If a person's instability is primarily caused by a perceptual deficit, simply training balance reactions will not address the main problem.

It would be preferable to view balance as an adaptable background to skill performance and to train it in the appropriate functional context, rather than emphasising the different groups of reactions (righting, equilibrium and protective) as being responsible for postural control.

Compensation

Compensation is another term which has different meaning for therapists, neurologists and movement scientists. If the nervous system is damaged in some way, then there will necessarily be compensation by the system for the damage sustained. This can take many forms, which may include plastic changes such as muscle adaptation and cortical reorganisation.

How the patient moves in response to their neurological reorganisation is another question. Shepherd & Carr (1991) suggest that the way in which the neurologically impaired person attempts to achieve a goal represents the best that can be done given the state of the neural and musculoskeletal systems. The questions we might ask are: How much does the person need to compensate? Can they function more efficiently and compensate less? For example, a stroke patient will prefer to use the unaffected side, only using the stroke-affected side when absolutely necessary and only if physically possible. However, the work of Bobath (1990) and evidence provided by Taub & Wolf (1997) has shown that by training of the stroke-affected side it is possible that, for some patients, fewer compensatory movements will be required because more effective movement is possible on the stroke side. No therapist should try and stop a patient moving in a certain way unless they can replace it with an alternative strategy which achieves the same goal. Concern for quality of movement needs to be realistic.

Associated reactions

Associated reactions (see Chapter 5) are another example of confusion in neurophysiotherapy and represent one of the greatest controversies and possibly mysteries in the neurological therapeutic world in the UK (Stephenson et al 1998).

Early positioning and the avoidance of effort were advocated by Bobath (1990) to reduce the effect of associated reactions which in the long-term might lead to contracture and reduce the potential for functional recovery. The main features of the management of these reactions in the more able client were:

- The client should be taught strategies to reduce them when they occurred. For example, using the sound arm to stretch out the affected side.
- To train more normal activity of the affected side to reduce effort and therefore the severity of the associated reactions. It was suggested that improving balance on the stroke-affected

side could lead to less effort in the maintenance of balance and less increase of tone in the upper limb associated with the need to balance.

However, there is no evidence to suggest that preventing a person who has had a stroke from moving in the early stages of recovery will influence spasticity and associated reactions; in fact, it may be detrimental to the client's potential for CNS recovery and thus functional recovery.

THE NATURE OF THE MOVEMENT DISORDER

It would seem that therapists have become so enthusiastic in the control of tone that other factors, such as weakness and dexterity, have assumed less importance. But a purely biomechanical view cannot be supported either. Neural damage that results in dysfunction of cortical and subcortical areas, particularly the descending tracts, reduces neural drive onto the motoneurone pool and results in reduced force generation which will not necessarily be regained. Thus there will always be a degree of weakness and loss of power. Muscle imbalance will be accompanied by muscle shortening, another contributor to lost ability to generate force – for example in walking (Ada et al 1998).

It has been shown in children with cerebral palsy (CP) that the inability selectively to activate muscles is in part due to a lack of synchronisation of muscles (Gibbs et al 1999). Axons usually branch to innervate several motoneurone pools to bring about the cooperative action of the muscles for a required task (Bremner et al 1991), or are activated synchronously if flexible strategies are required by the task (Gibbs et al 1995). This is one aspect of function of the corticospinal tract known to be disrupted when there is brain injury. Abnormal synchronisation of motor unit activity has been demonstrated in people with dystonia (Farmer et al 1998) and those with hemiplegic stroke (Farmer et al 1993, Nadler et al 1999), although the functional significance of this is unclear Another aspect of the movement disorder associated with spasticity in children is

co-contraction of antagonistic muscle pairs (Leonard et al 1991, Woollacott & Burtner 1996, Gibbs et al 1999). There are varying reports of co-contraction of antagonistic muscle pairs in adults with hypertonia, but the phenomenon seems less common. It is likely that weakness and altered viscoelastic properties of muscle are a more likely explanation of the stiffness experienced and felt in adult patients with increased tone (Gowland et al 1992, Davies et al 1996).

THE WAY FORWARD

Neuroplasticity

Plasticity underlies all skill learning and is a part of CNS function in healthy and brain-damaged individuals at any age (Leonard 1998).

The advent of imaging techniques such as PET and fMRI in conjunction with neurophysiological recordings in primates and humans has provided evidence of the plasticity of the CNS. In a study of monkeys following amputation of digit 3, it was shown that adjacent areas of the sensory cortex expanded to take over the representation of the lost digit (Merzenich et al 1984). Plasticity of the sensory cortex has also been induced through behavioural training. The tips of the second and third fingers were stimulated with a rotating disk, which resulted in an expansion of the sensory representation of those digits (Jenkins et al 1990). This suggests that sensory stimulation, if given effectively and often enough, can expand sensory areas of the cortex and may have implications for therapy.

Plastic changes have also been demonstrated in the motor system as a result of motor training. Recent work by Nudo and his group (Nudo et al 1992) has shown that training a hand expanded the cortical areas represented by the muscles executing that task. A later study by his group has shown that lesioning the motor cortex of a monkey and then training motor activity during recovery resulted in greater recovery of skill than the untrained group, and reduced loss of cortical tissue in the area surrounding the infarct (Nudo et al 1996). The effect of training of a novel motor skill in healthy human adults has also demonstrated changes in sensorimotor function (Nadler et al 1998). In this study subjects were trained to simultaneously flex the index finger (first dorsal interosseous; 1DI) and abduct the fifth finger (abductor digiti minimi; ADM). Before, during and after the training period, cutaneomuscular reflexes in response to stimulation of the digital nerves of the index finger were recorded. After a short period of training (2–3 days), the long-latency components of the reflex were significantly larger. This indicates that the sensory fields of the two muscles had expanded and come to lie closer together in the sensory cortex, so that the sensory input now reached the two muscles rather than just the 1DI. This correlate of Nudo's work in training motor skill in monkeys (Nudo et al 1992) suggests that motor training and skill learning can be detected using simple reflex testing and may be useful as a means of monitoring the effects of therapy in clients with neurological disability.

Skill learning

Practice is fundamental for motor learning and improving skill in both healthy and movement-impaired individuals (Taub et al 1993, Winstein et al 1997). Two other principles of equal significance are active participation and working to achieve meaningful goals. Therapy programmes should be based on these three principles and can be enhanced by 'preparation'.

The Bobath approach has been much criticised for its use of preparation for function (Shepherd 1995, Carr & Shepherd 1998), but this has been misunderstood. Preparation given as a treatment is of no value on its own, and must be incorporated into useful activity (Bobath 1965, unpublished notes). It includes the following:

- mobilisation of tight connective tissue and/or joints
- elongating muscles to enable activity from a better biomechanical advantage, to achieve better body alignment for more efficient balance and muscle activation
- practice of task-component parts to enable the patient to get the idea of the movement required

- practising in a functional task which the patient wants to achieve. To do this requires realistic goal setting.

Bobath (personal communication) suggested that it is what the neurologically impaired person can do with some assistance that is their potential. However, it is of little use to the person if these potentially achievable skills can only be practised with the therapist's help. When required, it is appropriate and important to enlist the help of others to enable the person to practise activities which are possible, with a little help, to achieve independently. Equally it is of no use to the person to be prevented from trying to practise activities because there is a danger of increasing spasticity through the occurrence of associated reactions. Indications are that early training will enable less secondary loss of cortical tissue and thus enable greater possibilities for recovery (Nudo et al 1996).

Can we predict outcomes?

Part of the realistic setting of goals (see Chapter 2) depends on having realistic expectations of the individual's optimal potential based on the therapist's expertise. However, neurophysiological tests such as TMS and reflex testing may also be used to predict recovery. Turton et al (1996) in their study were able to identify two patient groups (A = rapid recovery; B = slow and incomplete recovery) and further categorised them on the basis of EMG recordings and responses to TMS. While responses to TMS could be elicited from all muscles in group A from the outset, in the slow recovery group, the ability to elicit TMS responses was commensurate with the subsequent activation of hand muscles. In this way TMS provided a prognostic test for the return of muscle activity.

Nadler et al (1999b) studied the cutaneomuscular reflexes (see Jenner & Stephens 1982) of a small cohort of people who had a stroke. Their results suggest that those subjects in whom a large short-latency reflex response is recorded are unlikely to make a good recovery. Similarly, stroke patients who present with transient mirror movements early in recovery usually regain good function of that side (clinical observation).

However, not all therapy departments have access to these diagnostic and prognostic tools; therefore, for the moment, the clinical experience and the problem-solving ability of the therapist in the context of a knowledge and understanding of current research literature remains the main way to determine realistic goals for each client's management.

REFERENCES

Ada L, Vattanaslip W, O'Dwyer N J, Crosbie J 1998 Does spasticity contribute to walking dysfunction after stroke. Journal of Neurology, Neurosurgery and Psychiatry 64: 628–635

Basmajan J V, De Luca C J 1985 Muscles alive. Their functions revealed by electromyography. Williams and Wilkins, Baltimore, ch 10 and 11

Berger W, Quintern J, Dietz V 1982 Pathophysiology of gait in children with cerebral palsy. Electroencephalography and Clinical Neurophysiology 53: 538–548

Bernstein N 1967 The co-ordination and regulation of movements. Pergamon, Oxford

Bobath B 1985 Abnormal postural reflex activity caused by brain lesions, 3rd edn. William Heinemann Medical Books, London

Bobath B 1990 Adult hemiplegia: evaluation and treatment, 3rd edn. Heinemann Medical Books, London

Bobath B 1997 Bobath course notes (8-week paediatric course). The Bobath Centre, London

Bobath B, Bobath K 1964 The facilitation of normal postural reactions and movements in the treatment of cerebral palsy. Physiotherapy 50: 246–262

Bobath B, Bobath K 1975 Motor development in the different types of cerebral palsy. Heinemann Medical Books, London

Bourbonnais D, Van den Noven S 1989 Weakness in patients with hemiparesis. American Journal of Occupational Therapy 43: 676–685

Bremner F D, Baker J R, Stephens J A 1991 Correlation between the discharges of motor units recorded from the same and from different finger muscles in man. Journal of Physiology (London) 432: 355–380

Bryce J 1972 Facilitation of movement – the Bobath approach. Physiotherapy 58: 403–408

Capaday C, Lavoie B A, Barbeau H, Schneider C, Bonnard M 1999 Studies on the corticospinal control of human walking. 1. Responses to focal transcranial magnetic stimulation. Journal of Neurophysiology 81: 129–139

Carr J, Shepherd R 1998 Neurological rehabilitation – optimizing motor performance. Butterworth-Heinemann, Oxford

Datta A K, Harrison L M, Stephens J A 1989 Task-dependent changes in the size of response to magnetic brain stimulation in human first dorsal interosseous muscle. Journal of Physiology (London) 418: 13–23

Davidson I, Waters K 2000 Physiotherapists working with stroke patients: a national survey. Physiotherapy 86: 69–80

Davies J M, Mayston M J, Newham D J 1996 Electrical and mechanical output of the knee muscles during isometric and isokinetic activity in stroke and healthy adults. Disability and Rehabilitation 18: 83–90

Deecke L, Scheid P, Kornhuber H H 1969 Distribution of readiness potential, pre-motion positivity, and motor potential of the human cerebral cortex preceding voluntary finger movements. Experimental Brain Research 7: 158–168

Delcomyn F 1980 Neural basis of rhythmic behaviour in animals. Science 210: 492–498

Dietz V 1992 Human neuronal control of automatic functional movements: interaction between central programs and afferent input. Physiological Review 72: 33–69

Dietz V, Ketelsen U P, Berger W, Quintern J 1986 Motor unit involvement in spastic paresis. Relationship between leg muscle activation and histochemistry. Journal of Neurological Science 75: 89–103

Edstrom L 1970 Selective changes in the sizes of red and white muscle fibres in upper motor lesions and parkinsonism. Journal of Neuroscience 11: 537–550

Farmer S F, Swash M, Ingram D A, Stephens J A 1993 Changes in motor unit synchronization following central nervous lesions in man. Journal of Physiology (London) 463: 83–105

Farmer S F, Sheean G L, Mayston M J et al 1998 Abnormal motor unit synchronization of antagonist muscles underlies pathological co-contraction in upper limb dystonia. Brain 121: 801–814

Flament D, Goldsmith P, Buckley C J, Lemon R N 1993 Task dependence of responses in first dorsal interosseous muscles to magnetic brain stimulation in man. Journal of Physiology (London) 464: 361–378

Forrai 1999 Memoirs of the beginnings of conductive pedagogy and Andras Peto. Uj Aranyhid Budapest and the Foundation of Conductive Education, Birmingham

Forssberg H 1985 Ontogeny of human locomotor control. I. Infant stepping, supported locomotion and transition to independent locomotion. Experimental Brain Research 57: 480–493

Foster M 1985 A textbook of physiology. MacMillan, New York

Galea M G, Darian-Smith I 1997 Manual dexterity and corticospinal connectivity following unilateral lesion of the cervical spinal cord in the macaque monkey. Journal of Comparative Neurology 381: 307–319

Gatev P, Thomas S, Kepple T, Hallett M 1999 Feedforward ankle strategy of balance during quiet stance in adults. Journal of Physiology (London) 514: 915–928

Ghez C 1991 Muscles: effectors of the motor systems In: Kandel E R, Schwartz J H, Jessell T M (eds) Principles of neuroscience, 3rd edn. Elsevier, Amsterdam.

Gibbs J, Harrison L M, Stephens J A 1995 Organization of inputs to motoneurone pools in man. Journal of Physiology (London) 485: 245–256

Gibbs J, Harrison L M, Stephens J A 1999 Does abnormal branching of inputs to motor neurones explain abnormal muscle cocontraction in cerebral palsy? Developmental Medicine and Child Neurology 41: 465–472

Gowland C, de Bruin H, Basmajan J V, Plews N, Burcea I 1992 Agonist and antagonist activity during voluntary upper limb movement in patients with stroke. Physical Therapy 43: 624–633

Grillner S 1985 Neurobiological bases of rhythmic motor acts in vertebrates. Science 228: 143–149

Hamdy S, Rothwell J C, Quasim A, Singh K D, Thompson D G 1998 Long-term reorganisation of human motor cortex driven by short-term sensory stimulation. Nature Neuroscience 1: 64–68

Harrison L M, Mayston M J, Gibbs J, Stephens J A 1994 Central mechanisms underlying task dependence of cutaneous reflexes in man. Journal of Physiology 476: 18P

Horak F B 1992 Motor control models underlying neurologic rehabilitation of posture in children. In: Forssberg H, Hirschfeld H (eds) Movement disorders in children. Medicine and sport science series. Karger, Basel, Vol. 36, 21–30

Horak F B, Nashner L M 1986 Central programming of postural movements: adaptation to altered support-surface configurations. Journal of Neurophysiology 55: 1369–1381

Ito J, Araki A, Tanaka H, Tasaki T, Cho K, Yamazaki R 1996 Muscle histopathology in spastic cerebral palsy. Brain Development 18: 299–303

Jenkins W M, Merzenich M M, Ochs M T, Allard T, Guic-Robles E 1990 Functional reorganisation of primary somatosensory cortex in adult owl monkeys after behaviourally controlled tactile stimulation. Journal of Neurophysiology 63: 82–104

Jenner J R, Stephens J A 1982 Cutaneous reflex responses and their central nervous pathways studied in man. Journal of Physiology (London) 333: 405–419

Jueptner M, Weiller C 1998 A review of differences between basal ganglia and cerebellar control of movements as revealed by functional imaging studies. Brain 121: 1437–1449

Kabat H, Knott M 1954 Proprioceptive facilitation therapy for paralysis. Physiotherapy 40: 171–176

Kandel E R, Schwartz J H, Jessell 1991 Principles of neural science, chs 36–40, 3rd edn. Elsevier, Amsterdam

Keele S W 1968 Movement control in skilled motor performance. Psychology Bulletin 70: 387–403

Kristeva Feige R, Walter H, Lutkenhoner B et al 1994 A neuromagnetic study of the functional organization of the sensorimotor cortex. European Journal of Neuroscience 6: 632–639

Kuypers H G 1978 The motor system and the capacity to execute highly fractionated distal extremity movements. Electroencephalography and Clinical Neurophysiology Supplement 429–431

Lemon R N 1993 The G. L. Brown Prize Lecture. Cortical control of the primate hand. Experimental Physiology 78: 263–301

Leonard C T 1998 The neuroscience of human movement. Mosby, St Louis

Leonard C T, Hirschfeld H, Forssberg H 1988 Gait acquisition and reflex abnormalities in normal children and children with cerebral palsy. In: Amblard B, Berthoz A, Clarac F (eds) Posture and gait: development, adaptation and modulation. Elsevier Science (Biomedical Division), Amsterdam

Leonard C T, Hirschfeld H, Forssberg H 1991 The development of independent walking in children with cerebral palsy. Developmental Medicine and Child Neurology 33: 567–577

Loeb G E, Brown I E, Cheng E J 1999 A hierarchical foundation for models of sensorimotor control. Experimental Brain Research 126: 1–18

Martenuik R G, MacKenzie C L, Jennerod M, Athenes S, Dugas C 1987 Constraints on human arm movement trajectories. Canadian Journal of Psychology 41: 365–378

Massion J 1994 Postural control system. Current Opinions in Neurobiology 4: 877–887

Matthews P B 1991 The human stretch reflex and the motor cortex. Trends in Neuroscience 14(3): 87–89

Mayston M J 1992 The Bobath concept – evolution and application. In: Forssberg H, Hirschfeld H (eds) Movement disorders in children. Karger, Basel

Mayston M J 1996 Mechanisms underlying cocontraction during development and in pathology in man. PhD thesis, University of London

Mayston M J, Harrison L M, Stephens J A 1996 Co-contraction of antagonistic muscles during development and in children with cerebral palsy. Journal of Physiology 494: 67P

Mayston M J, Harrison L M, Quinton R, Krams M, Bouloux P-M G, Stephens J A 1997 Mirror movements in X-linked Kallmann's syndrome. I. A neurophysiological study. Brain 120: 1199–1216

Merzenich M, Nelson R J, Stryker M P, Cynader M S, Schoppmann A, Zook J M 1984 Somatosensory map changes following digit amputation in adult monkeys. Journal of Comparative Neurology 224: 591–605

Miall R 1995 In: Arbib M (ed) The handbook of brain theory and neural networks. MIT Press, Cambridge, Massachusetts, pp 597–600

Moore G P, Segundo J P, Perkel D H, Levitan H 1970 Statistical signs of synaptic interaction in neurons. Biophysics Journal 10: 876–900

Morris M E, Summers J J, Matyas T A, Iansek R 1994 Current status of the motor program. Physical Therapy 74: 738–748

Nadler M A, Harrison L M, Moore M, Townend E, Stephens J A 1998 Acquisition of a new motor skill is accompanied by changes in cutaneomuscular reflexes recorded from finger muscles in man. Journal of Physiology 511 P

Nadler M A, Harrison L M, Stephens J A 1999a Motor-unit synchronization between pairs of hand muscles is latered following stroke in man. Journal of Physiology 518P: 63P

Nadler M A, Harrison L M, Stephens J A 1999b Changes in cutaneomuscular reflexes following stroke in man: a two year longitudinal study. Society for Neuroscience Abstracts 52.14

Nudo R J, Jenkins W M, Merzenich M M 1992 Neurophysiological correlates of hand preference in primary motor cortex of adult squirrel monkeys. Journal of Neuroscience 12: 2918–2947

Nudo R J, Wise B M, SiFuentes F, Milliken G W 1996 Neural substrates for the effects of rehabilitative training on motor recovery after ischaemic infarct. Science 272: 1791–1794

Olivier E, Edgley S A, Armand J, Lemon R N 1997 An electrophysiological study of the postnatal development of the corticospinal system in the macaque monkey. Journal of Neuroscience 17: 267–276

Palmer F B, Shapiro B K, Wachtel R C et al 1988 The effects of physical therapy on cerebral palsy: a controlled trial in infants with spastic diplegia. New England Journal of Medicine 318: 803–808

Roland P E, Larsen B, Lassen N A, Skinhoj E 1980 Supplementary motor area and other cortical areas in organization of voluntary movements in man. Journal of Neurophysiology 43: 118–136

Rood M S 1954 Neurophysiologic reactions: a basis for physical therapy. Physical Therapy Review 34: 444–449

Rossignol S, Lund J P, Drew T 1988 The role of sensory inputs in regulating patterns of rhythmical movements in higher vertebrates. A comparison between locomotion, respiration and mastication. In: Cohen A H, Rossignol S, Grillner S (eds) Neural control of rhythmic movements in vertebrates. Wiley, New York

Rothwell J C 1994 Control of human voluntary movement, 2nd edn. Chapman Hall, London

Rothwell J C, Traub M M, Day B L, Obeso J A, Thomas P K, Marsden C D 1982 Manual motor performance in a deafferented man. Brain 105: 525–542

Sackley C M, Lincoln N B 1996 Physiotherapy for stroke patients: a survey of current practice. Physiotherapy Theory and Practice 12: 87–96

Schmidt R A 1991 Motor learning and performance: from principles to practice. Human Kinetics Publishers, Leeds

Schubert M, Curt A, Jensen L, Dietz V 1997 Corticospinal input in human gait: modulation of magnetically evoked responses. Experimental Brain Research 115: 234–246

Sears T A, Stagg D 1976 Short-term synchronization of intercostal motoneurone activity. Journal of Physiology (London) 263: 357–381

Shepherd R B 1995 Physiotherapy in paediatrics. Butterworth-Heinemann, Oxford

Shepherd R B, Carr J H 1991 An emergent or dynamical systems view of movement dysfunction. Australian Journal of Physiotherapy 37: 5–17

Sherrington C S 1906 The integrative action of the nervous system. Yale University Press, New Haven

Shibasaki H, Sadato N, Lyshkow H et al 1993 Both primary motor cortex and supplementary motor area play an important role in complex finger movement. Brain 116: 1387–1398

Shibasaki H, Nagae K 1984 Mirror movements: application of movement-related cortical potentials. Annals of Neurology 15: 299–302

Shumway-Cook A, Woollacott M 1995 Motor control – new models for rehabilitation Williams and Williams, Baltimore

Stephenson R, Edwards S, Freeman J 1998 Associated reactions: their value in clinical practice? Physiotherapy Research International 3: 69–78

Taub E, Wolf S L 1997 Constraint induced techniques to facilitate upper extremity use in stroke patients. Topics in Stroke Rehabilitation 3: 38–61

Taub E, Miller N E, Novack T A 1993 A technique for improving chronic motor deficit after stroke. Archives of Physical Medicine and Rehabilitation 74: 347–354

Turton A, Wroe S, Trepte N, Fraser C, Lemon R N 1996 Contralateral and ipsilateral EMG responses to transcranial magnetic stimulation during recovery of arm and hand function after stroke. Electroencephalography and Clinical Neurophysiology 101: 316–328

Voss D E 1967 Proprioceptive neuromuscular facilitation. American Journal of Physical Medicine 46: 838–898

Winstein C J, Merians A, Sullivan K 1997 Motor learning after unilateral brain damage. Neuropsychologia 37: 975–987

Woollacott M H, Burtner P 1996 Neural and musculoskeletal contributions to the development of stance control in typical children and children with cerebral palsy. Acta Paediatrica Scandinavica Supplement 416: 58–62

2

Assessment, outcome measurement and goal setting in physiotherapy practice

Jennifer A. Freeman

INTRODUCTION

In the past decade there has been an increasing demand on all health care professionals to provide evidence to support the effectiveness of their interventions and 'to make conscientious, explicit and judicious use of current best evidence to make decisions about the care of individual patients' (Sackett et al 1996). This concept of evidence-based practice is now widely considered to be best practice. Comprehensive assessment and outcome measurement are integral to this process.

There are two main aims of this chapter. The first is to describe the general principles of assessment, outcome measurement and goal setting. The second is to stress the importance of incorporating these principles in daily clinical practice. This chapter provides some guidelines on how to achieve this. For this purpose the chapter has been divided into three distinct sections. In reality, however, the three concepts are closely interrelated.

ASSESSMENT

Assessment is considered to be the first step in the process of rehabilitation (Wade 1998a). It is a continuous process by which information is gathered from a variety of sources, and then interpreted with the aim of identifying key problems and formulating a treatment plan relevant to the needs of the individual. In neurological physiotherapy its primary purpose is to describe the patient, and to objectively record and communicate findings about patients' movement disorders and activity levels (Bowers & Ashburn 1998).

Johnson & Thompson (1996) emphasise the importance of good quality assessment by stating that the 'quality of care given can only be as good as the assessment on which it is based. Effective physiotherapy management of disordered movement and function is therefore reliant upon accurate measurement and analysis of movement, posture and function (refer to Chapter 3). In neurological conditions, where the problems are often multiple, complex and interrelated, this not only requires considerable knowledge and skill about movement but also a willingness to consider a wide range of additional factors which may contribute to the problem. It requires the ability of therapists to recognise their own areas of expertise and limitations, and to refer to other professionals when indicated. There are many examples within clinical practice where an initial assessment may trigger referral to another professional to seek essential additional information to inform the planning of intervention. For example, referring for assessment of vision or blood pressure in the case of a person who is repeatedly falling but who has no apparent difficulties with movement; or to a psychologist when low mood appears to be impacting upon the patient's ability to participate in treatment. Just as we may depend upon other people for information, so too may our findings be beneficial in guiding the intervention of others. For example information about the ability of a patient to maintain a sitting posture will guide wheelchair and seating provision; assessment of tone and its response to pharmacological interventions (such as botulinum toxin or intrathecal baclofen) will guide optimal drug dosage. These examples highlight the necessity for collaborative multidisciplinary team working, an approach which is now widely considered fundamental to optimal patient management (Wood 1993).

Key elements of the assessment process

While there is little evidence to guide one on the most appropriate or efficient methods of assess-

ment (Wade 1998a), there appears to be general agreement with regard to the essential steps in the assessment process. These are outlined in the following sections.

Gathering background information

Background information from other relevant sources such as medical notes, investigations and psychology assessments informs the initial assessment process and minimises duplication of questioning and assessment.

The clinical interview

Interviewing the patient is an important aspect of the physiotherapy assessment. Table 2.1 provides a brief overview of important data to collect during the interview. It is not usually feasible to gather all of this information at a single session, and hence this process will be ongoing throughout treatment. Froelich & Bishop (1977) consider that there are a number of aims of the interview: to establish a relationship with the patient; gather information about their needs; and help them to understand their condition and the movement difficulties that arise from it. Croft (1980) believes that the ability of the therapist to create an open and communicative atmosphere, whereby information can be readily offered and received, is fundamental to achieving this aim.

The clinical examination

The purpose of the clinical examination is to gain information about the patient's movement disorder and functional status by observation and examination. An essential prerequisite for this is the ability of the therapist to analyse movement based on a knowledge of normal movement (refer to Chapter 3). Information collected by observation may be subjective and therefore open to error and bias since the descriptions and interpretations can differ widely according to the experience and expectations of the assessor and those who read the records (Bowers & Ashburn 1998). Such information can be made more reliable if it is structured, in some way, by techniques

Table 2.1   Example of a structured checklist for an initial assessment

Database Gathering information from relevant sources such as medical notes and psychology assessments:	Past medical history History of present condition Medications Results of specific investigations including X-rays, brain scans, EMG, cognitive assessments
Clinical interview Establishing the physical, psychological and social needs of the patient/carer through interview:	Perception of own problems/main concern Normal daily routine Social situation: family support, accommodation, employment, leisure Social service support Mobility with regard to indoor and outdoor mobility: home and work environment, methods of transport Other symptoms: continence, vision, hearing, swallowing, fatigue, pain Other ongoing treatment Past physiotherapy and response to treatment Expectations of treatment
Clinical examination Determining the quality of movement and the functional abilities of the patient through the interpretation of:	Posture and balance Volitional movement: range, strength, selectivity, coordination and endurance Abnormal tone Involuntary movement Muscle and joint range Sensation: tactile, stereognosis Sensory and perceptual disturbance: visual, auditory, vestibular Functional activities: bed mobility, transfers, upper limb function, gait, stairs Gait: pattern, distance, reliance on aids, orthoses, or assistance from others. Exercise tolerance/fatigue Cognitive status Respiratory status Swallowing difficulties

Adapted from ACPIN Standards of Physiotherapy Practice in Neurology (1995).

such as the use of checklists (for an example see Table 2.1), or standardised and objective assessment scales (such as the Motor Assessment Scale, Carr et al 1985).

Although standardised quantitative assessments provide valuable information the vast majority do not address the quality of performance of movement. Partridge & Edwards (1996) suggest that this is partly because of the difficulty in measuring quality in an objective manner. As a consequence, however, assessment of the quality of movement generally remains unstructured in format and subjective in content, relying upon the skill and experience of the therapist to detect and document key issues. This is unsatisfactory since evaluation of the quality of movement is

considered by many physiotherapists to be central in guiding their input, and evaluating their effectiveness in terms of outcome. Attempts have been made to improve this in areas such as gait analysis (for example Lord et al 1998); it is hoped that continued efforts such as these will help to resolve this problem.

Another area of the clinical examination which remains particularly problematic is the objective assessment and description of muscle tone. This is partly due to the paucity of standardised and objective assessment scales that are available for use within the clinical setting. Take for example the Modified Ashworth Scale, a subjective ordinal scale, based upon the assessment of the resistance to stretch imposed passively to the limb by the examiner (Bohannon & Smith 1987). Despite the fact that this is the most commonly used measure to assess 'spasticity' within the clinical setting, it lacks validity, since it fails to differentiate between the neural and non-neural elements of altered tone (Carr & Shepherd 1998) and to reflect the dynamic nature of tone which is felt by many to be critical to the impact it has on movement and function. Another method that has been used within clinical practice to grade 'spasticity' is the Associated Reactions Scale (Stephenson et al 1998). Unfortunately, despite reasonably widespread use (Haas 1994), this scale has not been evaluated in terms of its relia-

bility, validity, or responsiveness and therefore it is impossible to know whether the information provided is reliable and meaningful. Describing the distribution of abnormal tone has also proven difficult. One method used to achieve this is by means of a 'key point' diagram in which the severity and distribution of abnormal tone, and alignment, is broadly indicated (Fig. 2.1). A search of the literature, however, failed to reveal any evidence to determine the reliability or validity of this method.

Interpreting the findings and formulating a problem list

The power of assessment lies in the ability of the therapist to identify the key problems using a clinical reasoning process. In this process therapists must use their theoretical knowledge and clinical experience to analyse and interpret the assessment findings in the context of a wide range of factors, including the patient's diagnosis, age and co-morbidities. Such an analysis should enable the formulation of a problem list and treatment plan relevant to the patient's individual needs at the time of the assessment.

Discussing the findings and developing a treatment plan

Following assessment there should be a discussion of the assessment findings and an explanation of the resultant movement difficulties with patients, as well as with others involved in their care. This is a key point at which patients' perceptions of their problems, and their expectations with regard to intervention, can be clarified to ensure that the therapist, other members of the team and the patient are all working together towards a common goal. Discussing the findings with other team members is particularly important with regard to safe and effective methods of handling and moving the patient, and facilitating functional independence.

When developing the treatment plan it is essential to recognise that many issues relating to management impact directly, not only on the lifestyle of the patient but also on that of their

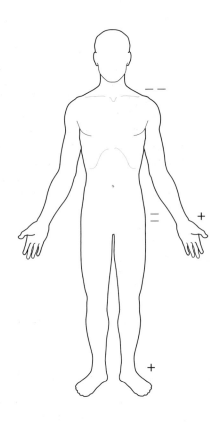

+ Mild hypertonicity   − Mild hypotonicity

++ Moderate hypertonicity   − − Moderate hypotonicity

+++ Severe hypertonicity   − − − Severe hypotonicity

Figure 2.1 Key point diagram describing the severity and distribution of abnormal tone.

family. From the patients' perspective their needs are always set in the context of their personal life objectives – and thus are intrinsically based on very different views to those of the professional staff concerned with them (Robinson et al 1996). Decisions may therefore become much more than simply a health issue; personal wishes and expectations, as well as social and environmental factors must be taken into account. In some cases this may indicate that no further intervention is required, whereas in others it may result in the development of an extensive and complex programme of care, involving a number of professionals from within and outside the health care system. This type of discussion begins to set the stage for involving the patient as an active learner and is likely to be beneficial in increasing their adherence to any treatment recommendations (Partridge 1997). The importance of taking the patient's perspective seriously is further emphasised by French (1997), who considers that it is only possible for rehabilitation to proceed successfully if some kind of a consensus between patient and therapist is reached.

Documenting the findings

Written evidence of the assessment findings in a clear, accurate and logical manner is fundamental to the assessment process. It 'is an essential and integral part of care and not a distraction from its provision' (UK Central Council for Nursing, Midwifery and Health Visiting 1993). Effective records not only provide a concrete history of the assessment and intervention programme, but also demonstrate the chronology of events, the factors observed, the response to treatment and the process of clinical reasoning related to the patient's care. This is necessary for a range of reasons that include communication between professionals; monitoring of standards; audit and quality assurance; and for medicolegal purposes.

The SOAP format is a widely used system of record keeping (Robertson 1991). SOAP stands for:

- **S**ubjective – how patients are feeling, what they tell the therapist

- **O**bjective – the objective examination undertaken by the therapist, and the treatment provided
- **A**ssessment – the therapist's assessment of her findings and of the effectiveness of the treatment undertaken; and
- **P**lan – what the therapist plans to do; whether the treatment will continue or will be changed.

It has been suggested that if this system is used effectively, it is extremely beneficial to the clinical reasoning process (Harris 1993) and enables the therapist to provide an adequate explanation of the nature of her contact with the patient for medicolegal purposes (Diamond 1999). Unfortunately there is no simple formula for deciding what to write or how much to write in the records; each individual must use their professional judgement to determine the most significant issues to document. It is likely that the provision of professional guidelines, together with regular auditing of records within departments, will help to ensure that records are clinically useful and meet the necessary professional standards for legal purposes.

Increasingly, health and social services are using 'shared records' in which all health professionals involved in the care of the patient make entries in a single record. In some situations this record may be held by the patient. This reflects the 'patient-centred team approach' that is now generally accepted as best practice. It presents a challenge to the physiotherapist to use non-jargon language that is easily understood by all those who read the record, be they professionals or lay people.

The importance of reassessment

It is easy to describe the need for an initial assessment, where the main purpose is to establish a set of baseline data and measurements against which improvement or deterioration may be judged at regular intervals, such as on discharge and follow-up. Less easy to translate is the notion of assessment being continually incorporated throughout intervention, a process wherein the therapist monitors and responds to the patient in a dynamic manner from moment to moment. In this approach the therapist is sensitive to both the physical and psychological needs of the patient at any point in time. The specifics of intervention may be altered throughout the session(s) in a variety of ways, such as the method of handling, the level of encouragement or reassurance given or the physical demands placed on the patient. This ongoing and continuous assessment, which enables effectiveness to be constantly evaluated, is fundamental to skilled intervention.

MEASURING OUTCOME

Health outcomes are the results, or effects, that can be attributed to health care interventions (Ware et al 1993). Measurement refers to the quantification of data, either in absolute or relative terms. It is now widely accepted that determining the effectiveness of an intervention by measuring its effect on outcome provides a basis for evidence-based clinical decision making (Sackett et al 1996). Hobart (1999) emphasises the importance of measuring outcome, stating that 'standardised methods of outcome measurement take the guesswork out of evaluation by offering objectivity, quantification, and a means of universal communication. In their absence we are left with only subjective appraisals and personal judgements upon which to base our decisions'.

There has been an increasing interest in the measurement of health outcomes since the 1980s. This was initially precipitated by extensive - technological developments that expanded all aspects of disease management, giving rise to an increase in the variations of clinical practice and escalating costs. As a direct consequence, there has been an ever-increasing demand on clinicians to demonstrate the benefits of their intervention. More recently, the need for evaluation has regained renewed momentum as an emphasis has been placed on actively involving patients in making decisions about their own health care provision (Hatch 1997). This process requires information to be available to an even wider group of people to enable informed decision making about the relative benefits of different health care interventions.

A framework for measurement

The World Health Organization's model of illness provides a useful framework and a common terminology for describing and measuring the consequences of diseases and the impact that rehabilitation interventions may have on them (WHO 1980). The original framework, termed *The International Classification of Impairments, Disabilities and Handicaps* (ICIDH), is now widely used as a basis for evaluation within both clinical and research practice. Recently it has been extensively reviewed in order to avoid a purely medical interpretation of disablements and to take into account the role of the environment in the disablement process (Ustam & Leonardi 1998). The new terminology of *The International Classification of Impairments, Activities and Participations* (ICIDH-2, WHO 1997) is:

- *Impairment* describes a loss or abnormality of body structure or of a psychological or physiological function.
- *Activities* describe the nature and extent of actual performance in functional activities, at the level of the person.
- *Participations* describe the nature and extent of a person's involvement in life situations in the actual context in which they live, at a societal level. It recognizes the complex relationship between a person's health condition, their impairments and activity restrictions.

Figure 2.2 illustrates how this framework may be applied to physiotherapy practice.

General principles of outcome measurement

The validity of outcome measurement is dependent upon the rigour of the measurement process and the validity of its measures (Rudick et al 1996). It is therefore necessary when undertaking an evaluation to consider a number of important factors. These are discussed in detail in the following sections.

Determining the purpose of the evaluation

When initially deciding what to measure it is important to be clear about the purpose of the evaluation and the information you wish to gain. This might be for a number of reasons. You might wish, for example, to routinely gather baseline and discharge data on all patients attending the service, regardless of their disorder, for the purpose of identifying key information about the individual, and for service evaluation and audit. Generic disability assessment scales such as the Barthel Index (Mahoney & Barthel 1965) or the Functional Independence Measure (Granger et al 1993) are commonly used for this purpose. On the other hand, you may wish to evaluate the impact of a specific intervention on an individual's specific problems. In this case the choice of measure (or combination of measures) may be quite different. For example, if the purpose was to evaluate the effectiveness of a splinting programme in a patient who presented with loss of joint range due to soft tissue shortening, the most relevant measure might be the measurement of a joint angle using a goniometer (Norkin & White 1975). It is likely that this would be combined with a measure of function relevant to the patient's particular problems, such as the ability to stand up or to walk. These two examples illustrate how the outcomes chosen may differ according to the purpose of the evaluation.

Although a combination of outcomes is often necessary to comprehensively evaluate your intervention, it is important to be selective, remembering that neither yourself nor the patient should be overburdened by excessive measurement. Research studies are better able, in most circumstances, to investigate the effectiveness of interventions in more detail and, where necessary, with more sophisticated equipment.

Selecting relevant outcomes to measure

In many neurological conditions long-term disability is the norm. For this reason outcome measurement can be broadly viewed in two ways: first, the extent to which stated aims of intervention are achieved; and, secondly, the extent to which adverse events might occur if the treatment is not given. The range of possible outcomes is presented schematically in Figure 2.3. Death is an easy outcome to measure, but this rarely has direct relevance to physiotherapy

OUTCOME			
CONCEPTUAL CONTINUUM			
Disease	Impairments	Activities	Participations
OPERATIONAL CONTINUUM			
Multiple sclerosis	Hypertonia Ataxia Weakness Poor memory	Difficulty with: Personal care Locomotion Transfers	Limitations with: Autonomy Occupation Social integration

Figure 2.2 The ICIDH: a conceptual and operational model for measuring outcome.

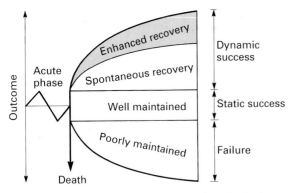

Figure 2.3 Range of possible outcomes following brain trauma (reproduced from Pope by kind permission).

management. More difficult to measure is the success or failure of the longer-term consequences of the disease with regard to morbidity. Pope (1992) refers to these in terms of 'dynamic success' (for instance the ability to walk again, to regain function, to get back to work); 'static success' (where the patient's condition is well maintained and where secondary complications do not occur); and 'failure' (for instance the development of pressure sores, contractures or pain). Bax et al (1988) illustrated the importance of static success in their study examining the health problems of a population of physically disabled young people in the community. Of the 104 subjects studied the secondary complications experienced included contractures of lower joints (59%), deformed feet (25%), urinary incontinence (59%) and pressure sores (33%). Many of these complications are avoidable and, hence, a successful outcome in terms of static success would have been attained if they had not occurred.

In the majority of cases, however, the aims of therapy are not simply to achieve static success but also to improve function and well-being. For this purpose it is important that the measurement of outcome is focussed at the level at which the intervention is intended to effect change. For example, interventions aimed to impact on impairments such as muscle weakness should measure strength; interventions aimed predominantly at improving function should measure function. To be successful, this requires the ther-

apist to have a thorough understanding of the intervention, and to be specific in identifying in advance what the intervention aims to achieve.

Selecting appropriate measures

In selecting which measure to use, a number of factors must be considered. It is not the purpose of this chapter to describe these in detail, but rather to provide an outline of the more important issues. Several textbooks (McDowell & Newell 1996, Wilkin et al 1992, Streiner & Norman 1995) and articles (Medical Outcomes Trust 1995, McDowell & Jenkinson 1996, Fitzpatrick et al 1998) address these issues comprehensively in a more detailed and technical manner.

In brief, in choosing an outcome measure, four key factors should be reviewed.

1. The purpose of the measure. The instrument should be relevant to the purpose of your evaluation.

2. Clinical utility. To be useful within the clinical setting the measure should be simple, easy to use, accessible and acceptable to the patient. A manual should be available, describing clearly and in detail the standardised procedure in which the measure should be used. Importantly, the measure should not take up more resources than are available, either in terms of its cost or the time taken.

3. Scientific properties. The measure should possess three scientific properties:

- reliability: the results produced should be accurate, consistent, reliable over time, and reproducible within and between raters
- validity: it should measure what it purports to measure, in the population and within the setting in which it is being used
- responsiveness: it should be able to detect clinically important change.

4. Standardisation. It is advantageous to choose a measure that is widely known (for example the Medical Research Council muscle strength grading system). Provided that the measure is used correctly, meaningful information can then be communicated within and between different professionals and different areas of service delivery. This enables uniform monitoring of the patient's condition over the longer term. This is particularly relevant to many neurological conditions where the person frequently accesses a wide variety of services over many years, and hence is reassessed by a number of different people in a diversity of settings.

Ideally, the outcome measure chosen should have been comprehensively evaluated and possess all of these attributes. Unfortunately, however, this is often not the case. To date, relatively few of the clinical measures available for measuring movement and function in neurological patients have been extensively and rigorously evaluated. It is the responsibility of clinicians and researchers to review critically the outcome measure chosen to determine how well it meets these criteria. This must be considered in the context of the population and the setting in which it will be used. This knowledge is essential to enable accurate interpretation of the information gained from the measure.

Ensuring the process of measurement is rigorous

The process of measurement must be rigorous if the results are to be credible. Measurement at the time of the initial assessment, before a treatment programme has commenced, is essential. The timing of subsequent measurements will vary according to the length of time that it is expected to take for a change to occur. To ensure reliability the assessments should be undertaken in accordance with operational guidelines and the measurement process should be clearly documented. It is important that the measurements are undertaken in similar circumstances if the comparisons made between evaluations are to be valid. For example, the assessment should be consistently undertaken prior to treatment rather than post-treatment when the patient's performance may be negatively affected by fatigue, or perhaps positively affected by the treatment which has just been given.

Interpreting the results

The primary reason for using outcome measures is to evaluate the success or failure of intervention, in a standardised and objective manner. It is essential that the information generated is used to inform practice. This requires the clinician to be clear about whether the outcome is attributable to the intervention given (Sackett et al 1996), and to reflect on and critically appraise the care given. Accurate and meaningful interpretation of the results must be based on a sound understanding of both the clinical context (e.g. the severity of the condition, the purpose of the intervention) and the measurement process (e.g. psychometric properties of the measures used, timing of the measurement).

Available measures

A large number of outcome measures are available for use in evaluating the outcome of physiotherapy and rehabilitation interventions. Table 2.2 lists some of the measures currently used within the clinical setting. For further information about these the reader is referred to the original articles and to a number of textbooks (for example Wade 1992, Bowling 1995) and reviews (for example McCulloch 1998, Sharrack et al 1999) which describe the measures in more detail.

GOAL SETTING

A goal is the object or aim of an action (Locke et al 1981). Goal setting is now widely accepted as a basic principle of rehabilitation practice, and is generally acknowledged as helping to focus the rehabilitation team on the needs of each individual patient (Duff et al 1999). It provides a structured and objective way of planning and documenting progress, and can aid multidisciplinary collaboration and communication (Schut & Stam 1994). It may be useful in involving and motivating the patient and carers to be active participants in the rehabilitation process. Furthermore, it is increasingly being recognised as a useful means of improving treatment effectiveness and as a method for measuring the effectiveness of interventions and for overall programme evaluation (Cott & Finch 1990).

Evidence to demonstrate the benefits of goal setting with regard to improved performance has

Table 2.2 Outcome measures frequently used within the clinical setting

Dimension	Outcome measure	Studies
Impairments		
(i) Muscle strength	Hand-held dynamometer	Bohannon et al 1995
	Medical Research Council Grades (MRC)	Medical Research Council 1976
(ii) Range of motion	Goniometry	Norkin & White 1975
(iii) Tone	Modified Ashworth Scale	Bohannon & Smith 1987
(iv) Sensation	Stereognosis	Lincoln & Edmans 1989
(v) Fatigue	Fatigue Severity Scale	Petajan et al 1996
Disability		
Global disability		
(i) Generic	Barthel Index	Mahoney & Barthel 1965
	Functional Independence Measure	Granger et al 1993
(ii) Disease-specific	Motor Assessment Scale for Stroke	Carr et al 1985
Focal disability		
(i) Gait	10-metre timed walking test	Wade 1992
	Hauser Ambulatory Index	Hauser et al 1983
(ii) Mobility	Rivermead Motor Assessment Scale	Lincoln & Leadbitter 1979
(iii) Balance	Functional Reach Test	Duncan et al 1990
	Timed get up and go test	Podsialo & Richardson 1991
(iv) Upper limb function	Nine-hole Peg Test	Mathiowetz et al 1985
	Action Research Arm Test	Crow et al 1989
	Frenchay Arm Test	Sunderland et al 1989
Handicap	London Handicap Scale	Harwood et al 1997
	Environmental Status Scale	Mellerup et al 1981
Quality of life		
(i) Generic	36-item Short Form Health Survey	Ware et al 1993
	Nottingham Health Profile	Hunt et al 1981
(ii) Disease-specific	39-item Parkinson's Disease Questionnaire	Peto et al 1995
	Functional Assessment of Multiple Sclerosis	Cella et al 1996

been demonstrated in a number of studies (Locke et al 1981, Williams & Stieg 1987, Malec et al 1991). Importantly, Duff et al (1999) showed that the majority of patients in their study considered that goal setting helped them to plan their rehabilitation.

General principles of goal setting

A number of factors have been identified in the literature as being important for effective goal setting. These are outlined in the following sections.

Involving the patient and family

In aiming to address the needs identified by patients it is key that patients are encouraged, from the outset, to participate actively in the goal-setting process (Haas 1993). This is essential to ensure that the goals set are relevant and motivating for the individual. Initially this may be a new and somewhat daunting prospect. The patient may, for example, lack knowledge about their condition, how it may be expected to change, and what physiotherapy has to offer. This may make it difficult for them to be specific about their goals of treatment. Other factors such as pain, depression or cognitive impairment may also make this process more challenging. In general, however, with experience patients usually develop a sense of how relevant their goals are to their needs and how they can become more actively involved in the process. It is the therapist's role to facilitate this by periodically reviewing, negotiating and adjusting the goals to assure their appropriateness throughout the rehabilitation process.

Formulating objective and measurable goals

The process of goal setting starts with a thorough understanding of the problems identified by the initial assessment. Based on this information, goals may generally be broken down into short- and long-term goals. Short-term goals indicate the first objectives to be met as a result of the immediate treatment plan, and provide a series of small specific steps which focus on achievement of the long-term goal. In contrast, the long-term goal generally indicates the expected level of function and independence that the patient will achieve in broader terms. It is important to recognise that patients do not always understand how short-term goals relate to the achievement of the long-term goal; it is often necessary for the therapist to reinforce this link. For example, the patient with an incomplete paraplegia may not recognise a link between a short-term goal of 'consistently achieving safe transfers independently using a sliding board' and their long-term goal of walking independently.

It has been suggested that goals should be appropriate, measurable, achievable and functional; i.e. goals should be SMART (Cott & Finch 1990). They should be formulated in small simple steps that are:

Specific – they should be specific and relevant to the individual and to the problem being addressed.

Measurable – the degree of accomplishment should be measurable.

Achievable – goals should be challenging but achievable. Locke et al (1981) in their comprehensive review of goal setting, provide a substantial body of evidence to demonstrate that goals can be a powerful motivating or demotivating force depending upon whether the goals set are specific, relevant and challenging (motivating) or are vague, easy, 'do best' goals (de-motivating).

Realistic – the difficulty of the goals should be determined within the limitations imposed by the neurological impairment and the person's wish and ability to change. It is also important to recognise that not all goals need be focused on improvement; goals might also relate to maintenance.

Time limited – a specific time frame for accomplishment should be agreed. The time frame should be reasonable; even a very relevant goal may become de-motivating if it takes a very long time to achieve.

Ensuring goals are clear and understandable

It is generally considered good practice to ensure that a written copy of the goals is easily accessible to the patient in language that is explicit and understandable. In many services a copy of the goals is given to the patient. Writing goals that fulfil the SMART criteria can be extremely challenging. A helpful framework is that each short-term goal should have four components:

- Who will perform the behaviour – this will usually be the patient, but could also be the carer.
- An observable behaviour – what they will do.
- How they will do it – to what standard the behaviour will be performed, the aids used, level of assistance required, consistency, the setting in which it will occur and the level of safety. These issues need to be specified to ensure the goal is measurable.
- The time scale for achievement with precise dates for achievement.

Awareness of factors which may impact on goal achievement

Factors such as cognitive and physical function, mood, fatigue, carer involvement and environmental factors are important to consider if realistic goals are to be set. By identifying and recording reasons for achievement and non-achievement of goals, the team is able to reflect on their practice and alter it as needed. In some services integrated care pathways have proven useful for ensuring that regular auditing of goals is incorporated within clinical practice (Rossiter et al 1998).

Providing feedback

There is evidence to suggest that feedback is important in improving performance (Locke et al

1981). This may be in the form of feedback about the achievement or non-achievement of goals, or feedforward about how hard the person will need to work to achieve the goal. There is no set formula for determining the frequency of feedback; a variety of different systems exist which are tailored to the needs of the service and to the individual (for example Malec et al 1991, Duff et al 1999). It is important, however, that members of the multidisciplinary team meet on a regular basis to review and set additional goals. In some departments this directly involves the patient, while in others it does not. Within the social science literature, the evidence remains equivocal as to whether direct participation in setting goals leads to better task performance or greater goal commitment (Locke et al 1981). Unfortunately, there is a paucity of research to determine whether this is the case in rehabilitation (Wade 1998b).

SUMMARY

The issues of measurement and outcome in physiotherapy are recognised as being one of the greatest challenges of the clinical effectiveness agenda (Bury & Mead 1998). This requires physiotherapists to incorporate objective standardised assessment, and rigorous evaluation of the effectiveness of interventions, as part of their daily clinical practice. It requires a willingness to keep an open mind, to remain objective and to take a risk in allowing our beliefs to be tested.

REFERENCES

Bax M C O, Smyth D P L, Thomas A P 1988 Health care of physically handicapped young adults. British Medical Journal 296: 1153–1155

Bohannon R W, Smith M B 1987 Interrater reliability of a modified Ashworth Scale of muscle spasticity. Physical Therapy 67: 206–207

Bohannon R W, Cassidy D, Walsh S 1995 Trunk muscle strength is impaired multidirectionally after stroke. Clinical Rehabilitation 9: 47–51

Bowers E, Ashburn A 1998 Principles of physiotherapy assessment and outcome measures. In: Stokes M (ed) Neurological physiotherapy. Mosby, London, p 43

Bowling A 1995 Measuring disease: a review of disease-specific quality of life measurement scales. Open University Press, Buckingham

Bury T, Mead J (eds) 1998 Evidence based healthcare: a practical guide for therapists. Butterworth-Heinemann, London

Carr J, Shepherd R 1998 Neurological rehabilitation: optimising motor performance. Butterworth-Heinemann, Oxford

Carr J H, Shepherd R B, Nordholm L, Lynne D 1985 Investigation of a new motor assessment scale for stroke patients. Physical Therapy 65: 175–180

Cella D F, Dineen K, Arnason B et al 1996 Validation of the functional assessment of multiple sclerosis quality of life instrument. Neurology 47: 129–139

Cott C, Finch E 1990 Goal-setting in physical therapy practice. Physiotherapy Canada 43(1): 19–22

Croft J J 1980 Interviewing in physical therapy. Physical Therapy 60(8): 1033–1036

Crow J L, Lincoln N B, Nouri F M, De Weerdt W 1989 The effectiveness of EMG feedback in the treatment of arm function after stroke. International Disability Studies 11: 155–160

Diamond B C 1999 Record keeping. In: Diamond B C (ed) Legal aspects of physiotherapy. Blackwell Science, London, pp 164–175

Duff J, Kennedy P, Swalwell E 1999 Clinical audit of rehabilitation: patients' views of goal planning. Clinical Psychology Forum 129: 34–38

Duncan P W, Weiner D K, Chandler J et al 1990 Functional reach: a new clinical measure of balance. Journal of Gerontology 45: 192–197

Fitzpatrick R, Davey C, Buxton M J, Jones D R 1998 Evaluating patient-based outcome measures for use in clinical trials. Health Technology Assessment 2(14)

French S 1997 Clinical interviewing. In: French S (ed) Physiotherapy a psychosocial approach, 2nd edn. Butterworth-Heinemann, Oxford, p 263

Froelich R E, Bishop F M 1977 Clinical interviewing skills. Mosby, St Louis

Granger C V, Cotter A C, Hamilton B B, Fiedler R C 1993 Functional assessment scales: a study of persons after stroke. Archives of Physical Medicine and Rehabilitation 74: 133–138

Haas J 1993 Ethical considerations of goal setting for patient care in rehabilitation medicine. American Journal of Physical Medicine and Rehabilitation 74(1): 16–20

Haas B M 1994 Measuring spasticity: a survey of current practice among health-care professionals. British Journal of Therapy and Rehabilitation 1(2): 90–95

Harris B A 1993 Building documentation using a clinical decision-making model. In: Stewart D L, Abelyn S H (eds) Documenting functional outcomes in physical therapy. Mosby, St Louis, pp 81–99

Harwood R H, Gompertz P, Pound P, Ebrahim S 1997 Determinants of handicap 1 and 3 years after a stroke. Disability and Rehabilitation 19(5): 205–211

Hatch J 1997 Building partnerships. In: Thompson A J, Polman C O, Hohlfeld R (eds) Multiple sclerosis: clinical challenges and controversies. Martin Dunitz, London, ch 26, p 345–351

Hauser S L, Dawson D M, Lehrich J R et al 1983 Intensive immunosuppression in progressive multiple sclerosis: a randomised, three arm study of high dose intravenous cyclophoshamide, plasma exchange, and ACTH. New England Journal of Medicine 308: 173–180

Hobart J 1999 Use of clinical scales. In: Thompson A J, McDonald W I (eds) Key advances in the effective management of multiple sclerosis. Royal Society of Medicine Press, London, pp 27–29

Hunt S M, McKenna S P, Williams J 1981 Reliability of a population survey tool for measuring perceived health problems: a study of patients with osteoarthritis. Journal of Epidemiology and Community Health 35: 297–300

Johnson J, Thompson A J 1996 Rehabilitation in a neuroscience centre: the role of expert assessment and selection. British Journal of Therapy and Rehabilitation 3(6): 303–308

Lincoln N B, Edmans J A 1989 A shortened version of the Rivermead Perceptual Assessment Battery. Clinical Rehabilitation 3: 199–204

Lincoln N B, Leadbitter D 1979 Assessment of motor function in stroke patients. Physiotherapy 65: 48–51

Locke E A, Shaw K N, Saari L M, Latham G P 1981 Goal setting and task performance: 1969–1980. Psychological Bulletin 90(1): 125–152

Lord S E, Halligan P W, Wade D T 1998 Visual gait analysis: the development of a clinical assessment and scale. Clinical Rehabilitation 12: 107–119

McCulloch K 1998 Standardised assessment tools for traumatic brain injury in physical therapy. Neurology Report 22(3): 114–125

McDowell I, Jenkinson C 1996 Development standards for health measures. Journal of Health Services Research and Policy 1(4): 238–246

McDowell I, Newell C 1996 Measuring health: a guide to rating scales and questionnaires. Oxford University Press, Oxford

Mahoney F I, Barthel D W 1965 Functional evaluation: the Barthel Index (BI). Maryland State Medical Journal 14: 61–65

Malec J F, Smigielski J S, DePompolo R W 1991 Goal attainment scaling and outcome measurement in postacute brain injury rehabilitation. Archives of Physical Medicine and Rehabilitation 72: 138–143

Mathiowetz V, Weber K, Kashman N et al 1985 Adult norms for the nine-hole peg test of finger dexterity. Occupational Therapy Journal of Research 5: 24–37

Medical Outcomes Trust 1995 Instrument review criteria. Medical Outcomes Trust Bulletin 3(4): 1–4

Medical Research Council 1976 Aids to the examination of the peripheral nervous system. HMSO, London

Mellerup E, Fog T, Raun N et al 1981 The socio-economic scale. Acta Neurologica Scandinavia 64: 130–138

Norkin C C, White D J 1975 Measurement of joint motion; a guide to goniometry. F A Davies, Philadelphia

Partridge C 1997 The patient as a decision maker (editorial). Physiotherapy Research International 2(4): 4–6

Partridge C, Edwards S 1996 The bases of practice–neurological physiotherapy. Physiotherapy Research International 1(3): 205–208

Petajan J H, Gappmaier E, White A T, Spencer M K, Mino L, Hicks R W 1996 Impact of aerobic training on fitness and quality of life in multiple sclerosis. Annals of Neurology 39: 432–441

Peto V, Jenkinson C, Fitzpatrick R, Greenhall R 1995 The development and validation of a short measure of functioning and well being for individuals with Parkinsons disease. Quality of Life Research 4: 241–248

Podsialo D, Richardson S 1991 The timed 'up and go': a test of basic functional mobility for frail elderly persons. Journal of American Geriatric Society 39: 142–148

Pope P M 1988 A model for evaluation of input in relation to outcome in severely brain damaged patients. Physiotherapy 74(12): 647–650

Pope P M 1992 Management of the physical condition in patients with chronic and severe neurological pathologies. Physiotherapy 78(12): 896–903

Robertson C 1991 Records and evaluation. In: Robertson C (ed) Health visiting in practice, 2nd edn. Churchill Livingstone, Edinburgh, pp 143–169

Robinson I, Robinson I, Hunter M, Neilson S (eds) 1996 A dispatch from the frontline: the views of people with multiple sclerosis about their needs. A qualitative approach. Brunel MS Research Unit, London

Rossiter D A, Edmondson A, Al Shahi R, Thompson A J 1998 Integrated care pathways in multiple sclerosis rehabilitation: completing the audit cycle. Multiple Sclerosis 4: 85–89

Rudick R, Antel J, Confavreux C et al (The Clinical Outcomes Assessment Force) 1996 Clinical outcomes assessment in multiple sclerosis. Annals of Neurology 40(469): 479

Sackett D L, Rosenberg W M, Gray J A M, Haynes R B, Richardson W S 1996 Evidence based medicine: what it is and what it isn't. British Medical Journal 312: 71–72

Schut H A, Stam H J 1994 Goals in rehabilitation teamwork. Disability and Rehabilitation 16(4): 223–226

Sharrack B, Hughes R A C, Soudain S, Dunn G 1999 The psychometric properties of clinical rating scales in multiple sclerosis. Brain 122: 141–159

Standards of Physiotherapy Practice in Neurology 1995 Association of Chartered Physiotherapists Interested in Neurology. The Chartered Society of Physiotherapy, London

Stephenson R, Edwards S, Freeman J 1998 Associated reactions: their value in clinical practice? Physiotherapy Research International 3(1): 69–75

Streiner D L, Norman G R 1995 Health measurement scales: a practical guide to their development and use, 2nd edn. Oxford University Press, Oxford

Sunderland A, Tinson D, Bradley L, Langton Hewer R 1989 Arm function after stroke. An evaluation of grip strength as a measure of recovery and a prognostic indicator. Journal of Neurology, Neurosurgery and Psychiatry 52: 1267–1272

United Kingdom Central Council for Nursing, Midwifery and Health Visiting 1993. Standards for Records and Record Keeping, London

Ustu T B, Leonard M 1998 The revision of the International Classification of Impairments, Disabilities and Handicaps (ICIDH-2). European Journal of Neurology 5 (Suppl. 2): S31–S32

Wade D T 1992 Measurement in neurological rehabilitation. Oxford University Press, Oxford

Wade D T 1998a Evidence relating to assessment in rehabilitation (editorial). Clinical Rehabilitation 12: 183–186

Wade D T 1998b Evidence relating to goal planning in rehabilitation (editorial). Clinical Rehabilitation 12: 273–275

Ware J E, Snow K K, Kosinski M et al 1993 SF-36 Health Survey: manual and interpretation guide. The Health Institute, New England Medical Centre, Boston, Massachusetts

WHO 1980 International classification of impairments, disabilities and handicaps. World Health Organisation, Geneva

WHO 1997 ICIDH-2 International classification of impairments, activities and participations. A manual of dimensions of disablement and functioning. Beta-1 draft for field trials. World Health Organisation, Geneva

Wilkin D, Hallam L, Doggett M 1992 Measures of need and outcome for primary health care. Oxford University Press, Oxford

Williams R C, Stieg R L 1987 Validity and therapeutic efficacy of individual patient goal attainment procedures in a chronic pain treatment centre. Clinical Journal of Pain 2: 219–228

Wood R 1993 The rehabilitation team. In: Greenwood R, Barnes M P, McMillan T M, Ward C D (eds) Neurological rehabilitation. Churchill Livingstone, Edinburgh, pp 41–49

3

An analysis of normal movement as the basis for the development of treatment techniques

Susan Edwards

INTRODUCTION

Normal movement or activity may be considered to be a skill acquired through learning for the purpose of achieving the most efficient and economical movement or performance of a given task and is specific to the individual. Motor control concerns the nature and cause of movement and is dependent upon the interaction of both perceptual and action systems, with cognition affecting both systems at many levels (Shumway-Cook & Woollacott 1995).

The purpose of this chapter is to describe aspects of posture and movement which relate to the normal adult population. Many components of movement are consistent and these form the basis of this analysis of normal behaviour. Similarities and differences which arise within the normal adult population will be discussed throughout this chapter as they relate to specific postures or movement components.

The emphasis on regaining 'normal movement' following neurological damage has been challenged by Latash & Anson (1996). Their provocative but fascinating article suggests that the restoration of function is an adaptive process, dependent upon the residual capability of a damaged nervous system. Comparison is made between each end of the spectrum of 'normal movement', highlighting the disparity between the clumsy individual and the elite sports person. Although ordinary mortals may admire the athlete capable of high jumping in excess of 6 feet, how many 'normal' individuals consider a

Fosbury flop, the high jump technique, to be a fundamental part of their physical repertoire?

A knowledge of normal movement has been described by many authors as a basis for treatment of the neurologically damaged patient (Davies 1985, Carr & Shepherd 1986, Galley & Forster 1987, Bobath 1990, Davies 1990, Lynch & Grisogono 1991). A wide range of different clinical presentations exist in patients with neurological dysfunction and, consequently, different aspects of movement impairment will be demonstrated. For example, a patient with acquired brain injury or one with multiple sclerosis may present with hypertonus or ataxia or indeed a combination of the two. The clinical presentation and selection of the most appropriate treatment intervention may only be accurately assessed on (a) the basis of an extensive knowledge of normal movement and (b) recognition of the severity and duration of the neurological damage which may necessitate compensatory strategies.

The main remit of physiotherapy is to enable patients to attain their optimal level of function with regard to effectiveness and efficiency of movement. In the acute stage of management emphasis is on the recovery of normal movement strategies, with the patient regaining the ability to perform tasks in the same way as prior to the onset of their neurological damage. However, for patients with more chronic, established conditions, compensatory/alternative strategies, may need to be adopted to accomplish the task.

It is not within the scope of this chapter to discuss the neuropsychological impairment which may be an integral component of the patient's disability. The implications of behavioural, perceptual, cognitive or memory dysfunction are described in Chapter 4, and movement cannot be considered to be a separate entity from these aspects. Lack of emphasis on these neuropsychological aspects in this chapter in no way reflects any lack of recognition of their importance in the total picture of neurological rehabilitation.

FEATURES OF NORMAL MOVEMENT

Normal movement is dependent upon a neuromuscular system which can receive, integrate and respond appropriately to multiple intrinsic and extrinsic stimuli. It is controlled not only by central commands and spinal activity but also by functional and behavioural aspects which influence posture and movement. The central and peripheral systems interact extensively during the execution of motor plans and comprise sets of feedforward commands for complex motor actions. These are learned from successful, previous motor performance (Brooks 1986). In order for this interaction to be effective in producing normal movement, key components should be considered.

Normal postural tone

Both neural and non-neural mechanisms contribute to the generation of muscle tone or stiffness in individual muscles. In the assessment of patients with neurological impairment, neurologists define muscle tone in an operational manner as the resistance to movement when the patient is in a state of voluntary relaxation (Davidoff 1992). Perhaps more appropriately for therapists, postural tone or the activity in muscles when counteracting the force of gravity, has been described as the state of readiness of the body musculature in preparation for the maintenance of a posture or the performance of a movement (Bernstein 1967).

Normal postural tone enables an individual to:

- maintain an upright posture against the force of gravity
- vary and adapt to a constantly changing base of support
- allow selective movement to attain functional skills.

Postural tone is adaptable and varies throughout different parts of the body in response to desired goals. Brooks (1986) describes the intricacy of the golf swing to illustrate the synchronous coordination of posture and movement. The stance of the golfer must be such as to afford stability during the arm swing by setting the stance muscles at the proper steady tensions, while at the same time setting the readiness to respond to stretch of contracting muscles. The tone of the trunk and lower limbs must provide adequate postural support for the moving parts before a successful swing can be accomplished.

From this example of a golf swing it can be seen that the distribution and intensity of postural tone can be influenced by the size of the base of support. From a mechanical perspective, this is the area within the boundaries of each point of contact with the supporting surface. However, of relevance to patient treatment is the ability of the individual to respond and interact appropriately with this support, as described in Chapter 6. The larger the base of support and the lower the centre of mass in relation to the supporting surface, the less effort is required to maintain position and stability. For example, lying provides a far greater base of support than does standing and therefore is the more stable position. Postural tone is therefore normally lower in lying than in standing.

Clinical application

These factors are relevant in the choice of position in which to treat a patient. Many patients following neurological damage spend a considerable proportion of time in lying and, depending on the extent of their disability, may be unable to stand independently. Recruitment of muscle activity in lying, particularly for patients with low tone, is often difficult. Considerable effort is required to overcome the force of gravity and, in functional terms, it is a position which, in normal circumstances, is rarely used for activities of daily life. For this reason, it is often more appropriate for the patient with low tone to be placed in a more upright position with a reduced base of support and the centre of mass higher in relation to the supporting surface. However, careful preparation is essential before placing these patients in standing. Effective support must be given to ensure alignment of body parts and thus minimise inappropriate and unnecessary compensation.

Reciprocal innervation

According to Bobath (1990) reciprocal innervation is the graded and synchronous interaction of agonists, antagonists and synergists throughout the body. Marsden (1982) describes this interaction when:

> starting from an initial posture, the limb or digit is repositioned in space by activation of the prime moving muscle, the agonist; at the same time, the activity of antagonists must be adjusted, and the actions of both the agonists and antagonists around a joint must be complemented by appropriate changes in activity in synergistic muscles. Not only do simple synergies fixate a joint to allow action of the prime movers, there must also be appropriate contraction of proximal fixating muscles so as to adjust the trunk to maintain balance.

The physiological basis of reciprocal innervation is described in Chapter 1. Reciprocal innervation occurs during discrete, selective movements, for example of the fingers during fine manipulation, and also in postural control. It may be considered to be an integral part of balance. The constant postural adjustments and interaction between muscle groups provides the automatic adaptation of the body in response to the functional goal and to changes in the environment.

When standing, the interaction of muscle groups, primarily those of the pelvis, trunk and legs, is dynamic with constant adjustments occurring to enable mobility within the base of support. This dynamic feature frees the arms for selective movement. It is suggested that the nervous system combines independent, though related, muscles, into units called muscle synergies. This is the functional coupling of groups of muscles such that they are constrained to act together as a unit, thereby simplifying the control demand of the CNS (Shumway-Cook & Woollacott 1995).

The postural adjustments that occur automatically, prior to, during and after the performance of a movement provide:

- equilibrium by maintaining the centre of gravity within the base of support; these adjustments occur during the performance of a selective movement such as reaching forwards with the arm and when there is an application of an external force to the body (a perturbation)
- body stability; that is the postural adjustments govern the position of given segments such as

the head or trunk (Massion 1992, Soechting & Flanders 1992).

Potentially destabilising movement is preceded by activation of postural muscles, called anticipatory postural adjustments, which serve to compensate in advance for changes in equilibrium or posture caused by the movement. These preparatory postural responses occur both to preserve balance in standing (Cordo & Nashner 1982) and to stabilise posture before an arm movement (Massion & Woollacott 1996, Wing et al 1997).

Clinical application

Patients with abnormal tone following neurological damage illustrate impaired reciprocal innervation. This may be as a result of hypotonus causing inadequate stability due to reduced activity, or of hypertonus where there is excessive and stereotyped activity preventing these tonal adaptations. In the latter case, co-contraction may become static and constant. Dominance of the hypertonic muscles prevents interaction between the opposing and complementary muscle groups, resulting in a static fixation rather than a dynamic stability (Massion 1984).

The ability to co-activate agonist and antagonist muscles is also important in terms of trunk control. Functional tasks such as eating and dressing require constant adaptation of muscular activity with regard to the trunk and pelvis. Reaching to pick up a cup from a table requires stability within the trunk and of the pelvis in order to transfer weight and accomplish the task most efficiently (Moore et al 1992). A disabled person with a neurological impairment adversely affecting trunk and pelvic stability may be able to adapt and perform the function, but the effort required may be substantially greater and compensatory strategies may be used.

Altered reciprocal innervation is a feature in patients with cerebellar lesions. Complex motor programmes involving postural adjustment in support of the focal movement of the limb are impaired (Diener et al 1990, 1992). This is illustrated in the finger–nose test which is used to determine the severity of ataxia. It is often considerably easier for the patient to coordinate arm movement with the body supported and the elbow resting on a firm surface than with the body and arm unsupported (Haggard et al 1994). In this way, the movement is broken down to the more simple task of elbow flexion and extension and is therefore less dependent on proximal stability.

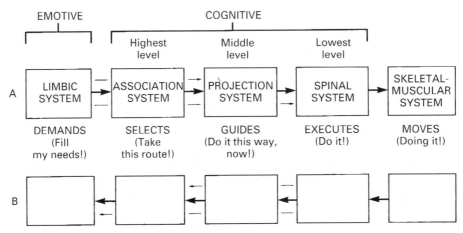

Figure 3.1 Cartoon summary highlighting the motivational function of the limbic system in motor control. Direct connections are indicated by heavy arrows and indirect connections by light arrows. Feedforward connections are represented in (A) and feedback between equivalent systems in (B). (Reproduced from Brooks 1986 The neural basis of motor control, Oxford University Press, with kind permission.)

Sensorimotor feedback and feedforward

Postures and movements are guided by a mixture of motor programmes and sensory feedback. Motor programmes have been described as a set of muscle commands which are structured before a movement sequence begins and that allow the entire sequence to be carried out uninfluenced by peripheral feedback (Keele 1968). Feedback brings the programme commands up to date with their execution and corrects errors (Brooks 1986) (Fig. 3.1).

Control of posture and movement requires initiation and planning at the highest level, control and updating from the middle level and execution and regulation of the task at the lowest level. However, it must be stressed that interaction between these levels is constant and ongoing, providing information in both directions (see Chapter 1).

Movement skills are constantly reinforced and refined by variable repetition, the CNS being ever sensitive to both intrinsic and extrinsic sensory information, which is assimilated to produce effective activity. Motor learning is therefore an active process. This is of particular relevance in the treatment of patients with neurological disability. Patients who are unable to move cannot reinforce their motor programmes and the maxim 'use it or lose it' may therefore apply. There is evidence of extensive functional and structural plasticity in the adult cerebral cortex. Functional maps in sensory and motor cortex are dynamically maintained by use and are altered by central and peripheral pathophysiological disturbances (Nudo 1999).

Everyday activities such as walking and getting out of bed require little conscious effort once they become established movement patterns. The objective is to achieve a functional goal, as opposed to having to consider how one accomplishes each stage of the task. In contrast, the learning of new skills, such as how to drive a car, will initially involve considerable concentration until the movement patterns become established, after which time the task becomes relatively automatic (Schmidt 1991a).

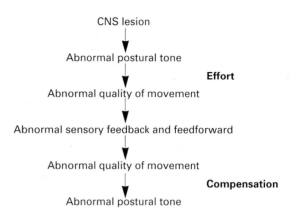

Figure 3.2   Pattern of response following CNS lesion (Bryce 1989).

Normal movement is dependent upon constant interaction of neural structures within the CNS. This neural activity may be considered a cyclical event during the performance of normal movement which reinforces movement patterns. Any interruption in this cycle of events will affect the outcome. If there is abnormal postural tone as a result of neurological damage, there may be disordered movement or a limited movement repertoire, producing an abnormal sensory input to the CNS. This may give rise to a response which is produced by effort and/or compensation, which in turn produces abnormal movement and abnormal postural adaptation (Fig. 3.2).

Clinical application

Sensory-motor integration in terms of continual feedback and feedforward is essential in the learning experience of any individual. By enabling the patient to move in a more normal way, effective motor programmes may be regained.

Motor learning is a set of processes associated with practice or experience, leading to relatively permanent changes in the capability for skilled performance (Schmidt 1991b). The only way motor learning may be clinically observed is in a change in the patient's functional capability. The performance at the end of practice is not an indicator of the degree of learning. In fact certain factors which improve performance at the end of practice do not necessarily lead to long-term learning or carry-over (Schmidt 1988).

Shumway-Cook & Woollacott (1995) provide an excellent review of the theories of motor control. They propose that movement emerges from an interaction between the individual, the task and the environment in which the task is being carried out and that movement is the result of a dynamic interplay between perceptual, cognitive and action systems.

Balance reactions

Postural or equilibrium control is a sensorimotor task requiring the coordination of sensory information with motor aspects of postural control and is the foundation for all voluntary skills. Almost every movement is made up of both postural components which stabilise the body and the prime mover components which relate to the particular movement goal (Massion & Woollacott 1996).

For the purpose of assessment and treatment, Bobath (1990) differentiated between three groups of automatic postural reactions. These were referred to as righting, equilibrium and protective/saving reactions. Although many therapists continue to make use of this terminology, there is some confusion, particularly with regard to righting reactions. As discussed in Chapter 1, the righting reactions are observed only in developing infants and in specific animal preparations. In the mature adult, they become integrated into more complex equilibrium reactions (Bobath 1990) and division between the two is impossible (Bryce 1972).

Clinicians refer to righting reactions as they relate to the alignment of body segments to each other and to the environment and in the performance of sequences of movement such as rolling, sitting up and lying down (Davies 1985, Edwards 1998). However, when considering posture and balance in a broader context, this may be considered to be an artificial divide.

Key tasks have been attributed to postural control:

- The maintenance of the alignment of body posture with a vertical relationship between body segments to counteract the forces of gravity to attain an upright stance.
- The maintenance of equilibrium by keeping the body's centre of mass within the base of support while a movement or task is being performed.
- The interaction between perception and action systems to maintain bodily orientation to the environment. This provides an internal postural image or postural body schema, which is monitored by multisensory inputs.
- The organisation of body segments according to the function of the task and the dynamic adjustment of joint stiffness during the movement (Massion & Woollacott 1996).

Unpredictable forces that disturb equilibrium in standing produce automatic, coordinated responses of muscles across a number of body segments that serve to maintain posture. The anticipatory postural adjustments have been described above in the context of reciprocal innervation (see page 38). This 'pre-tuning' of sensory and motor systems for postural demands is based on previous experience and learning and is more variable the slower the movement (Horak et al 1984). As less stabilisation is required during slower movement, the preparatory muscle activity is not programmed as consistently as with more rapid movement. In addition, if a perturbation is applied in standing when the hand is in contact with a fixed support, the automatic postural response includes activation of the muscles of the arm and hand to help to restore balance (Cordo & Nashner 1982). This adaptive postural control therefore involves modifying sensory and motor systems in response to changing and environmental demands (Shumway-Cook & Woollacott 1995).

Characteristic patterns of synergic muscle activity have been described which underlie movement strategies critical for postural control in standing (Nashner 1977, Horak & Nashner 1986). These are referred to as the ankle, hip and stepping strategies and are used in both a feedback and feedforward (anticipatory) manner to maintain balance.

The ankle strategy is that which is used during quiet stance, when the perturbation to equilibrium is small and the support is firm. The hip strategy is used when the perturbation to balance is faster and greater and when the support surface is pliant or smaller than the feet, such as when standing on a beam. Movement at either the ankle or hip is dependent upon full range of movement and strength of muscles acting over these joints. The stepping strategy is called into play when the perturbation is such as to displace the centre of mass outside the base of support and a step or hop is required to restore alignment.

In addition to the ability to generate force to control the position of the body in space, effective postural control is dependent upon sensory information from visual, somatosensory and vestibular systems. Visual inputs provide a reference for verticality and head motion; the somatosensory system provides information regarding the body's position in space with reference to the supporting surface and the relationship of body segments to each other; and the vestibular system provides information about the position and movement of the head. It is suggested that the nervous system might 'weight' the importance of somatosensory information for postural control more heavily than visual or vestibular inputs (Shumway-Cook & Woollacott 1995).

Clinical application

When a movement is performed, postural control is provided by segmental adjustments which compensate for the displacement of the centre of mass caused by the moving segments (Massion 1992). Changes in the location of the centre of mass necessitate preparatory and continuous postural adjustments during any movement, and even the smallest alteration has to be countered by modifications of tone throughout the body musculature (Bobath 1990).

Although the limbs frequently adopt a position of asymmetry in relation to each other, there is invariably predominant symmetry of the trunk, pelvis and shoulder girdles. It is important to recognise that, although many positions are asymmetrical in normal movement, this asymmetry is transient and interchangeable through symmetry. In contrast, patients with neurological disability are observed to have asymmetry imposed by weakness or abnormal movement strategies. For example, if a patient with a dense left hemiplegia attempts to roll towards the right side, the affected side may be unable to initiate or participate in the movement and tends to be left behind. Realignment of body segments on completion of the movement is often impaired.

The increased variability in the anticipatory postural adjustments with slower movements and the use of motor pathways controlling arm and hand movement when support is provided has implications in the treatment of patients with neurological damage. Many patients will be unable to move as quickly as normal subjects and changes in the postural adjustments may be related more to the speed of movement as opposed to the pathology. Similarly, some patients may require assistance or mechanical aids to enable them to stand and walk. The support offered by the therapist or, for example, a walking frame will influence the postural adjustments. While it is important to facilitate a more normal posture or movement, it may be of equal value to give the patient the opportunity to correct his own posture. If the therapist constantly supports the patient, the postural adjustments will always be dependent on this support (Edwards 1998).

Postural control requires all degrees of reciprocal innervation through the coordinated response of neuromuscular excitatory and inhibitory control to enable postural holding patterns and those for selective movement to operate effectively (Mink 1996). This interaction between opposing and complementary muscle groups is the basis for the maintenance of posture and the performance of selective movement. The ability to maintain equilibrium in a great variety of positions provides the basis for all the skilled movements that are required for self-care, work and recreation (Davies 1985).

Nerve–muscle interaction

Control of movement is dependent upon the interaction between the nervous system and the musculoskeletal system. While the central nervous system generates patterns of movement or motor programmes, their effectiveness is dependent upon the viscoelastic properties of muscles and the anatomical alignment of bones and joints. This section discusses the nerve–muscle interaction which may be affected by neurological impairment.

Neural components

The motor unit. The combination of the motoneurone, its axon and the muscle fibres that it innervates is known as the motor unit or 'final common pathway'. It is activated according to the sum of excitatory and inhibitory inputs and it is through this route that all processing in the CNS is finally transformed into movement (Rothwell 1994, Vrbova et al 1995).

Each muscle fibre is supplied by only one motoneurone but each motoneurone supplies many muscle fibres. The number of fibres supplied by a single motoneurone is referred to as the innervation ratio. Smaller muscles such as the intrinsic hand muscles have a lower innervation ratio – each motoneurone supplying fewer muscle fibres – and it is suggested that there is at least a moderate correlation between innervation ratio and the ability to finely grade muscle force (Enoka 1995).

Muscle fibre type. Skeletal muscles are composed of a variety of functionally diverse fibre types. They are dynamic structures capable of changing their phenotypic profile according to the functional demands placed upon them. This adaptive responsiveness is the basis of fibre type transitions (Pette & Staron 1997).

There are three basic fibre types:

- Slow-twitch oxidative (SO) or type I. These are innervated by small motoneurones and have a small fibre diameter. They are slow to contract, generate a small force and are very resistant to fatigue.

- Fast-twitch oxidative glycolytic (FOG), or type IIA. These have a medium–small fibre diameter, are fast contracting, generate an intermediate force and have some resistance to fatigue.

- Fast-twitch glycolytic (FG) or type IIB. These have motoneurones with large cell bodies and have large-diameter axons. They are fast contracting, generate a large force and fatigue readily (Rothwell 1994).

The characteristics of the three main fibre types are summarised in Table 3.1.

However, other fibre types have been reported in both animal and human studies. There are reports of an intermediate type IID/X in skeletal muscle (Vrbova et al 1995, Pette & Staron 1997) and it is suggested that a considerable percentage of hybrid fibres are present in normal adult muscles (Pette & Staron 1997).

It may be that there is some misclassification of fibre types in human muscles in that type IIB fibres are more similar to the rat IIX than to the rat type IIB (Ennion et al 1995, Pette & Staron 1997, Goldspink 1999a). Hill (1950 as cited by Ennion et al 1995) hypothesised that because the muscles in larger animals are longer, with more sarcomeres in series, their intrinsic velocities of shortening would have to be lower than those of small animals; otherwise, the rate of force development would be unsustainable. It is suggested that the type IIB fibre type expressed in rodents is associated with too high an intrinsic velocity for humans and is therefore not expressed. This difference between type IIB fibre type in rats as compared to humans was described most succinctly by Goldspink (1999b). If humans moved at the same speed as rodents, the ballistic movements of the limbs would be so extreme as to cause them to become detached from the torso.

Table 3.1 The characteristics of different types of skeletal muscles (from Rothwell 1994, Table 3.1, with kind permission)

Fibre type	I SO	IIA FOG	IIB FG
Motor unit type	Slow(S)	Fast fatigue resistant (FR)	Fast fatiguable (FF)
Fibre diameter	Small	Medium–small	Large

A muscle does not consist of a homogenous population of muscle fibres; there are several different fibre types within a muscle, each of which has different mechanical properties. The range of operation of the whole muscle is extended beyond that of any one fibre type alone. A predominance of one fibre type gives the muscle its characteristic properties (Rothwell 1994).

Muscles with predominantly SO fibres participate in longer-lasting but relatively weak contractions, such as in postural control, whereas those with predominantly FG fibres generate large forces but are more readily fatigued. A sporting analogy is to compare the marathon runner with the sprinter. The marathon runner has endurance, due to a predominance of SO fibres, whereas the sprinter, with predominantly fast-twitch muscles, demonstrates explosive power but which is of short duration and therefore cannot be sustained.

Gene expression/fibre type determination. Fibre phenotype is dependent not only on neural activity but also to a large extent on mechanical factors, specifically a combination of stretch and muscle activity (Lin et al 1993, Goldspink 1999a). All muscles stay phenotypically fast unless they are subjected to stretch and force generation. For example, in rats, soleus, with predominantly slow oxidative fibres, if immobilised in a shortened position, subjected to hypogravity or denervated by spinalisation, reverts to expressing the fast gene (Goldspink et al 1992). Furthermore, experiments have shown that the number of SO fibres in the rat soleus muscle increases after birth as the animal uses this muscle for support. If this supporting function is negated by hind limb suspension, the increase in slow-twitch fibres is arrested or fails to occur. A similar finding results following tenotomy of soleus preventing it from being stretched. The contractile speed of the tenotomised muscle becomes fast although the innervation is unchanged (Vrbova et al 1995, Pette & Staron 1997). The main regulation in the expression of the slow phenotype seems to depend on the repression of the fast-type as much as activation of the slow-type genes (Goldspink et al 1992).

Development, innervation, increased and decreased neurological muscular activity, over-

Increased neuromuscular activity/overloading

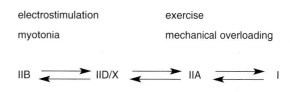

| electrostimulation | exercise |
| myotonia | mechanical overloading |

Decreased neuromuscular activity/unloading

denervation	immobilisation
spinal cord transection	hindlimb suspension
detraining	microgravity

Figure 3.3 Schematic representation of major factors affecting sequential fibre-type transitions. (From Pette & Staron 1997 with permission.)

loading and under-loading, hormones and ageing have all been shown to be influential in determining the phenotypic expression of skeletal muscle fibres. In general, activity and loading result in fast-to-slow fibre type transition and decreased neuromuscular activity or load cause transitions from slow-to-fast (Pette & Staron 1997, Pette 1998) (Fig. 3.3).

Certainly in animal muscle, on which most experiments have been conducted, this fibre type transition is a graded event (Vrbova et al 1995)

The nerve has a powerful influence on the properties of muscle fibres. Nerve transfer in animals shows fast muscles supplied by a slow nerve become slow contracting, and slow muscles supplied by a fast nerve become fast acting, although the cross-innervated muscles are not as slow or as fast as predicted and this nerve transfer does not produce a complete change in phenotype (Vrbova et al 1995).

Muscles may alter their characteristics depending on their usage (Dietz 1992). FG muscles will readily hypertrophy when they are recruited and overloaded during sustained exercise training, as under normal conditions, compared with the SO muscles, they are recruited relatively infrequently. Conversely, although the SO muscles may also hypertrophy, this will be to a lesser extent as they already participate to a more maximal degree in postural control (Rothwell 1994). However, exercise alone cannot radically change fibre type composition or contractile characteristics. During exercise, the motor units are still recruited in an orderly fashion although activated more often and the sequence of recruitment of motor units remains the same, there being no evidence that the motoneuronal properties which influence the pattern of firing are changed by increased use (Vrbova et al 1995).

Recruitment order. The recruitment order of a motor unit depends on the size of its motoneurone. Motoneurones with the smallest axons are excited before those with larger axons: i.e. in the order SO > FOG > FG (Henneman et al 1965 as cited by Rothwell 1994). In this way skeletal muscles are well designed and matched for highly specific functions in the orchestration of any movement by the CNS (Rothwell 1994, Vrbova et al 1995). Postural muscles, which are made up predominantly of SO muscle fibres and participate in long-lasting but relatively weak contractions, are recruited before those which are predominantly fast-twitch and generate larger forces but are more readily fatigued.

For example, it has been shown with electromyographic (EMG) studies that postural muscle fibres such as those of soleus, are activated almost continuously during standing and walking whereas fibres in other skeletal muscles are activated only 5% of the time (Goldspink 1999a). With a common input to the medial gastrocnemius and soleus motoneuronal pools, soleus, which has a predominance of SO muscle fibres, is always recruited before gastrocnemius, which has a greater percentage of fast-twitch fibres. It is not only active during tonic contractions: even in jumping, soleus is maximally active but, in this case, the gastrocnemius produces the most force (Rothwell 1994).

Non-neural components

Contractile properties of muscle. Skeletal muscle fibres are gathered together into bundles called fascicles which are surrounded by a connective tissue sheath. The internal structure of the muscle fibre is complex, with the main elements

being the myofibrils which constitute the contractile machinery of the muscle. Each myofibril consists of longitudinally orientated filaments called myofilaments, the bulk of which are composed of two proteins, actin and myosin. Actin and myosin filaments overlap in the sarcomeres when a muscle contracts. This is referred to as the 'sliding filament' hypothesis. The critical stage of force generation is rotation of the myosin head. This causes the filaments to slide over one another if they are free to move, producing an isotonic contraction, or otherwise an isometric force is generated.

At rest, the concentration of calcium in the sarcoplasmic reticulum is very low, so the majority of actin–myosin bonds remain unformed. The release of neurotransmitter at the neuromuscular junction initiates an action potential along the cell membrane of the muscle fibre, causing a release of calcium from the sarcoplasmic reticulum into the sarcoplasm. This process allows for the formation of actin–myosin bonds. Calcium is then actively pumped back into the sarcoplasmic reticulum and the contraction ceases.

Mechanical properties of muscle. There are three elements in the mechanical behaviour of muscle. The contractile element has its own mechanical properties, viscosity and stiffness, which change with the level of muscle contraction. The contractile mechanism resides in the interaction between the actin and myosin filaments. The series elastic element lies in the tendinous insertions of the muscle and in the actin and myosin cross-bridges themselves, and transmits the force of contraction. The parallel elastic element resides in the sarcolemma of the muscle cells and in the surrounding connective tissue. This both distributes the forces associated with passive stretch and maintains the relative position of fibres (Goldspink & Williams 1990, Rothwell 1994). The contractile element actively generates muscle force, whereas the series and parallel elastic elements are passive components, acting as mechanical springs.

There are two important relationships which influence the control of muscle contraction. The first is the length–tension relationship whereby, as the muscle length is increased, the force exerted rises. The tension is due not only to the activity of the contractile element but also to passive stretch of the non-contractile elements. The force produced therefore differs depending on the muscle length, maximum work being performed by a muscle shortening at intermediate muscle lengths. The example cited by Rothwell (1994) is the extended position of the wrist while the fingers flex powerfully on to an object in the palm of the hand. The power of the grip is substantially weakened with a more flexed wrist position. This may be significant following stroke, where flexor hypertonia is often predominant in the upper limb. Many people are unable to extend the wrist, with a resultant decrease in grip strength and impairment of manipulation skills.

The second is the force–velocity relationship in that the rate at which a muscle can shorten depends upon the force exerted: the greater the resistance to movement, the more the velocity of movement is decreased.

The length–tension and force–velocity contribute to compensation for unexpected disturbances. A sudden increase in load can produce increased muscle tension not only through reflex pathways but also by the nature of the length–tension characteristics of the muscle. Even in the deafferented man, the force output adjusts although not to the same extent as normal (Rothwell 1994).

The elastic compliance of muscle is dependent upon the concentration of collagen, a major component of intramuscular connective tissue. This concentration is higher in slow-twitch as opposed to fast-twitch muscle and is reflected in the passive length–tension curves which show that fast-twitch muscle has a higher compliance. Experiments with rats have shown that slow-twitch postural muscles are particularly sensitive to immobilisation. The intramuscular connective tissue increased more rapidly in the immobilised soleus than in gastrocnemius, which is composed primarily of fast-twitch fibres, and this was more prevalent when the muscles were held in a shortened position (Given et al 1995).

The force generated by a muscle is dependent upon the number of cross-bridges which can be engaged between actin and myosin filaments and this in turn depends on the overlap of these filaments in the sarcomere. The number of sarcomeres in series determines the distance through which a muscle can shorten and regulation of the sarcomere number is considered to be an adaptation to changes in the functional length of muscle. If a muscle is immobilised in a shortened position, there is a reduction in the number of sarcomeres and conversely, if a muscle is immobilised in a lengthened position, there is an increase in the number of sarcomeres (Herbert 1988, Goldspink & Williams 1990). However, in animals, the changes in sarcomeres have been shown to be age dependent, the young adapting to a fixed lengthened state by lengthening the tendon as opposed to adults adapting with sarcomeres growing longer under the same conditions (Whitlock 1990).

The interaction between the actin and myosin filaments gives the muscle a certain resting tension and short-range dynamic stiffness. This plastic behaviour or stiffness within the muscle fibre itself is known as thixotropy (Hagbarth 1994); this is an engineering term which is used to describe the dynamic viscosity of fluids. When applied to muscle, thixotropy has been attributed to abnormal cross-bridges between actin and myosin filaments, producing an inherent muscle stiffness (Sheean 1998).

Clinical implications

Neural activity is a major factor in influencing the characteristic properties of skeletal muscles (Dietz 1992). Changes in function imposed by neurological impairment may produce muscle fibre type transformation and/or change in muscle fibre type distribution that is dependent upon the amount and the pattern of neuronal input (Jones & Round 1990, Cameron & Calancie 1995). Within the upper motor neurone syndrome both fibre type transitions have been reported (see Chapter 5).

Prevention or reversal of denervation atrophy depends on the capacity of the nerves of surviving motoneurones to sprout and reinnervate as many denervated fibres as possible. As a result of sprouting, each motoneurone supplies an increased number of muscle fibres. The innervation ratio is therefore increased, each motoneurone supplying more muscle fibres, leading to a decrease in selective movement (Gordon & Mao 1994).

Although exercise to improve muscle strength is recommended, strenuous activity of partially denervated muscle can lead to an irreversible increase in weakness (Bennett & Knowlton 1958). It is suggested that, in order to avoid overwork weakness, there must be:

- a balance between rest and activity
- an emphasis on submaximal intensities of exercise
- the development of preventative muscular strengthening programmes specific to the patterns of weakness
- the creation of endurance training programmes for normal cardiovascular responses to exercise (Curtis & Weir 1996).

In patients with neurological disability, muscles may be constrained in a shortened position due to the prevalence of abnormal tone. There is loss of sarcomeres and a reduction in muscle fibre length with an increased resistance to passive stretch. This alters both the length–tension and force–velocity relationships of muscle contraction, and optimal force production is impaired. Sustained stretch of shortened structures may go some way to improving the biomechanical advantage and enabling more effective activation of muscle, a factor noted in clinical practice. Many patients automatically elongate shortened muscles and report greater ease of movement following sustained stretch. Splinting may also be used as a means of imposing sustained stretch. The advantages and disadvantages of this intervention are described in Chapter 10.

AN APPROACH TO THE ANALYSIS OF POSTURE AND MOVEMENT

This section aims to identify key components relating to the analysis of positions and of movement sequences.

Rotation of body segments

Rotation may be described as the coordinated response between flexion and extension in all planes of movement. The importance of rotation in the maintenance of posture and performance of movement is discussed by many authors (Knott & Voss 1968, Galley & Forster 1987, Bobath 1990). Certainly, loss of rotation and arm swing are noticeable aspects of impaired movement, characterised in, for example, the patient with Parkinson's disease (Marsden 1984, Rogers 1991).

This interplay between flexion and extension can be illustrated when observing the development of rolling in children. At birth, the child is predominantly flexed, with some extension at the neck allowing for rotation of the head. Slowly over a period of 3–4 months, the child learns to lift his head when in prone, support on his forearms and, by 6 months, push up on to extended arms, developing extensor activity throughout the body. The initial movement of the child from prone to supine is a crude, gross movement rather than a controlled activity. As the child becomes more confident in pushing up on to extended arms, he begins to look around, and in so doing transfers his weight from side to side. Over-exuberance takes the centre of gravity outside of the base of support and he falls on to his back. This first experience of movement from prone to supine is an illustration of the innate lack of coordination between extension and flexion. Over the following months, rolling from prone to supine and from supine to prone, is refined as a direct integration of extensor and flexor activity. The weight-bearing side actively works against the surface as the body rotates around its axis, providing stability for the movement (Alexander et al 1993). The more intricate skill, of getting from the floor up into sitting, is only achieved when the child has developed the necessary level of neuromuscular control.

Rotation within the trunk and of the prime movers in the limbs is fundamental for the performance of functional skills such as eating, dressing, writing and walking. Any alteration in the distribution of tone, either excessive flexion or extension, will result in impaired rotation and subsequent impoverishment of movement.

Postural sets

'Postural sets' is a term used by Bobath (1990) to describe adaptations of posture or adjustments which precede and accompany a movement. They can be viewed as anticipatory postural adjustments which occur prior to the disturbance of posture and equilibrium resulting from the movement (Massion 1992).

When considering these responses in relation to activity of the arm, Cordo & Nashner (1982) observed that, with a voluntary arm movement, the leg muscles involved in postural control are activated prior to the prime movers. The duration of the anticipatory postural adjustments increases with the load to be raised by the arm (Lee et al 1987). These authors suggest that the preparatory adjustments are not specifically related to balance control but that they also directly provide additional force for performing the movement. These anticipatory postural adjustments also serve to stabilise the position of segments such as the head, trunk or limbs during movement performance (Massion 1992).

A practical example of this preparation for movement and the control during performance of the movement is in jumping into the deep end as opposed to the shallow end of a swimming pool. When jumping into deep water, contact with the bottom is cushioned by the volume and depth of the water. The legs tend to be held straight as the feet search for the bottom of the pool. Conversely, when jumping into shallow water, the legs remain slightly flexed in preparation for the impact of hitting the bottom. On making contact with the bottom of the pool, the knees give, cushioning the effects of the impact. Providing the individual is aware of the depth of the water, the body is pre-programmed to respond appropriately. However, if an individual jumps into shallow water thinking it to be considerably deeper, then the correct adjustments are not made and injury may result.

There are an infinite number of postural sets relating to both the posture which an individual assumes and the preparatory adjustments made in advance of movement. For example, no one individual will consistently assume or maintain repeatable positions in standing. Equally, the means by which a person attains the standing position will vary according to the starting position and the reason for standing. For any given task from a given position, postural adjustments are felt to be uniform but flexible to change with changing task (Hansen et al 1988, Horak et al 1994).

Key points of control

Key points of control are described as areas of the body from which movement may be most effectively controlled (Bobath 1990). Proximal key points are the trunk, head, shoulder girdles and pelvis and distal key points are the hands and feet.

The choice of key point from which to influence movement is determined by the ability of the individual to respond to facilitation of movement (Fig. 3.4A&B). For example, if the therapist facilitates movement using the patient's hand as a key point, there must be adequate postural tone within the trunk to make an appropriate response. If proximal control is lacking, attempts to bring the patient forwards from this key point may traumatise the shoulder joint. It is for this reason that the proximal key points tend to be utilised more frequently to ensure stability within the trunk prior to facilitating movement of the limbs.

Midline – the alignment of body segments

The midline is an abstract reference point against which alignment of the aforementioned key points, particularly the trunk, shoulder girdles and pelvis, can be compared. It may be considered a dividing line that serves as a point of reference for analysing body alignment and movement in either the sagittal, coronal or horizontal planes. Taylor et al (1994) describe the midline as an imaginary line that bisects the body into a right and left sector in the sagittal plane. This definition, which is limited to one plane, enables the physiotherapist to assess and describe body alignment in terms of lateral symmetry when observing the patient from in front or behind. The midline should also be considered as a point of reference in the coronal and transverse planes which provides a means of

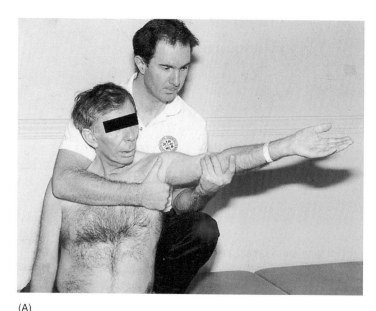
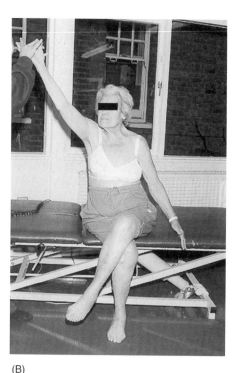

(A)
(B)

Figure 3.4 (A) Proximal key point control. (B) Distal key point control.

describing the anteroposterior relationships of body structures and alignment with regard to rotation.

The perception of body orientation in space depends on multisensory evaluation of visual, vestibular and proprioceptive sensory input (Karnath et al 1994). The concept of midline has physiological significance as it seems, at least for the upper limb, that some movements are programmed to occur relative to the midline (Soechting & Flanders 1992).

ANALYSIS OF SPECIFIC POSITIONS

It is useful to analyse positions because it provides a baseline for determining differences which may arise due to pathology. It is important to recognise that very few normal subjects demonstrate the exact characteristics identified in this analysis. Many will show variability such as excessive flexion at the shoulders, an increased lumbar lordosis in supine or a greater degree of

lateral rotation in one leg than the other. This variability may ultimately prove to be irrelevant but one may question whether or not there is a reason for this discrepancy.

The analysis of tonal influences in certain positions may be based on observation of the relationship between the trunk and the proximal key points and the limbs. This relationship may be used to enable the therapist to determine the overall influence of extension or flexion in each particular position.

Supine lying

An individual generally adopts a symmetrical position in relation to the supporting surface (Fig. 3.5).

When lying supine, the influence of gravity and the reduction in the level of postural activity result in the shoulder girdles falling into retraction. The ability to accept the base of support will vary considerably, depending upon the level of

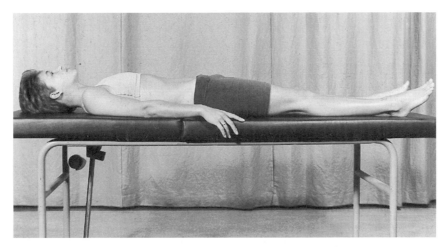

Figure 3.5 Supine lying.

tonus and biomechanical properties of soft tissue structures.

The upper limbs tend to adopt a position of lateral rotation with some abduction, the degree being determined by the individual's inherent level of postural tone. In general, the lower the tonus, the greater the degree of lateral rotation and abduction.

The pelvis tends to tilt posteriorly with increased extension at the hips. The extent of this pelvic movement is determined by the anatomical structure of the individual, in particular the alignment of the pelvis with the lumbar spine and the bulk of the gluteal region. The legs usually adopt a position of lateral rotation with some degree of abduction.

This is a position of predominant extension; movement out of this position requires flexor activity, most commonly observed in conjunction with rotation.

Prone lying

The individual generally adopts a symmetrical position in relation to the supporting surface, but with the head turned laterally (Fig. 3.6).

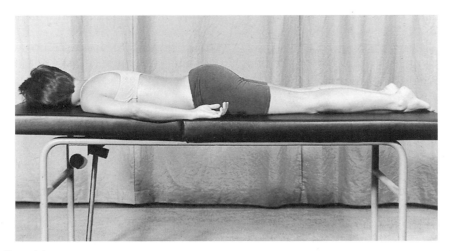

Figure 3.6 Prone lying.

When prone, the shoulder girdles protract and the upper limbs rest in a position of flexion, medial rotation and adduction; the degree of adduction is determined by the amount of flexion.

The pelvis tends to tilt anteriorly, producing a degree of flexion at the hips. The legs are extended, adducted and medially rotated and the feet plantar flexed.

This is a position of predominant flexion. Movement out of this position requires extensor activity with a rotational component determined by the side to which the head is turned.

As prone is a position with a predominant flexor influence, it is not necessarily the position of choice for management of those with flexor hypertonus. However, if the patient is able to accommodate to this position, it may be useful for preventing or correcting hip flexion contractures. Standing, which has a greater influence of extension, may be more effective in managing this problem.

Side-lying

This is a position in which a degree of asymmetry between the two sides of the body is invariably present. Figure 3.7 illustrates one posture which may be adopted by an individual when asked to assume this position.

Certain characteristics may be noted. The weight-bearing side of the body is more extended and elongated than the non-weight-bearing side which is side flexed. This position is influenced by the anatomical structure of the individual; the greater the pelvic girth, the greater is the side flexion of the non-weight-bearing side.

There are many variations of the side-lying position. One such variation is bilateral flexion of the legs where the individual takes up a modified foetal position.

The position of the shoulder is determined by the tendency to lie towards prone or supine. Only those with bilateral leg flexion will lie with one side of the body virtually in alignment with the other. People who lie towards supine tend to protract the supporting shoulder, whereas those who lie towards prone tend to lie with the

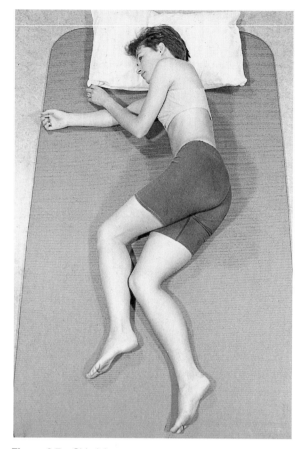

Figure 3.7 Side-lying.

supporting shoulder retracted. Accordingly, the degree of trunk rotation varies in respect of the position of the shoulders and their relationship with the pelvis.

The weight-bearing side provides stability, through its acceptance of and interaction with the base of support, to allow for selective movement of the non-weight-bearing side. Impairment resulting in inactivity or inappropriate activity of the weight-bearing side may disrupt or prevent functional movement of the non-weight-bearing side.

This is a position widely used and recommended in the positioning of patients with neurological disability (Bobath 1990, Davies 1994). The relative asymmetry of this position enables 'the break up' of either predominant flexor or extensor hypertonus. It is also recommended as a position whereby coordination, postural control and sensory reintegration of the weight-bearing side may be facilitated through functional movement of the non-weight-bearing side.

Sitting

Analysis of this position is complex due to the varying amount and type of support offered. This posture is described in terms of unsupported and supported sitting.

Unsupported sitting with the hips and knees at 90 degrees

Anti-gravity control in unsupported sitting (Fig. 3.8) is recruited primarily through extensor

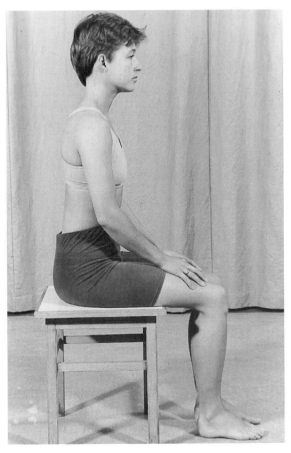

Figure 3.8 Unsupported sitting.

activity at the pelvis and lumbar spine. In the absence of full support this anti-gravity, extensor activity is essential for dynamic maintenance of an upright posture. Consideration of the base of support in relation to the feet is discussed when analysing moving from sitting to standing.

The shoulder girdles are protracted with medial rotation and adduction of the shoulders. This reflects the relative lack of activity required by the upper limbs to maintain this posture.

The position of the pelvis depends upon the degree of upright or slumped sitting assumed by the individual. There is an element of extensor activity observed primarily at the lumbar spine and reflected in the degree of anterior pelvic tilt.

The degree of pelvic tilt influences the position of the lower limbs and vice versa. It is observed that the starting position affects associated limb movements. With the hips and knees at 90 degrees or more flexion, the greater the anterior tilt, the more pronounced will be the degree of lateral rotation and abduction. However, if the subject is seated on a higher chair with the hips and knees at an angle of less than 90 degrees, an increase in the anterior pelvic tilt tends to produce medial rotation and adduction. Conversely, if a patient has limited hip flexion, this is combined with posterior pelvic tilt and flexion of the lumbar spine.

Unsupported sitting is a position of predominant flexion with recruitment of extensor activity arising primarily at the lumbar spine, pelvis and hips.

Supported sitting

The amount and type of support offered varies considerably between, for example, a dining chair and a lounge chair. The dining chair is a more rigid structure and therefore most individuals are less likely to relax and depend on it for full support. In many respects, the posture taken up by an individual sitting on a dining chair is no different from that of unsupported sitting.

Conversely, the lounge chair, depending upon the degree of comfort, the angle of recline and the provision or otherwise of a head support, affords more support to the individual (Fig. 3.9). The

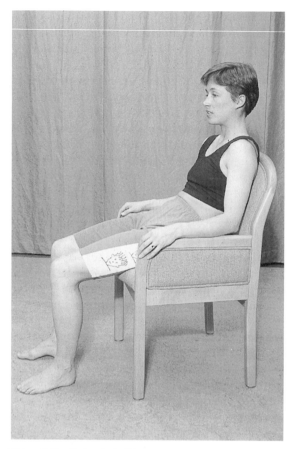

Figure 3.9 Supported sitting.

The distribution of tone is also dependent on the extent of support. This support is substantially increased if the individual leans forward, resting the arms on a table such as when writing. In this posture there is a marked reduction in the anti-gravity activity within the trunk and pelvis. The size and distribution of the base of support are changed significantly with more weight being taken through the upper limbs, and hence the requirement for dynamic postural stability within the trunk and pelvis is reduced.

Clinical application

This analysis of sitting assists with the planning of treatment interventions. For example, for patients with hypertonus, it may be more effective to provide an increased base of support in sitting to facilitate tone reduction. Conversely, for those with hypotonus, where the aim of treatment is to increase tone, less support should be provided by the therapist, thereby facilitating activity within the trunk. This analysis is also relevant to the provision of wheelchairs and the correct positioning of the patient in the chair. The position of the pelvis will have a direct influence on the posture of the lower limbs. Equally, the use of upper limb support, such as a tray attached to a wheelchair, will have a direct effect on trunk and pelvic activity.

Standing

Standing requires extensive anti-gravity activity to sustain the upright position over a relatively small base of support.

Muscle relaxation tends to accentuate the lumbar, thoracic and cervical curvatures and the pelvis tilts anteriorly. This posture may be seen in particularly lethargic individuals and in women in the later stages of pregnancy (Kapandji 1980).

Normal subjects may demonstrate flattening of spinal curvatures commensurate with their level of tonus (Fig. 3.10). This is initiated at the level of the pelvis. The anterior tilt of the pelvis is counterbalanced by the activity, primarily of gluteus maximus and the hamstrings, restoring the horizontal alignment of the interspinous line

body conforms to the chair with a posterior pelvic tilt and the shoulder girdles protracted. The arms and legs rest in various and diverse positions. Movement away from this position of full support initially requires flexor activity closely followed by extension to provide the proximal stability essential for the achievement of function such as reaching for a cup or preparing to stand.

Supported sitting in a lounge chair is a position of predominant flexion, there being no necessity to recruit anti-gravity activity, given the extended base of support offered by the chair back and arms.

In contrast, the amount of activity when sitting on a dining chair depends upon the position of the pelvis: the degree of anterior or posterior tilt and whether it is forwards on the edge of the chair or positioned at the back of the chair.

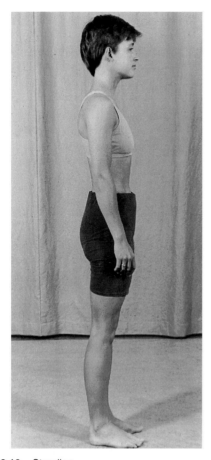

Figure 3.10 Standing.

It may be postulated that the position of the pelvis determines the extent of activity at the shoulder girdles and upper limbs. An anterior pelvic tilt introduces an element of flexion at the hips counteracted by increased extensor activity in the trunk, shoulder girdles and upper limbs. A neutral position of the pelvis or a slight posterior tilt produces a more mechanically efficient position as the iliofemoral ligament provides anterior stability which complements the extensor activity at the hips and pelvis.

Activity within the foot musculature varies according to the size of the base of support. There is less activity in stride standing than when standing with a smaller base of support when the feet are closer together. The constant adjustments by the lower limbs and feet in response to any change in weight distribution serve to maintain the centre of gravity within the supporting surface. For this activity to be effective, adequate mobility within the feet and in the muscles acting over the ankle joint is essential.

In clinical practice it is observed that the majority of patients with abnormal tone affecting the feet lose some and, in severe cases, all of this mobility and as a result their balance in standing is impaired. Unless the problem of immobility of the feet is first addressed, rehabilitation of standing balance will be compromised.

ANALYSIS OF MOVEMENT SEQUENCES

Although adults may be consistent in their performance, they have the ability to vary the movement patterns used in order to accomplish the task. It is this potential for variability that characterises normality (VanSant 1990a).

Analysis of movement in clinical practice is based primarily on observation and knowledge of what is considered to be within normal limits. The movements of lying to sitting, sitting to standing and walking are discussed in a clinical perspective to identify certain features of these movement sequences. Although there will be significant variability in these movement sequences depending upon age, gender, body build, the height of the bed and the firmness of the sup-

between the anterior superior iliac spine and the posterior superior iliac spine. The abdominal muscles contract in conjunction with the gluteus maximus to flatten the lumbar curvature. From this position the paravertebral muscles can act effectively to pull back the upper lumbar vertebrae and extend the vertebral column (Kapandji 1980).

In standing, the upper limbs adopt a position of medial rotation with the shoulder girdles protracted. Providing the centre of gravity remains within the base of support, the upper limbs are not essential for the maintenance of balance. This state of relative inactivity enables freedom of movement of the arms for the performance of functional tasks.

porting surface, the characteristics described are those which may be considered to be within normal limits.

Moving from supine lying to sitting

Initiation of movements from supine have been discussed in part in the previous analysis of the position of supine lying. The large base of support and low centre of mass demand significant effort on the part of the individual to move away from this position. The movement sequence will differ significantly between sitting up from lying on the floor and sitting up and placing the legs over the side of a bed. For relevance to treatment, it is the latter sequence which will be analysed. An assumption is made that the height of the bed is such that the individual can sit with the hips and knees at 90 degrees on completion of the movement and the surface of the bed is firm.

How is this movement from lying initiated? Bobath (1990) states that turning commences with the upper part of the body. It is observed that the majority of individuals flex forwards at the head and shoulders with varying degrees of rotation towards the side to which they are moving. However, others may initiate the movement with propulsion from the leg opposite to the side to which they are moving. Here the initial movement is one of flexion prior to pushing through the limb to generate the movement. The movement of the leg is then followed almost simultaneously by flexion of the head and trunk.

The fulcrum of movement is at the pelvis. As the individual brings the upper trunk forwards off the bed, the legs move towards the side of the bed. As the subject pivots over the pelvis to sit with the legs over the side of the bed, the weight-bearing side is elongated with contralateral side flexion of the opposite side of the trunk. During the course of the movement, the pelvis tends to be in a position of posterior tilt, but this will vary depending on the strength and control of the abdominals. Having attained this end position, the trunk is then realigned with more equal weight-bearing over the ischeal tuberosities with an anterior pelvic tilt.

To move from lying into sitting requires that the abdominal muscles move or hold the weight of the trunk against the pull of gravity and control the speed at which it moves (Davies 1990). As with all movement, the speed at which the sequence is carried out influences the co-ordination and degree of effort entailed. Young agile individuals will move more quickly and fluently than those of an older age group. The slower the speed at which the movement is carried out, the greater the effort required and the greater the likelihood of dependence on the arms.

Clinical application

In clinical practice, impairment of this sequence of events is observed in a wide variety of cases. For example, in patients following surgery to the lumbar spine, pain inhibits movement and there is a loss of flexibility at the operation site. This disturbs the balance of activity and grading of movement within the trunk, most noticeably through the relative inactivity of the abdominals. Characteristically, these patients break up the movement sequence into specific components with an absence of rotation to minimise movement at the operation site. They first turn on to their side, often initiating the movement with one or both legs. They then move the legs over the side of the bed at virtually the same moment as they push up on their arms with little or no interplay within the trunk and pelvis as described above. The psoas muscle seems to be more active, compensating for the inhibition of the abdominals, in that the pelvis is held in a position of anterior tilt throughout the movement. A further illustration of the relationship between abdominal control and arm support is in people with a high thoracic cord lesion with paralysis of the abdominals. They are only able to attain the sitting position independently by means of a forced ballistic type movement of the upper limbs to initiate movement out of supine, and arm support to maintain themselves once in sitting.

Moving from sitting to standing

Standing from sitting is an activity which is performed frequently in daily life. In a review of the literature, Kerr et al (1991) categorised the research relating to rising from a chair into four major areas:

- biomechanical investigations
- kinematic studies
- investigations of muscle activity
- general studies of the functional aspects of seating for disabled people.

Many variables have been shown to influence getting up from a chair. These include the height of the chair, use of the arms, speed of movement, the direction of movement, placement of the feet and the age and sex of the individual. An example of the complexity of analysis of this movement sequence may be found in a study which demonstrated that in a sample of 10 young adults, five different arm patterns, three different head and trunk patterns and three different leg patterns were found to occur (Francis et al 1988 as cited by VanSant 1990b).

While producing definitive numerical data on moments of force generated at the joints and muscles of the lower extremity during rising, many of the biomechanical studies have demonstrated substantial complexity in study design, involving highly sophisticated technical equipment and considerable manipulation of subjects. This may preclude the application of such procedures to large samples of disabled subjects (Kerr et al 1991). The following analysis discusses the key components of sitting to standing and their significance to clinical practice.

The initial base of support is relatively large and includes the surface area of the chair with which the body is in contact, the floor area within the base of the chair and the area within and posterior to the foot position. A key component of this movement is the transference of weight from a relatively large base of support to one which is significantly smaller – the feet alone.

Many studies identify two distinct phases in moving from sitting into standing – initial forward trunk lean and upward extension (Nuzik et al 1986, Schenkman et al 1990).

On clinical observation, the movement forwards of the trunk varies. In some individuals the trunk moves forwards on the pelvis prior to the pelvis tilting anteriorly, whereas in others the trunk is held more rigidly extended and the trunk and pelvis move forwards simultaneously. This trunk and pelvic movement enables the weight to be transferred forwards over the feet. It may also be necessary for the individual to move the buttocks forwards, depending upon the initial position in the chair.

As the trunk and pelvis move forwards, the head extends and the knees move forwards over the feet so as to facilitate the transference of weight during upward extension. The knees move forwards over the feet producing dorsiflexion at the ankle, the maximum range of dorsiflexion occurring as the buttocks are lifted from the seat of the chair. The legs extend as the individual moves into the upright position with a decreasing amount of activity in quadriceps as the knee angle approaches zero (Schuldt et al 1983). The anterior tilt of the pelvis is at its maximum as the buttocks are lifted off the chair and reduces as the sequence progresses, with extension of the hips on completion of the movement. Similarly, the position of the head adjusts relative to the trunk throughout the sequence, moving from a more extended position at the beginning of the movement to one of relative flexion.

Clinical application

Many people with neurological disability have difficulty with this complex movement sequence. Treatment strategies vary depending on the different reasons for the problem. Such problems may include restricted joint range at the foot and ankle or abnormal tone within the trunk and pelvis, both of which may preclude or impair the initial forward lean.

In clinical practice, the height of the chair or plinth is seen to be a critical factor in performance of the activity. Increasing seat height and the use of arms decreases muscle and joint forces at the hips and knees (Burdett et al 1985, Arborelius et al 1992) and also decreases energy expenditure (Didier et al 1993). Many patients benefit from first practising the movement from a higher seat and gradually reducing the height as they become more proficient.

Walking

The purpose of this analysis is to consider aspects of normal gait in relationship to pathological gait of neurological origin. Throughout this section the terms 'walking' and 'gait' are used interchangeably, although Whittle (1991) defines gait as the manner or style of walking rather than the walking process itself. There are many definitions of gait, which include:

- a series of controlled falls (Rose et al 1982)
- a method of locomotion involving the use of the two legs, alternately, to provide both support and propulsion, at least one foot being in contact with the ground at all times (Whittle 1991)
- a highly coordinated series of events in which balance is being constantly challenged and regained continuously (Galley & Forster 1987).

There are numerous studies which have described aspects of gait in detail. These include Saunders et al (1953), Murray et al (1964) and Whittle (1991). Saunders et al (1953) identified the primary determinants of human locomotion in respect of the behaviour of the centre of gravity of the body. In normal level walking, this follows a smooth, regular sinusoidal curve in the plane of progression which enables the human body to conserve energy.

Murray et al (1964) recorded the displacements associated with locomotion and established the ranges of normal values for many components of the walking cycle. These were considered in respect of the speed and timing of gait and stride dimensions, sagittal rotation of the pelvis, hip, knee and ankle and vertical, lateral and forward movement of the trunk and the transverse rotation of the pelvis and thorax.

The gait cycle

The gait cycle is the time interval between two successive occurrences of one of the repetitive events of walking (Whittle 1991). The cycle comprises two component parts, the stance and swing phases. The stance phase is the portion of the cycle where the foot is in contact with the floor and the swing phase is where the leg is off the ground moving forwards to take a step. There are two periods during the cycle when both feet are in contact with the ground. The proportion as a percentage of the walking cycle is 60% stance and 40% swing. The duration of the supportive phases of the walking cycle decreases with increased walking speeds (Smidt 1990).

Common characteristics of gait

Step and stride length. The step length is the distance between successive points of floor-to-floor contact of alternate feet; the stride length is the linear distance between successive points of floor-to-floor contact of the same foot. The step and stride length are related to the height of the individual, shorter subjects taking shorter steps and taller subjects longer steps, and to age, subjects over 60 having a shorter step length than those of a younger age group (Murray et al 1964, Prince et al 1997).

The stride width or walking base. This is the side-to-side distance between the line of the two feet, usually measured at the midpoint of the heel (Whittle 1991). It is directly related to the lateral displacement of the pelvis produced by the horizontal shift of the pelvis or relative adduction of the hip (Saunders et al 1953). This allows the stride width to remain within the pelvic circumference throughout the gait cycle, and Murray et al (1964) observed that the midpoint of one foot may even cross over the other. The stride width is not related to age or height nor does it correlate significantly with foot length, bi-acromial or bi-iliac measures (Murray et al 1964). Murray identified an increase in the foot angle (outward placement) of subjects over 60 years of age and suggested this to be their means of achieving additional lateral stability as the neuromuscular system begins to decline. The foot angle is also increased at slower walking speeds. An increase in the stride width is a notable feature in people with impaired balance. The degree to which it occurs depends on the extent of the damage to the CNS.

Cadence and velocity. The cadence is the number of steps taken in a given time and the

Table 3.2 Normal ranges for gait parameters

Approximate range (95%) limits for general gait parameters in free-speed walking by normal *female* subjects of different ages (reproduced from Whittle 1991 with kind permission)

Age (years)	Cadence (steps/min)	Stride length (m)	Velocity (m/s)
13–14	103–150	0.99–1.55	0.90–1.62
15–17	100–144	1.03–1.57	0.92–1.64
18–49	98–138	1.06–1.58	0.94–1.66
50–64	97–137	1.04–1.56	0.91–1.63
65–80	96–136	0.94–1.46	0.80–1.52

Approximate range (95%) limits for general gait parameters in free-speed walking by normal *male* subjects of different ages

Age (years)	Cadence (steps/min)	Stride length (m)	Velocity (m/s)
13–14	100–149	1.06–1.64	0.95–1.67
15–17	96–142	1.15–1.75	1.03–1.75
18–49	91–135	1.25–1.85	1.10–1.82
50–64	82–126	1.22–1.82	0.96–1.68
65–80	81–125	1.11–1.71	0.81–1.61

velocity of walking is the distance covered in a given time. The normal ranges for gait parameters are given in Table 3.2.

Greater velocities of locomotion are achieved by the lengthening of the stride rather than by an increase in cadence (Saunders et al 1953) and this depends to a great extent on the functional objective. For example, strolling along the promenade is more leisurely than walking quickly knowing one is late for an appointment. Balance modification is directly related to speed; enforced reduction in the natural cadence will require increased postural adaptation.

The muscle activity required to step forwards differs in accordance with the speed of movement. For example, a step from a standing position requires greater hip flexor activity than a step taken as part of the gait cycle at the individual's natural cadence. Similarly, the initiation of a step from a standing position produces a backward displacement of the body to counter the extended lever anteriorly, whereas the body is more upright in the natural gait cycle. These are important considerations for the physiotherapist when re-educating gait. In many instances, treatment of necessity takes the form of re-education of the component parts, but it must be appreciated that fluidity and economy of movement are dependent upon the many factors associated with the gait cycle, not least cadence and speed. Re-education of gait at slow speeds often makes performance more difficult (Mauritz & Hesse 1996).

Rotation. The pelvis and thorax rotate simultaneously in the transverse plane during each cycle of gait, the pelvis and shoulders rotating in opposite directions. Murray (1967) suggested that one of the functions of arm swing is to counteract excessive trunk rotation in the transverse plane. Maximum rotation occurs at the time of heel contact and the greater speed, the greater the degree of rotation and subsequent arm swing. The enhanced amplitude of rotation is achieved mainly by increased shoulder extension on the backward end of the arm swing (Murray 1967). There is a decreased amplitude of rotation in the elderly which may be related to a more flexed posture (Elble et al 1991).

With increasing speed, either walking as quickly as possible or when running, the arm swing becomes more vigorous to help in both generating pace and in maintaining balance. An example is that of a sprinter in action. As the speed increases, so too does the pumping action of the arms combined with increased extension of the thoracic spine, perfectly illustrated as the athlete crosses the finishing line.

Disability resulting in an imbalance of the inter-reaction between flexor and extensor activity may impair rotation. An example of this is illustrated in the person with Parkinson's disease (Rogers 1991). The main observable features are those of increased flexion and lack of rotation with the characteristic shuffling gait. In the past, therapists were taught to work for improved rotation by facilitating arm swing. Little attention was paid to the inherent loss of extensor activity. It is now widely accepted in clinical practice that rotation can only be facilitated on the basis of appropriate inter-reaction between flexion and extension within the trunk. Hence, in this instance, improving extension must occur before rotation is possible.

Vertical displacement. This occurs twice during the gait cycle and is approximately 50 mm (Whittle 1991). The summit of these oscillations occurs during the middle of stance phase and the centre of gravity falls to its lowest level during double stance when both feet are in contact with the ground (Saunders et al 1953). The magnitude of the vertical excursion correlates with the length of stride because when the step lengths are longer the lower limbs are more obliquely situated (Murray et al 1964). This characteristic ascent and descent of the body mass is altered in patients with hemiplegia. The movement is dependent upon sufficient muscle activity to maintain stability of the pelvis and hip joint during stance phase. Patients with hemiplegia often have inadequate or inappropriate activity to provide this stability. This gives rise to the characteristic unilateral Trendelenburg gait whereby the vertical displacement occurs only during stance phase of the unaffected leg (Wagenaar & Beek 1992).

Muscle activity and joint range associated with gait

Normal walking is dependent upon the continual interchange between mobility and stability (Perry 1992) with more than 1000 muscles moving over 200 bones around 100 movable joints (Prince et al 1997). Box 3.1 provides a summary of normal muscle activity and function during gait. These muscles do not have one single action but may work concentrically, eccentrically or isometrically at different stages of the gait cycle.

This is of particular relevance when considering the use of muscle (botulinum toxin) or nerve (phenol) blocks. For example, the role of the plantar flexors is to contribute to knee stability, provide ankle stability, restrain the forward movement of the tibia on the talus during stance phase and minimise the vertical oscillation of the whole body centre of mass (Sutherland et al 1980). Therefore, while muscle or nerve blocks may reduce excessive or poorly timed calf muscle activation (Hesse et al 1994, Richardson et al 2000), they may also lead to knee and ankle instability and increased energy expenditure.

The foot and ankle

Efficient transfer of weight from one leg to the other is partly dependent upon the ability of the feet to respond and adjust effectively to the base of support, be it a firm surface or over rough ground. The ankle and intrinsic foot musculature make constant adjustments to adapt appropriately to provide the dynamic stability essential for this acceptance of, and movement over, the base of support. The mobility of the foot and ankle is therefore essential for effective transfer of weight. The total range of dorsiflexion and plantar flexion varies between about 20 and 35 degrees, with foot clearance being only 0.87 cm in mid-swing (Gage 1992). Any restriction in this mobility will necessitate compensatory adjustments – for example, increased knee flexion or hip hitching.

The muscle action occurring at the ankle is primarily that of dorsiflexion controlling the placing of the foot on the supporting surface following heel strike and plantar flexion to propel the body forwards (Winter 1987, Kameyama et al 1990).

The knee

The range of movement at the knees is between approximately 70 degrees during the swing phase and full extension at the moment of heel strike and in mid-stance (Whittle 1991). In normal locomotion, the body moves forwards over the leg while the knee joint is flexed, the knee extending during stance and then once more flexing to carry the non-weight-bearing limb forwards. Saunders et al (1953) refer to the knee being 'locked in extension' during heel strike and during mid-stance but, on clinical observation, it would seem that this only occurs with pathology.

The hip

Movement at the hip is between approximately 30 degrees flexion and 20 degrees extension (Whittle 1991). The predominant activity during stance phase is that of extension and abduction as the

---

Box 3.1 A summary of normal muscle activity and function during gait (after adaptation by Gage 1991, with permission from MacKeith Press)

Terminal swing
Muscle function. Ends swing and prepares limb for stance.
- Hip flexors – these muscles are usually not active at this time
- Hamstrings – eccentric action decelerates the forward swing of the thigh and leg
- Quadriceps – concentric action to extend knee for stance
- Tibialis anterior – ankle dorsiflexion supports the ankle at neutral to prevent foot drop

Initial contact
Muscle function. Acts to allow smooth progression and stabilizes joints while simultaneously decelerating the body's inertia.
- Gluteus maximus – controls flexor moment produced by ground reaction forces (GRFs)
- Hamstrings – inhibit knee hyperextension and assist in controlling flexion moment at hip
- Tibialis anterior – initiates the heel rocker

Loading response
Muscle function. Acts to allow smooth progression and stabilizes joints while simultaneously decelerating the body's inertia.
- Hamstrings – concentric action unlocks the knee
- Tibialis anterior – decelerates foot fall by eccentric contraction and pulls the tibia anterior to the body's weight line which results in knee flexion
- Quadriceps – eccentric contraction to decelerate knee flexion and absorb shock of floor contact
- Gluteus maximus – concentric action to extend hip and accelerate trunk over femur. Its action through the iliotibial band contributes to knee extension
- Adductor magnus – concentric action to advance and internally rotate pelvis on stance limb
- Gluteus medius – eccentric action to abduct hip and stabilize pelvis to minimize contralateral pelvic drop

Midstance
Muscle function. Acts to allow smooth progression over a stationary foot while controlling position of the GRF referable to hip and knee.
- Soleus – eccentric action to decelerate ankle dorsiflexion over the planted foot during the period of the second rocker

- Quadriceps – stabilizes flexed knee. Action ceases when GRF vector passes in front of knee
- Gluteus maximus – ceases action when GRF becomes posterior to hip

Terminal stance
Muscle function. Acts to provide acceleration and adequate step length.
- Soleus – intensity of action increases to limit dorsiflexion. Also acts as invertor of subtalar joint to provide stability
- Gastrocnemius – concentric action to stop forward motion of tibia and begin plantarflexion of ankle
- Tibialis posterior – stabilizes the foot against eversion forces
- Peroneals – stabilize the foot against inversion forces
- Long toe flexors – stabilizes metatarsophalangeal (MTP) joints to augment forefoot support

Pre-swing
Muscle function. Muscle control ends stance and prepares limb for swing.
- Gastrocnemius – may unlock the knee so that it may resume flexion
- Adductor longus – concentric action advances the thigh
- Rectus femoris – eccentric action at knee to decelerate the inertia of the shank. Concentric action at hip to augment hip flexion

Initial swing
Muscle function. Provides ability to vary cadence and maintain foot clearance.
- Hip flexor group (iliacus, adductor longus, sartorius, gracilis) – concentric action to advance thigh and works in conjunction with shank inertia to create knee flexion
- Biceps femoris (short head) – augments knee flexion during slow gait when inertial forces are inadequate
- Tibialis anterior – concentric action to dorsiflex foot
- Long toe extensors – concentric action with tibialis anterior to dorsiflex foot

Mid-swing
Muscle function. Little muscle action necessary because inertial forces are propelling the limb.
- Tibialis anterior – concentric action to prevent foot drop

---

body moves forwards over the supporting foot. Prior to initiation of swing phase, the extended position at the hips is dependent upon the ability of the hip flexors to lengthen, thereby allowing this transference of weight. During swing phase, the primary activity is again that of extension acting as a deceleration force as the leg moves forwards through momentum prior to heel strike (Whittle 1991). The leg initially flexes, with adduc-

tion and medial rotation at the hips. As the knee begins to extend in preparation for heel contact, the leg becomes more laterally rotated.

The pelvis

The pelvis provides the dynamic stability essential for coordinating the activity of the lower limbs and the control and alignment of the trunk.

Many authors refer to rotation of the pelvis although it may be more appropriate, as the pelvis is a rigid structure, to consider rotation in relation to the hips and the thoracolumbar spine. Palpating the anterior superior iliac spines while walking at one's natural pace reveals little discernible movement, the rotational movement being approximately 4 degrees on either side of the central axis, the lateral movement approximately 5 degrees (Saunders et al 1953) and the anterior/posterior movement approximately 3 degrees (Murray et al 1964).

As the body moves forwards over the supporting leg, the pelvis maintains its stability predominantly through the action of gluteus maximus and medius. The maintenance of a neutral or slight posterior tilt of the pelvis is also determined by this activity.

Neural control

Control of locomotion is extremely complex. Leonard (1998) highlights this complexity in his analysis of human gait:

the CNS somehow must generate the locomotor pattern; generate appropriate propulsive forces; modulate changes in centre of gravity; coordinate multi-limb trajectories; adapt to changing conditions and changing joint positions; coordinate visual, auditory, vestibular and peripheral afferent information; and account for the viscoelastic properties of muscles. It must do all of this within milliseconds and usually in conjunction with coordinating a multitude of other bodily functions and movements.

Central pattern generators (CPGs) within the spinal cord generate the locomotor rhythm, but whereas cats with totally transected spinal cords still maintain the ability to walk, humans depend upon supraspinal control. It is suggested that descending systems integrate with spinal cord circuitry to fractionate lower limb movement and provide greater adaptability to changing afferent conditions (Dietz 1997, Leonard 1998).

Clinical application

For normal subjects, walking is goal-oriented and automatic with no consideration given to the component parts necessary to propel them on their way. In contrast, many patients with neurological impairment may have to consider every aspect of movement in walking. Conscious thought about how to put one foot forward in front of the other and maintain balance in order to achieve a functional goal is both physically and mentally demanding.

There are many assumptions within physiotherapy regarding the re-education of gait, the majority of which are unsubstantiated. Quality of movement is considered to be of the essence and yet, with a damaged nervous system, is it possible to regain normal activity (Latash & Anson 1996)? There is widespread reluctance by physiotherapists to recommend the use of walking aids (Sackley & Lincoln 1996). However, Tyson (1999) found that these did not adversely affect walking ability and, although Hesse et al (1998) reported a more balanced walking pattern immediately following gait facilitation by Bobath therapists as opposed to walking with or without an aid, no carry-over could be demonstrated 1 hour after treatment. Hesse et al (1998) concluded that 'hesitant prescription' of walking aids for hemiplegic patients was not justified.

Significant improvements in gait have also been reported with the use of treadmill training with supported body weight. This means of gait training has been used for both incomplete spinal cord injured patients (Dobkin 1994, Dietz et al 1995) and for those with hemiplegia (Hesse et al 1995). For patients with spinal cord damage, it is suggested that this means of enhancing lower limb movement may prove useful in guiding and strengthening functional synapses of regenerating axons to maximise their contribution towards restoring function (Muir & Steeves 1997).

Summary

In summary, gait is an holistic motor goal of enormous complexity. There is only partial agreement between investigators as to what is the 'normal' pattern of muscle usage during gait (Whittle 1991). It is an automatic function whereby there is continual adaptation of postural tone in response to the constantly changing base of support. Any impairment, particularly of the trunk, pelvis or lower limbs, may produce compensatory strategies, thereby disturbing the rhythm and economy of movement. However, Dietz (1997) suggests that the simpler regulation of muscle tension following spinal or supraspinal damage may be beneficial in that it enables the patient to support the body weight and achieve mobility. Although rapid movements are impaired due to the inability to modulate muscle activity, the altered regulation of 'spastic gait' may be considered as optimal for the given state of the motor system.

It is important that physiotherapists do not become too focused on using principles of their preferred treatment approaches to the detriment of others (Lennon 1996). For example, preventing patients with a pathological gait from walking until they have acquired a more normal pattern must be weighed against the advantages of early ambulation, namely to the musculoskeletal, cardiovascular, pulmonary and renal systems (Mauritz & Hesse 1996). Therapists must be aware of new developments and take these on board as possible treatment modalities in the functional re-education of gait.

Upper limb function

Selective movement of the upper limb is dependent upon, not only normal neuromuscular innervation of the muscles of the arm but also the musculature of the shoulder girdle, trunk and legs. The shoulder is the most mobile joint of the body, being dependent primarily on muscle activity for its stability (Lippitt & Matsen 1993) and it is for this reason that it is so vulnerable to trauma. Following neurological impairment, weakness, abnormal tone and impaired coordination of movement will have devastating effects on the glenohumeral joint.

In order to fully understand the functional problems which occur as a result of neurological impairment, it is first important to review the anatomy of the shoulder girdle. For this purpose, the shoulder mechanism is best considered in the context of thoracoscapular–humeral articulation. There are seven joints which provide this articulation (Fig. 3.11):

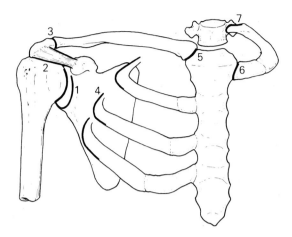

Figure 3.11 Composite drawing of the shoulder girdle (reproduced from Cailliet 1980 with kind permission). Key: 1 = glenohumeral; 2 = suprahumeral; 3 = acromioclavicular; 4 = scapulocostal; 5 = sternoclavicular; 6 = costosternal; 7 = costovertebral.

- glenohumeral
- suprahumeral (a functional joint as opposed to a true articulation)
- acromioclavicular
- scapulocostal
- sternoclavicular
- costosternal
- costovertebral.

Relationship between shoulder girdle structures

Each joint is dependent on the others for the stability and control required in the performance of selective movement.

The angular alignment of the glenoid fossa and its resultant position in relation to the head of humerus, provides a degree of stability described by Basmajian (1979) as 'the locking mechanism' of the shoulder.

The positioning of the scapula is of importance in providing the degree of stability described by Basmajian. In normal subjects, if the arm is slightly abducted and then displaced downwards, there is greater laxity at the glenohumeral joint than when this force is applied with the arm close in to the side of the body. Conversely, if the scapula rests in a more medially rotated position around the chest wall, this produces an increased range of abduction at the glenohumeral joint with the potential for instability in the same way as that described above.

Prevost et al (1987) dispute Basmajian's description of the scapula position in producing 'a locking mechanism'. In their study of 50 subjects following cerebrovascular accident (CVA), they found that there was a greater degree of downward facing of the glenoid fossa in the non-affected arm of these subjects than in the affected arm. They concluded that 'the glenoid fossa has a downward orientation in most normal shoulders and that Basmajian's generalisation that the normal angle faces upward and the suggestion of a "locking mechanism" should be questioned'.

It may be hypothesised that following CVA the sound side becomes stronger to compensate for the impaired movement of the affected side. On observation, it seems that the greater the development of the shoulder girdle musculature, the greater the degree of medial rotation of the scapula.

Functional movement of the upper limb is also dependent upon thoracic joint motion. Increased thoracic mobility in younger subjects is related to a large range of arm elevation, whereas an increased kyphosis in older subjects is related to a reduced range of arm elevation (Crawford & Jull 1993). O'Gorman & Jull (1987) also revealed significant changes in the angle of kyphosis after the fifth decade and that the range of thoracic spine movement decreased with age. This relationship between thoracic and glenohumeral movement is of significance when treating patients who are wheelchair dependent. The constant adoption of a flexed posture will consequently reduce extensor activity within the trunk.

When sitting or standing, anti-gravity muscle activity is recruited primarily in the trunk, pelvis and lower limbs; the shoulder girdles are relatively inactive in the maintenance of balance. This proximal stability is a prerequisite for upper limb function. Anticipatory postural adjustments precede arm movements and appear to be pre-programmed (Friedli et al 1984).

Prehension/reaching and grasping

A prehensile act can be considered as two co-ordinated functional components that allow the hand eventually to establish the required contact with the object for manipulation to ensue.

The *transport component* is responsible for bringing the hand/wrist system into the vicinity of the object to be grasped, and the *grasp component* is responsible for the formation of the grip (Bootsma et al 1994). The transport component is that of a high velocity, ballistic movement, involving primarily the proximal musculature of the shoulder and elbow to place the hand in the correct spatial location. The grasp component, the low-velocity phase, involves the musculature of the hand and forearm and serves to:

- orientate the hand and fingers to the structural characteristics of the object
- ready the hand by forming an appropriate grasping shape
- capture the object by closing the fingers about it (Marteniuk et al 1990).

These components occur at the same time and are thought to be independently programmed processes with visuomotor links (Jeannerod 1984). During visually guided movements, the CNS must convert information originating in visual brain regions into a pattern of muscle activity that moves the hand towards the target (Kalaska & Crammond 1992). Not only does vision direct placement of the arm during reach, it also influences the speed of the movement (Leonard 1998).

The theory of independence of the transport and grasp components is strengthened by the different times at which they develop (Rosenbaum 1991, Gordon 1994), the fact that each can be solely affected by brain insult (Jeannerod 1994) and the different reaction times of the two components to a perturbation (Jeannerod et al 1991).

Inevitably the two components must be coordinated in some way in that the hand must open before contact with the object if prehension is to be achieved (Marteniuk et al 1990). This coordination is felt to be task specific, the exact temporal relationship between the two depending on the requirements of the task (Marteniuk et al 1990, van Vliet 1993, Wier 1994).

The velocity of the transport component is asymmetrical, there being a sharp rise to its peak and then a less steep deceleration. There is a break point in the deceleration after approximately 70–80% of the movement where the velocity becomes constant.

The grasp component occurs at the same time as the transport component. The grip size rapidly increases to a maximum aperture, the fingers then flex and the grip size decreases to match the size of the object. The finger grip opens wider than required so that the index finger can turn around the object to achieve the proper orientation of the grip. The index finger seems to contribute most to the grip formation with the thumb position remaining constant (Jeannerod 1984).

Prehension is influenced by many factors. These include:

- vision (Jeannerod 1984, Marteniuk et al 1990)
- proprioception (Jeannerod 1984, Gentilucci et al 1994)
- touch (Wier 1994)
- object properties relating to:
  - substance: size and width (Jeannerod 1984, Marteniuk et al 1987, Bootsma et al 1994)
  - structure: weight, texture and fragility (Marteniuk et al 1987, Wier 1994)
- function (van Vliet 1993, Ada et al 1994).

In the context of re-education of upper limb function it is important to take these factors into account. Retraining should be functional as information about the environment and the task appears to influence movement organisation (van Vliet 1993). The postural adjustments accompanying reaching and grasping, either in sitting (Moore et al 1992) or standing (Lee 1980, Friedli et al 1984, Horak et al 1984), must also be

addressed (Shepherd 1992). Brain-damaged patients may have difficulty eliciting any muscle activity in the early stages (Shepherd 1992, Ada et al 1994) or in controlling that activity in the presence of increased tone.

Compensatory motor patterns may emerge as a result of several factors, which include:

- the effects of the lesion
- the mechanical characteristics of the musculo-skeletal linkage
- the environment in which the action is performed (Shepherd 1992).

These must be considered in respect of positioning and appropriate treatment strategies to modify the demands placed upon the neuromuscular system when attempting to re-educate prehension.

CONCLUSION

Analysis of 'normal movement' is recognised as an essential prerequisite for the assessment of patients with impairment of movement. It is this analysis that provides the basis for the problem-solving approach to treatment. Improved understanding and awareness of movement enables the therapist to identify how a posture or movement differs from the normal and why an individual may have difficulty with functional skills.

It is inappropriate to imply that individuals must move or take up positions in a certain way to be considered normal. People with physical disability resent the implication that they are in some way abnormal merely because, through necessity, they use compensatory strategies and no longer function in the way they did before the onset of their disability.

Subsequent chapters will use this analysis in determining appropriate treatment strategies which may be adopted in the management of patients with neurological disability.

REFERENCES

Ada L, Canning C, Carr J, Kilbreath S, Shepherd R 1994 In: Bennett K, Castiello U (eds) Insights into the reach and grasp movement. Elsevier Science, London

Alexander R, Boehme R, Cupps B 1993 Normal development of functional motor skills. Therapy Skill Builders, Arizona

Arborelius U, Wretenberg P, Lindberg F 1992 The effects of arm rests and high seat heights on lower-limb joint load and muscular activity during sitting and rising. Ergonomics 35(11): 1377–1391

Basmajian V J 1979 Muscles alive: their function revealed by electromyography, 4th edn. Williams & Wilkins, London

Bennett R, Knowlton G 1958 Overwork weakness in partially denervated skeletal muscle. Clinical Orthopaedics 12: 22–29

Bernstein N 1967 The co-ordination and regulation of movements. Pergamon, Oxford

Bobath B 1990 Adult hemiplegia: evaluation and treatment, 3rd edn. Heinemann Medical Books, Oxford

Bootsma R, Marteniuk R, MacKenzie C, Zaal F 1994 The speed accuracy trade-off in manual prehension: effects of movement amplitude, object size and object width on kinematic characteristics. Experimental Brain Research 98: 535–541

Brooks V 1986 The neural basis of motor control. Oxford University Press, Oxford

Bryce J 1972 Facilitation of movement – the Bobath approach. Physiotherapy 58: 403–408

Bryce J 1989 Lecture: the Bobath concept. International Bobath Tutor's Meeting, Nijmegen, Holland

Burdett R, Habasevich R, Pisciotta J, Simon S 1985 Biomechanical comparison of rising from two types of chairs. Physical Therapy 65(8): 1177–1183

Cailliet R 1980 The shoulder in hemiplegia, 5th edn. F A Davis, Philadelphia

Cameron T, Calancie B 1995 Mechanical and fatigue properties of wrist flexor muscles during repetitive contractions after cervical spinal cord injury. Archives of Physical Medicine and Rehabilitation 76: 929–933

Carr J H, Shepherd R B 1986 Motor training following stroke. In: Banks M (ed) Stroke. Churchill Livingstone, London

Cordo P J, Nashner L M 1982 Properties of postural adjustments associated with rapid arm movements. Journal of Neurophysiology 47: 287–302

Crawford H J, Jull G A 1993 The influence of thoracic posture and movement on range of arm elevation. Physiotherapy Theory and Practice 9(3): 143–148

Curtis C L, Weir J P 1996 Overview of exercise responses in healthy and impaired states. Neurology Report, American Physical Therapy Association 20: 13–19

Davidoff R A 1992 Skeletal muscle tone and the misunderstood stretch reflex. Neurology 42: 951–963

Davies P M 1985 Steps to follow: a guide to the treatment of adult hemiplegia. Springer-Verlag, Berlin

Davies P M 1990 Right in the middle. Springer-Verlag, Berlin

Davies P M 1994 Starting again: early rehabilitation after traumatic brain injury or other severe brain lesions. Springer-Verlag, Berlin

Didier J, Mourey F, Brondel L et al 1993 The energetic cost of some daily activities: a comparison in a young and old population. Age and Ageing 22: 90–96

Diener H-C, Dichgans J, Guschlbauer B, Bacher M, Rapp H, Langenbach P 1990 Associated postural adjustments with body movements in normal subjects and patients with parkinsonism and cerebellar disease. Revue Neurologie (Paris) 146: 555–563

Diener H-C, Dichgans J, Guschlbauer B, Bacher M, Rapp H, Klockgether T 1992 The coordination of posture and voluntary movement in patients with cerebellar dysfunction. Movement Disorders 7: 14–17

Dietz V 1992 Human neuronal control of automatic functional movements: interaction between central programs and afferent input. Physiological Reviews 72(1): 33–69

Dietz V 1997 Neurophysiology of gait disorders: present and future applications. Electroencephalography and Clinical Neurophysiology 103: 333–355

Dietz V, Colombo G, Jensen L, Baumgartner L 1995 Locomotor capacity of spinal cord in paraplegic patients. Annals of Neurology 37: 574–578

Dobkin B H 1994 New frontiers in SCI rehabilitation. Journal of Rehabilitation 8: 33–39

Edwards S 1998 The incomplete spinal lesion. In: Bromley I (ed) Tetraplegia and paraplegia: a guide for physiotherapists, 5th edn. Churchill Livingstone, London

Elble R J, Sienko Thomas S, Higgins C, Colliver J 1991 Stride-dependent changes in gait of older people. Journal of Neurology 238: 1–5

Ennion S, Sant'ana Pereira J, Sargeant A J, Young A, Goldspink G 1995 Characterisation of human skeletal muscle fibres according to the myosin heavy chain they express. Journal of Muscle Research and Cell Motility 16: 35–43

Enoka R M 1995 Morphological features and activation patterns of motor units. Journal of Clinical Neurophysiology 12: 538–559

Friedli W, Hallett M, Simon S 1984 Postural adjustments associated with rapid voluntary arm movements 1. Electromyographic data. Journal of Neurology, Neurosurgery and Psychiatry 47: 611–622

Gage J R 1991 Gait analysis in cerebral party. MacKeith Press, London

Gage J R 1992 An overview of normal walking. In: Perry J (ed) Gait analysis: normal and pathological function. Slack, New Jersey

Galley P M, Forster A L 1987 Human movement, 2nd edn. Churchill Livingstone, London

Gentilucci M, Toni I, Chieffi S, Pavesi G 1994 The role of proprioception in the control of prehension movements: a kinematic study in a peripherally deafferented patient and in normal subjects. Experimental Brain Research 99: 483–500

Given J D, Dewald J P A, Rymer W Z 1995 Joint dependent passive stiffness in paretic and contralateral limbs of spastic patients with hemiparetic stroke. Journal of Neurology, Neurosurgery and Psychiatry 59: 271–279

Goldspink G 1999a Changes in muscle mass and phenotype and the expression of autocrine and systemic growth factors by muscle in response to stretch and overload. Journal of Anatomy 194: 323–334

Goldspink G 1999b Lecture to ACPIN Conference, London

Goldspink G, Williams P 1990 Muscle fibre and connective tissue changes associated with use and disuse. In: Ada L, Canning C (eds) Key issues in neurological physiotherapy. Butterworth-Heinemann, Oxford

Goldspink G, Schutt A, Loughna P T, Wells D J, Jaenicke, Gerlach G F 1992 Gene expression in skeletal muscle in response to stretch and force generation. American Journal of Physiology 262: R356–R363

Gordon A 1994 In: Bennet K, Castiello U (eds) Insights into the reach and grasp movement. Elsevier Science, London

Gordon T, Mao J 1994 Muscle atrophy and procedures for training after spinal cord injury. Physical Therapy 74: 50–60

Hagbarth K-E 1994 Evaluation of and methods to change muscle tone. Scandinavian Journal of Rehabilitation Medicine Suppl 30: 19–32

Haggard P, Jenner J, Wing A 1994 Coordination of aimed movements in a case of unilateral cerebellar damage. Neuropsychologia 32(7): 827–846

Hansen P, Woollacott M, Debu B 1988 Postural responses to changing task conditions. Experimental Brain Research 73: 627–636

Herbert R 1988 The passive mechanical properties of muscle and their adaptations to altered patterns of use. Australian Journal of Physiotherapy 34: 141–149

Hesse S, Luecke D, Malezic M et al 1994 Botulinum toxin treatment for lower limb extensor spasticity in chronic hemiparetic patients. Journal of Neurology, Neurosurgery and Psychiatry 57: 1321–1324

Hesse S, Bertelt C, Jahnke M T et al 1995 Treadmill training with partial body weight support compared with physiotherapy in non-ambulatory hemiparetic patients. Stroke 26: 976–981

Hesse S, Jahnke M T, Schaffrin A, Lucke D, Reiter F, Konrad M 1998 Immediate effects of therapeutic facilitation on the gait of hemiplegic patients as compared with walking with and without a cane. Electroencephalography and Clinical Neurophysiology 109: 515–522

Horak F, Nashner L 1986 Central programming of postural movements: adaptation to altered support surface configurations. Journal of Neurophysiology 55: 1369–1381

Horak F, Esselman P, Anderson M, Lynch M 1984 The effects of movement velocity, mass displaced and task certainty on associated postural adjustments made by normal and hemiplegic individuals. Journal of Neurology, Neurosurgery and Psychiatry 47: 1020–1028

Horak F, Shupert C, Dietz V, Horstmann G 1994 Vestibular and somatosensory contributions to responses to head and body displacements in stance. Experimental Brain Research 100: 93–106

Jeannerod M 1984 The timing of natural prehension movements. Journal of Motor Behaviour 16(3): 235–254

Jeannerod M 1994 Object orientated action. In: Bennett K, Castiello U (eds) Insights into the reach and grasp movement. Elsevier Science, London

Jeannerod M, Paulignan Y, MacKenzie C, Marteniuk R 1991 Parallel visuomotor processing in human prehension movements. Experimental Brain Research Suppl 16: 27–44

Jones D A Round J M 1990 Histochemistry, contractile properties and motor control. In: Jones D A, Round J M (eds) Skeletal muscle in health and disease: a textbook of muscle physiology. Manchester University Press, Manchester

Kalaska J F, Crammond D J 1992 Cerebral cortical mechanisms of reaching movements. Science 255: 1517–1523

Kameyama O, Ogawa R, Okamoto T, Kumamoto M 1990 Electric discharge patterns of ankle muscles during the normal gait cycle. Archives of Physical Medicine and Rehabilitation 71: 969–974

Kapandji I A 1980 The physiology of joints. Volume 3 The trunk and the vertebral column. Churchill Livingstone, London

Karnath H-O, Sievering D, Fetter M 1994 The interactive contribution of neck muscle proprioception and vestibular stimulation to subjective 'straight-ahead' orientation in man. Experimental Brain Research 101: 140–146

Keele S W 1968 Movement control in skilled motor performance. Psychology Bulletin 70: 387–403

Kerr K M, White J A, Mollan R, Baird H E 1991 Rising from a chair: a review of the literature. Physiotherapy 77(1): 15–19

Knott M, Voss D 1968 Proprioceptive neuromuscular facilitation. Harper & Row, New York

Latash M L, Anson J G 1996 What are 'normal movements' in atypical populations? Behavioral and Brain Sciences 19: 55–106

Lee W 1980 Anticipatory control of posture and task muscles during rapid arm flexion. Journal of Motor Behaviour 12(3): 185–196

Lee W A, Buchanan T S, Rogers M W 1987 Effect of arm acceleration and behavioural conditions on the organisation of postural adjustments during arm flexion. Experimental Brain Research 66: 257–270

Lennon S 1996 The Bobath concept: a critical review of the theoretical assumptions that guide physiotherapy practice in stroke rehabilitation. Physical Therapy Review 1: 35–45

Leonard C T 1998 The neuroscience of human movement. Mosby, London

Lin J-P, Brown J K, Walsh E G 1993 Physiological maturation of muscles in childhood. Lancet 343: 1386–1389

Lippitt S, Matsen F 1993 Mechanisms of gleno-humeral joint stability. Clinical Orthopaedics and Related Research 291: 20–28

Lynch M, Grisogono V 1991 Strokes and head injuries. John Murray, London

Marsden C D 1982 The mysterious motor function of the basal ganglia: the Robert Wartenberg lecture. Neurology 32: 514–539

Marsden C D 1984 Motor disorders in basal ganglia disease. Human Neurobiology 2: 245–250

Marteniuk R, MacKenzie C, Jeannerod M, Athenes S, Dugas C 1987 Constraints on human arm movement trajectories. Canadian Journal of Psychology 41: 365–378

Marteniuk R, Leavitt J, MacKenzie C, Athenes S 1990 Functional relationships between grasp and transport components in a prehension task. Human Movement Science 9: 149–176

Massion J 1984 Postural changes accompanying voluntary movements. Normal and pathological aspects. Human Neurobiology 2: 261–267

Massion J 1992 Movement, posture and equilibrium: interaction and coordination. Progress in Neurobiology 38: 35–56

Massion J, Woollacott M 1996 Posture and equilibrium. In: Bronstein A M, Brandt T, Woollacott M (eds) Balance posture and gait. Arnold, London

Mauritz K-H, Hesse S 1996 Neurological rehabilitation of gait and balance disorders. In: Bronstein A M, Brandt T, Woollacott M (eds) Balance posture and gait. Arnold, London

Mink J W 1996 The basal ganglia: focused selection and inhibition of competing motor programmes. Progress in Neurobiology 50: 381–425

Moore S, Brunt D, Nesbitt M, Juarez T 1992 Investigation of evidence for anticipatory postural adjustments in seated subjects who performed a reaching task. Physical Therapy 72(5): 335–343

Muir G D, Steeves J D 1997 Sensorimotor stimulation to improve locomotor recovery after spinal cord injury. Trends in Neuroscience 20: 72–77

Murray M P 1967 Patterns of sagittal rotation of the upper limbs in walking. Physical Therapy 47(4): 272–284

Murray M P, Drought A B, Kory R C 1964 Walking patterns of normal men. Journal of Bone and Joint Surgery 46A(2): 335–359

Nashner L M 1977 Fixed patterns or rapid postural responses among leg muscles during stance. Experimental Brain Research 30: 13–24

Nudo R J 1999 Recovery after damage to motor cortical areas. Current Opinion in Neurobiology 9: 740–747

Nuzik S, Lamb R, VanSant A, Hirt S 1986 Sit to stand movement pattern. Physical Therapy 66(11): 1708–1713

O'Gorman H J, Jull G A 1987 Thoracic kyphosis and mobility: the effect of age. Physiotherapy Practice 3: 154–162

Perry J 1992 Pathological gait. In: Perry J (ed) Gait analysis: normal and pathological function. Slack, New Jersey

Pette D 1998 Training effects on the contractile apparatus. Acta Physiologica Scandinavica 162: 367–376

Pette D, Staron R S 1997 Mammalian skeletal muscle fibre type transitions. International Review Cytology 170: 143–223

Prevost R, Arsenault A B, Dutil E, Drouin G 1987 Rotation of the scapula and shoulder subluxation in hemiplegia. Archives of Physical Medicine and Rehabilitation 68: 786–790

Prince F, Corriveau H, Herbert R, Winter D A 1997 Gait in the elderly. Gait and Posture 5: 128–135

Richardson D, Greenwood R, Sheean G, Thompson A, Edwards S 2000 Treatment of focal spasticity with botulinum toxin: effect on the 'positive support reaction'. Physiotherapy Research International 5: 62–70

Rogers M 1991 Motor control problems in Parkinson's disease. In: Lister M (ed) Contemporary management of motor control problems. Foundation for Physical Therapy, Alexandria, VA

Rose G K, Butler P, Stallard J 1982 Gait: principles, biomechanics and assessment. Orlau Publishing, Oswestry, UK

Rosenbaum D 1991 Human motor control. Academic Press, London

Rothwell J 1994 Control of human voluntary movement, 2nd edn. Chapman & Hall, London

Sackley C M, Lincoln N B 1996 Physiotherapy treatment for stroke patients: a survey of current practice. Physiotherapy Theory and Practice 12: 87–96

Saunders J, Inman V, Eberhart H 1953 The major determinants in normal and pathological gait. Journal of Bone and Joint Surgery 35A: 543–558

Schenkman M, Berger R, O'Riley P, Mann R, Hodge W 1990 Whole-body movements during rising to standing from sitting. Physical Therapy 70(10): 638–648

Schmidt R A 1988 Motor control and learning: a behavioural emphasis, 2nd edn. Human Kinetics Publishers, Leeds

Schmidt R A 1991a Motor learning and performance: from principles to practice. Human Kinetics Publishers, Leeds

Schmidt R A 1991b Motor learning principles for physical therapy. In: Lister M (ed) Contemporary management of motor control problems. Foundation for Physical Therapy, Alexandria, VA

Schuldt K, Ekholm J, Nemeth G, Arborelius U, Harms-Ringdahlk K 1983 Knee load and muscle activity during exercises in rising. Scandinavian Journal of Rehabilitation Medicine 9(Suppl): 174–188

Sheean G L 1998 Pathophysiology of spasticity. In: Sheean G (ed) Spasticity rehabilitation. Churchill Communications, Europe, London

Shepherd R B 1992 Adaptive motor behaviour in response to perturbations of balance. Physiotherapy Theory and Practice 8: 137–143

Shumway-Cook A, Woollacott M 1995 Motor control. Theory and practical applications. Williams & Wilkins, London

Smidt G 1990 Rudiments of gait. In: Smidt G (ed) Clinics in physical therapy. Gait in rehabilitation. Churchill Livingstone, London

Soechting T F, Flanders M 1992 Moving in three dimensional space: frames of reference, vectors and coordinate systems. Annual Reviews of Neuroscience 15: 167–191

Sutherland D H, Cooper L, Daniel D 1980 The role of the ankle plantar flexors in normal walking. Journal of Bone and Joint Surgery 62A: 354–363

Taylor D, Ashburn A, Ward C D 1994 Asymmetrical trunk posture, unilateral neglect and motor performance following stroke. Clinical Rehabilitation 8: 48–53

Tyson S F 1999 Trunk kinematics in hemiplegic gait and the effect of walking aids. Clinical Rehabilitation 13: 295–300

van Vliet P 1993 An investigation of the task specificity of reaching: implications for retraining. Physiotherapy Theory and Practice 9: 69–76

VanSant A F 1990a Life span development in functional tasks. Physical Therapy 70(12): 788–798

VanSant A F 1990b Commentary. Physical Therapy 70(10): 648–649

Vrbova G, Gordon T, Jones R 1995 Nerve–muscle interaction. Chapman & Hall, London.

Wagenaar R C, Beek W J 1992 Hemiplegic gait: a kinematic analysis using walking speed as a basis. Journal of Biomechanics 25(9): 1007–1015

Whitlock J A 1990 Neurophysiology of spasticity. In: Glen M B, Whyte J (eds) The practical management of spasticity in children and adults. Lea & Febiger, London

Whittle M 1991 Gait analysis: an introduction. Butterworth-Heinemann, Oxford

Wier P L 1994 Object property and task effects on prehension. In: Bennet K, Castiello U (eds) Insights into the reach and grasp movements. Elsevier Science, London

Wing A M, Flanagan J R, Richardson J 1997 Anticipatory postural adjustments in stance and grip. Experimental Brain Research 116: 122–130

Winter D A 1987 The biomechanics and motor control of human gait. University of Waterloo Press, Waterloo, Ontario

4

Neuropsychological problems and solutions

Dawn Wendy Langdon

Many neurological conditions involve the cerebral hemispheres and thus have an impact on higher cortical function. A patient's cognitive function can have a great influence on the direction, efficiency and success of a physiotherapy treatment. Sometimes this can be at a basic level, for example where a patient's memory dysfunction or inability to initiate action means that she cannot present herself for treatment appointments and hence the physiotherapist must escort her to and from the treatment area. On other occasions the influence of cognitive dysfunction might be at a more complex level, where, for example, a patient with multiple sclerosis (MS) who has the physical potential to walk is nevertheless unsafe to do so, because of a marked disinhibition and impulsivity in his actions, and thus physiotherapy may target wheelchair techniques because they provide a safer form of mobility.

Research has shown that cognitive impairment can affect the outcome of therapy. Even in a fairly disabled group of MS patients undergoing intensive inpatient multidisciplinary therapy, their cognitive characteristics influenced how much independence they gained in everyday motor tasks (Langdon & Thompson 1999). However, functional independence can improve, even in the context of unchanging cognitive impairment (Langdon & Thompson 2000).

Neuropsychology attempts to understand the relationship between brain and behaviour. In a clinical setting, this means determining the pattern of neuropsychological impairment that a patient has suffered. The consequent cognitive profile is then related to clinical observations of the patient's disability. Behaviours to be targeted in treatment are identified and agreed. A treatment programme is designed taking account of the patient's cognitive profile. Lastly, mechanisms for evaluation of treatment and for making programme adjustments are put in place. Thus the approach does not differ substantially in structure from that of a physiotherapist except, understandably, cognitive function is considered in a more explicit and detailed manner and, correspondingly, physical aspects receive much less attention. These differences in emphasis and experience between the two disciplines make collaborative work essential with many neurological patients.

Neuropsychologists have a wealth of validated measures and research findings to inform their clinical work. However, the purpose of this chapter is not to explore theoretical aspects in detail, and copious referencing has been avoided. Similarly, no consideration is given to diagnostic groups or anatomical correlates. There are many excellent neuropsychology texts that cover this ground (Obrzut 1986, Ellis & Young 1988, McCarthy & Warrington 1990).

Interested readers are advised to consult these authors for discussion of cognitive models of neuropsychological syndromes, anatomical considerations and for standard references. This chapter will focus on how acquired neuropsychological deficits affect the function of adult neurological patients and ways in which these deficits can be identified and overcome in therapy. This is a less well researched area and is, therefore, approached from a clinical context.

The remainder of this chapter is arranged under 10 main headings: general intellectual function; memory function; attention; language function; visual perception; spatial processing; praxis; executive functions; insight; and emotional distress. These sections reflect the areas that might concern a neuropsychologist in the assessment and treatment of a patient. Each section is divided into three parts. First, one or two measures devised by neuropsychologists to delineate the deficit are described. This part aims to give a flavour of neuropsychological testing

and also a clearer impression of the impairment under consideration. Secondly, clinical observations and therapeutic problems that typically relate to the cognitive deficit are described. With the assistance of a neuropsychologist, the clinical observations can be related to test findings and a clear profile of the patient's cognitive abilities may emerge. If you are relying on your own professional skill to determine cognitive impairment, then the part on clinical observation offers a brief description of how the cognitive deficit might manifest itself in therapy and pointers towards clinical assessment. Thirdly, some basic treatment strategies and options are discussed in relation to the cognitive deficit.

Admittedly, in most clinical practices it is rare to see patients with a single, or 'focal', cognitive deficit: however, this way of considering neuropsychological dysfunction tends to be the clearest. It is also the most convenient arrangement for those seeking to locate specific information relevant to a particular clinical problem.

GENERAL INTELLECTUAL FUNCTION

Neuropsychological tests of general intellectual impairment

The most widely used test of individual general intellectual level is the Wechsler Adult Intelligence Scale – Revised (WAIS-III; Wechsler 1997). It comprises subtests, which are divided into verbal and performance subscales. The verbal subtests include:

- Information, which tests general knowledge
- Comprehension, which examines common sense and social competence
- Vocabulary, which requires the subject to define a graded list of words
- Similarities, which asks the subject to say how pairs of words are alike
- Arithmetic, a graded set of arithmetic problems
- Digit Span, requiring the repetition of strings of digits either forwards or backwards.

The performance subtests utilise pictorial and spatial materials and include:

- Digit Symbol, a recoding task which requires the subject to write appropriate abstract symbols under printed numbers
- Picture Completion, where the subject must indicate which important part is missing from each of 21 line drawings
- Picture Arrangement, where small groups of drawings are laid on a desk in scrambled order and the subject must rearrange them to make a sensible story
- Object Assembly, where the subject must assemble a complete two-dimensional object from the several flat fragments scattered before her on the desk.

The verbal subtest scores are summed as part of the calculation of the Verbal IQ and, similarly, the performance subtests are added together to obtain the Performance IQ. The Verbal, Performance and Full Scale IQs are derived by reference to normative data. As well as for the three IQs, age-referenced norms are also tabulated for each of the subtests. The classification and distribution of IQ scores are given in Table 4.1.

The WAIS-III gives a good indication of the patient's current level of intellectual function, a cognitive 'snapshot'. However, in order to detect intellectual deterioration, it is necessary to compare current function with how good a person's intellect has been in the past, which is termed their pre-morbid optimum. For some patients, their education or occupational history will provide a pointer to their pre-morbid optimum, but this can at best only give a broad indication. A more precise estimate of pre-morbid intellect can be obtained from a patient's reading, for example on the National Adult Reading Test – Revised (NART-R; Nelson & Willison 1992). Reading scores are less affected in dementia than other cognitive skills (Nelson & McKenna 1975, Nelson & O'Connell 1978).

The NART-R consists of 50 printed words whose correct pronunciation is irregular, in the sense that the usual English spelling-to-sound rules do not apply. For example, a person who was to read the word 'debt' for the first time would probably sound the 'b' as part of the word and thus read it aloud incorrectly. However, people familiar with the word 'debt' pronounce it correctly. Their previous knowledge of the word allows them to pronounce it. Because all the words in the NART-R are similarly irregular, they are unlikely to be guessed correctly. Only words already in a patient's reading vocabulary will be accurately read aloud. By comparing a patient's current IQ with the NART-R, it is possible to determine whether any significant loss of general intellectual function has occurred.

Tests of cognitive ability which were originally developed for general population use, such as the WAIS-III, often include task demands which can be inappropriate for neurological patients. For example, the Picture Arrangement subtest requires the patient to study between three and six cards, each of which carries a detailed line drawing (none greater than 5 cm square) and then to rearrange them so that they tell a story. Good manual dexterity and visual acuity are required, in addition to reasoning skills. Clearly, peripheral neurological dysfunction can handicap a patient on this subtest. If a patient with poor acuity and poor dexterity does badly, it is not clear whether peripheral deficits, cognitive deficits, or some mixture of both are to blame. The interpretation of the test results becomes problematic.

Many tests have been developed especially for neurological populations, although none have attained the dominance of the WAIS-III. An example of one designed to assess the general

Table 4.1 The classification and distribution of IQ scores. From the manual of the Wechsler Adult Intelligence Scale – Revised. Copyright © 1981 by The Psychological Corporation. Reproduced by permission. All rights reserved.

IQ	Classification	% included	
		Theoretical normal curve	Control sample
130 and above	Very superior	2.2	2.6
120–129	Superior	6.7	6.9
110–119	High average	16.1	16.6
90–109	Average	50.0	49.1
80–89	Low average	16.1	16.1
70–79	Borderline	6.7	6.4
69 and below	Mentally retarded	2.2	2.3

intellectual level of neurological patients is the Verbal and Spatial Reasoning Test (VESPAR; Langdon & Warrington 1995). The VESPAR tests three types of inductive reasoning: categorisation, analogy and series completion. The problems are arranged in three matched sets of 25 verbal and 25 spatial items. The matched design allows fairly clear conclusions to be drawn if either verbal or spatial stimuli lead to poor performance, because the difference is unlikely to be due to different test procedures or task demands and most likely to be due to a specific deficit in either verbal or spatial processing.

The stimuli were selected for their appropriateness for neurological patients. The verbal items use common, or high-frequency, words which are less vulnerable to acquired language deficits. The spatial items are all clearly drawn and their solution does not depend on fine visual acuity or shape discrimination, faculties which may be compromised by neurological disease (Fig. 4.1). No manual dexterity is required of the patient. The forced choice format means that a variety of output modalities are possible. There are no penalties for slow performance. Thus the VESPAR attempts to minimise the effects of peripheral neurological deficits that may confound patients' performance on traditional reasoning tests, which attempt to measure central cognitive processes.

Clinical observations of general intellectual loss

The clinical detection of a dementia can often be problematic, particularly in the early stages. This is especially true of Alzheimer's disease, where

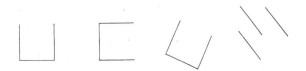

Figure 4.1 Sample item from the verbal (A) and (B) spatial odd-one out sections of the VESPAR. (From Langdon D W, Warrington E K 1995 The VESPAR: a verbal and spatial reasoning test. Reprinted by permission of Lawrence Erlbaum Associates Ltd., Hove, UK.)

typically social skills are preserved and a casual conversation will not reveal anything amiss; or of MS, where typically language skills are unaffected and even an in-depth conversation will not reveal anything untoward. In general, patients who have suffered a widespread cognitive deterioration will find new information difficult to absorb and retain. They may require a great deal of prompting and repetition. Their powers of abstraction will be weakened and they will tend to see the world (and themselves) in rather concrete terms. This may result in their failing to bring problems to your attention or realise the implications of medical or treatment developments.

Their reduced cognitive capacity may have forced them to withdraw from established activities, although patients may explain the change in terms of peripheral physical causes. For example, a patient whose reasoning powers fell to a level where they could no longer carry her through a knitting pattern, explained that she had given up knitting due to failing eyesight.

Treatment strategies for patients with general intellectual loss

A good recent summary of psychological treatment approaches to patients with dementia can be found in Holden & Woods (1995). In general, the poor abstracting abilities of these patients make it necessary for information to be provided in clear and concrete terms using short sentences and everyday words. For example a patient with a significant intellectual loss, who spends most of the day in a wheelchair and long periods immobile in bed, may not appreciate the need for a pressure care regime. The reasons why a pressure care regime will prevent pressure areas developing may not be obvious to the patient. Similarly, the results of developing a pressure sore may need to be spelt out in graphic detail, because the logical outcome of failing to implement pressure care may well escape the patient. A written account in clear, concrete terms can pay dividends both as a prompt and as an aid to understanding.

This patient group requires as much structure as possible in their physiotherapy programme and follow-up. They may need to be oriented at the start of each therapy session as to its purpose and content; to have their progress summarised at regular intervals; and to receive help, and perhaps explicit practice, in transferring techniques to new settings. If they have a home exercise programme, a diary or weekly chart to follow can be very helpful.

MEMORY FUNCTION

Neuropsychological tests of memory function

Memory function is the registration and retrieval of information of all kinds. A detailed review of the neuropsychology of memory in clinical practice may be found in Kapur (1988). The basic principles of assessing memory function require a valid and systematic procedure in which a person remembers certain pieces of information in response to standard instructions. A memory test in widespread clinical use is the Recognition Memory Test (RMT; Warrington 1984). Fifty everyday words are presented to the patient at a rate of one every three seconds. The patient is required to say whether she likes each word, as a way of ensuring her attention. Next the patient is shown 50 pairs of everyday words. Each pair includes one word from the original single showing. The patient must say which of the two words she has just seen. A visual version, using photographs of male faces, follows the same procedure. The RMT is a relatively pure test of memory function, placing few demands on other cognitive skills. It was designed as a diagnostic test, to detect minor degrees of memory dysfunction across a wide range of the adult population.

Wilson et al (1985) devised a test to evaluate everyday memory function. It includes a number of procedures:

- remembering a name associated with a face after 25 minutes
- remembering to ask for an item and where it was hidden, after 25 minutes
- remembering to question the examiner after 20 minutes

- recognising 10 pictures
- recognising five faces
- orientation
- immediate and delayed recall of a story and a route.

There are four parallel forms, allowing change in patients' performance on the test to be monitored, unconfounded by the patient remembering stimuli from previous testing. The Rivermead Behavioural Memory Test samples a range of memory functions. It is a useful tool for both clinical screening and monitoring change.

Clinical observations of memory dysfunction

A patient with memory dysfunction may fail to remember many kinds of information. Perhaps the most common demonstration in therapy is a failure to carry over techniques from a previous session, or to apply techniques to everyday life that have been rehearsed in therapy. However, a patient with a dense amnesic syndrome can exhibit far more extensive and disabling memory dysfunction. For example, if a therapist leaves an amnesic patient for a few minutes to answer a telephone, the amnesic patient may well be bewildered when the therapist returns and ask who the therapist is. In the few minutes the therapist spent answering the telephone, all recall of the therapist, the therapy session and the location has vanished.

Discrepancies in different types of memory function can be observed. For example, a patient may have difficulty remembering words and other verbal material, but remain competent at remembering pictures and other visual material. This can be elucidated by discrepancies on the verbal and visual sections of the RMT (Warrington 1984), if a neuropsychological assessment is available. Otherwise, a simple test of telling the patient his appointment time (a verbal strategy) for one session and then showing him a picture of a clock set at the time of his appointment (a visual strategy) for the next session and observing the patient's attendance, might well indicate which memory system is the most efficient.

Apart from a general memory dysfunction for either verbal information or visual information, memory for certain types of verbal and visual information can be selectively impaired. For example, although a patient may be able to perceive an object efficiently (i.e. her visual perceptual processes are intact), she may not be able to remember any knowledge about the object, for example its purpose. In the pure form, this impairment is termed visual agnosia. This syndrome can have devastating results in everyday life, because patients may not be able to recognise a door handle or a toothbrush. In therapy, they may not be able to recognise a wheelchair brake and it will be hard for them to plan their movements in relation to objects if they are uncertain what they will operate or how to manipulate it.

Similarly, aspects of visual memory can be affected in isolation. Some patients can have a particular difficulty in recognising faces, a syndrome termed prosopagnosia. Others may have a selective impairment in remembering routes within the hospital or around their home locality, which is termed topographical memory dysfunction. Patients who cannot find their way around are clearly seriously disadvantaged when trying to improve their mobility.

As well as different types of memory being selectively impaired, different ways of remembering can be affected to varying degrees. For example, the RMT (Warrington 1984) requires patients to recognise words or faces that they have just seen and is thus a test of recognition memory. The test stimuli act as a prompt or a cue to help the patient remember. Patients remember far more words in this recognition format than they would if they were asked to recite all the words that they had just been shown, that is to recall the words without cue or prompt. For patients with memory dysfunction, the difference between their ability to recall information unaided and their ability to remember information aided by a cue or a prompt can be very great.

As well as recall and recognition memory procedures, another format is paired-associate memory. Pairs of words are shown to the patient; then the first word of each pair is shown and the patient is required to produce the second word that was its associate in the previously seen pair. The association can be strong (e.g. tea–cup) or so weak as to be simply that they were two unrelated words that had been previously seen together (e.g. gate–carpet). The importance of this format is its apparent link to everyday memory function (Wilson et al 1985).

When assessing a patient's ability to remember information in therapy, it is important to be alert to how much prompting and cueing the patient is receiving. A patient may be able to recite perfectly the procedures for transferring safely from a wheelchair, in response to a series of questions, but that procedure assesses his prompted verbal memory function. The memory function required to perform transfers safely at home is recall performance memory, which could be assessed by observing the patient perform unprompted.

Treatment strategies for patients with memory dysfunction

A detailed account of neuropsychological treatments of memory dysfunction can be found in Wilson & Moffat (1984) and Wilson (1987). The first step to devising treatment strategies to overcome memory dysfunction is to assess the nature and extent of the patient's difficulties. If verbal memory function appears to be generally more efficient than visual memory function, then a written protocol for wheelchairs could be devised. It should be tested by observing the patient transferring when following the written protocol. If any further prompts or explanation are required from the therapist, then these should be added as amendments to the protocol or extra steps. Once the patient has demonstrated step 1 – independent transfers using the protocol (which includes remembering to use the protocol) – then it may be possible for her to learn the protocol by heart and recite it aloud to guide her transfers; this is step 2. Step 3 would be for the patient to rehearse the protocol silently during the transfer. Even if a patient's general intellectual function means that she can never move beyond using the written protocol, she has still achieved independence in that task.

Conversely, if visual memory function appears to be generally more efficient than verbal memory function, then pictures and other visual material may be used to good effect. The pictured information can be used explicitly, for example a set of drawings to prompt each item in a home exercise programme. Or it may be implicit, for example encouraging a patient to visualise striking images that link his therapist to the day of the week when he must attend for his out-patient treatment. The use of visual imagery is extensively reported by Wilson (1987).

The first general principle is, therefore, to identify and utilise competent areas of memory function.

The second principle is to reduce the memory load for the patient at any one time. A task is broken down into components, each of which is sufficiently small for the patient to grasp immediately. Each component is practised extensively, as a single movement with many repetitions. This increases the chances of the component being learnt in the long term. Sometimes this is termed 'overlearning', which indicates the large number of repetitions of a single component that may be required to consolidate the learning, before proceeding to the next component. This breaking down of an activity into separate, smaller components does not fit comfortably with the idea of educating a patient to perform normal movements. However, some patients' memory deficits may be so severe that practising an activity as a whole will never register sufficiently for adequate carry-over and, if they are to make essential functional gains, then the task may need to be broken down into component actions ('chunking') with separate practice of each activity component.

The third principle is 'errorless learning', a technique whereby the patient is taught to perform correctly from the start and not left to arrive at a correct solution by trial, error and feedback. As in the chunking approach described above, errorless learning goes some way against the grain of conventional therapy wisdom, which usually advocates observing the patient and giving feedback concerning the good and bad aspects of the patient's movement. In most therapy situations it clearly makes sense to dis-cover where a patient is going wrong so that effort and expertise can be targeted efficiently.

However, for patients with severe memory dysfunction, there is evidence that once they have tried an incorrect manoeuvre, it is very difficult for their compromised memory systems to erase the incorrect manoeuvre from their plan of that activity. An incorrect manoeuvre can include an omission. For example, patients transferring for the first time from a wheelchair to a bed may move their hands straight from the wheels to the bed, omitting to put on the wheelchair brakes. Their learnt manoeuvre is to move their hands from the wheels to the bed. It would be very hard for patients with severe memory problems to then 'unlearn' that sequence and insert the 'brakes on' manoeuvre into their recorded plan of activity. Errorless learning is probably most useful for patients with very severe memory dysfunction. Some detailed experiments which demonstrate how errorless learning benefits amnesic patients are described by Wilson et al (1994).

ATTENTION

Neurological tests of attention

In some ways the most fundamental cognitive faculty, attention underpins all other cognitive activities. If patients cannot concentrate, they cannot employ any other cognitive function effectively, however efficient their other cognitive processes may be. Attention must be directed and sustained if more (apparently) sophisticated cognitive systems are to be brought to bear on either external information or internal processing. A review of assessments of attention in the context of traumatic brain injury gives a useful overview (Kinsella 1998). Perhaps the best-known and most widely used clinical test of attention is the Digit Span subtest of the WAIS-III (Wechsler 1997), discussed above. The repetition of random digit strings will be compromised if the patient has an attentional deficit. It appears that repetition of lists of unrelated items can be achieved with very little additional processing of the items. For most patients, it is a relatively pure test of attention. Sometimes, Digit Span is mistakenly thought of as a general memory test. Because it does not necessarily involve the registration and remembering processes of memory, it is best thought of as a test of attention.

A test of attention which illustrates this emphasis on concentration and relatively low demands on other processing is the Paced Auditory Serial Addition Task (Gronwall 1977). The patient listens to single digits spoken aloud on an audio tape. There are various rates of presentation: for example, one digit every second or one digit every 4 seconds. The patient's task is to add together the last two digits he or she has heard. For example, the number 1 might come first, followed by 4. The correct response from the patient is 5. Then the patient hears the next number in the series on the tape, which is 7. The last two numbers that the patient has heard are now 4 and 7 and the correct response is 11. Clearly, the arithmetic demands are small: just the addition of pairs of single digits. However, the attentional demands are very exacting, requiring the patient to remain alert to the two digits which constitute the last pair heard while performing the simple serial additions correctly.

Robertson et al (1994) have developed the Test of Everyday Attention (TEA), which samples selective attention (the ability to filter out unnecessary information), sustained attention and attention switching. The tasks utilise both visual and auditory stimuli: for example, searching a telephone directory for specified symbols and counting tones from an audio tape. There are three parallel versions. The TEA allows three types of attention to be assessed separately and any change in attention skills to be monitored.

Clinical observations of attentional deficits

In therapy, the most common and disruptive attentional deficit will probably be distractibility, i.e. a failure to ignore irrelevant stimuli. This occurs when the selective function of attention is compromised. Think for a moment of all the detail and activity in a hospital ward or treatment gym. All humans filter out vast amounts of information in their immediate environment so that the stimuli they process are of manageable quantity and appropriate type. The distractible patient, however, may not be able to exclude the conversation that another therapist is having with a patient on the next mat. It may intrude into his processing and prevent him fully comprehending your comments and suggestions.

Pointers towards poor selective attention are that patients may fail to respond appropriately, or at all, in conversation. They may look away, towards another conversation or a sudden activity in another part of the room, when you would expect them to be maintaining eye contact with you as you speak. A detailed qualitative and quantitative account of attentional problems experienced by patients following head injury is given by Gronwall (1977).

Sustained attention deficits will manifest themselves as poor concentration. After a brief, successful period at the start of a therapy session, things will rapidly deteriorate. Movements which were performed efficiently at the start become inconsistent or even impossible. A law of diminishing returns has clearly set into the session. Another stumbling block in therapy can be the patient's inability to switch attention. For example, a patient working hard to preserve her midline while practising indoor mobility may topple over as she opens a door, because she had been concentrating on her midline to the exclusion of the balance requirements of opening doors.

Treatment strategies for patients with attentional deficits

Studies of treatment for attentional deficits have tended to use computers for training and evaluation and for research purposes, and the tasks have been abstract (e.g. Gray et al 1992). However, one home-based programme to improve attention in reading has been described (Wilson & Robertson 1992). Broadly, there are two possible approaches which are likely to reduce the effect of a patient's selective attention deficits on therapy. The first method is to change the therapeutic environment. A quiet, single treatment room is probably an unobtainable ideal in most hospital settings but can often be easily achieved in a patient's home. It may be best to speak only when you have the patient's eye contact and discontinue when it is broken. Talking patients through a task may help to keep them focused. The second way to minimise the effects of selective attention deficits is for the patients to implement strategies themselves. These can range from imagery-guided techniques to verbal commentaries, which can either be spoken aloud or rehearsed internally.

Difficulties in sustaining attention are usually best tackled by simple pacing techniques. Rest periods can be scheduled during a therapy session to allow patients to refocus their concentration, or a number of short sessions may be spaced throughout the day. Switching attention can be facilitated by verbal prompts or commentaries from either the therapist or patient.

LANGUAGE FUNCTION

Neuropsychological tests of language

A detailed historical introduction to the assessment of language dysfunction is given by Howard & Hatfield (1987). A widely used clinical test of naming is the Graded Naming Test (GNT; McKenna & Warrington 1983). It consists of 30 black and white line drawings. The objects depicted range from those which everyone in the normal sample could name ('kangaroo') to rare items that only a small percentage of the normal sample were able to name. It is the less frequently used words which are most vulnerable to neurological disease. It is often necessary to test patients to the limits of their naming vocabulary in order to discount or demonstrate a naming difficulty. The graded difficulty of the test allows a level of performance to be recorded at any point across the normal range. Thus even mild naming difficulties can be identified.

The Graded Naming Test is a useful diagnostic screening tool; however, sometimes a more detailed assessment of language dysfunction is required. The Psycholinguistic Assessments of Language Processing in Aphasia (PALPA; Kay et al 1992) is based on theoretical models of language function. It comprises 60 tests of different aspects of language such as writing, grammar, speech and comprehension. Tests can be selected according to the pattern of language difficulty a particular patient experiences.

Clinical observation of language dysfunction

Any aspect of a patient's language processing can be affected by neurological disease. Patients may have difficulty in pronouncing words correctly or in finding the right words to say; understanding spoken or written words; or they may be unable to spell. Patients will sometimes attribute difficulties in reading and writing to peripheral or physical problems, such as failing eyesight or stiff fingers. The terminology is not clear cut for the acquired language disorders. Generally, in cases where the difficulties are attributed to disease or damage of the cerebral cortex:

- difficulties with speaking or the spoken word are termed 'aphasias'
- difficulties with reading are termed 'dyslexias'
- difficulties with writing are termed 'dysgraphias'.

In therapy, the patients' difficulties in conversation are likely to be the most problematic. If patients can only partially understand what is being said to them, they may find it hard either to appreciate the reasons for particular exercises or to grasp what changes and modifications of movement are being required of them. If patients cannot express themselves clearly and fluently, then their perceptions and sensations may be hard for the therapist to appreciate fully. Discussion of the home situation will also be limited.

Treatment strategies for patients with language dysfunction

The aim of any strategy employed with a patient with acquired language deficits is to optimise communication. A review of specialised aphasia therapy can be found in Howard & Hatfield (1987). If patients have serious speech problems, they may be able to write information that you need to know. If comprehension problems are known or suspected, then using everyday words in short sentences with pauses at the end may help. It may also be the case that the patient's reading comprehension is less affected. If no verbal input is satisfactory, however modified, then pictures, photographs and drawings may be helpful.

It is a concern that the use of simple words and pictures may lead the patient to feel patronised. Every effort should be made to avoid this. It is a natural reaction to raise the volume of speech if a patient fails to understand first time, but it is important to keep the voice even toned when repeating or explaining information. Similarly, any stationery, such as folders used to organise written information or pictures, should be as businesslike as possible.

VISUAL PERCEPTION

Neuropsychologicial tests of visual perception

Neurological disease and damage can result in the disruption of any aspect of visual processing. In rare cases, single aspects such as colour or acuity may be selectively compromised. The breakdown of these early visual processes has been studied in detail by Warrington (1986). Sometimes basic visual information such as colour and form may be processed well, but the integration of these components into an object that can be recognised may be weak. A model of how objects are seen as integrated wholes was devised by Marr (1982).

The Visual Object and Space Perception Battery (VOSP; Warrington & James 1991) includes four tests which are widely used in the clinical evaluation of visual perception. They have been designed to place minimal reliance on other cognitive skills, for example by only requiring simple responses from the patient. The tests are to:

- identify single, black capital letters, whose form has been degraded by a random scatter of small white squares

- identify rotated silhouettes of animals and household objects, which thus have an atypical outline
- select which of four black shapes represents the rotated silhouette of an everyday object
- identify two objects, which are each presented as a series of rotated silhouettes which become progressively more typical (and thus easier to identify).

Clinical observations of visual perceptual deficits

Weak visual perceptual skills can result in subtle problems in therapy, which may not be immediately apparent to either the patient or the clinician. It is likely that the patient's interactions with objects will be clumsy and ill-judged. Overlapping objects may pose special difficulties, because the full outline of each object is not in direct sight and, therefore, only partial visual information on each object is available, which can pose too great a challenge to weakened object perception processes. In general, such patients will exhibit difficulty in making sense of the world around them.

Treatment strategies for patients with visual perceptual deficits

Patients are likely to be helped by objects and equipment being presented in a typical view. For example, they could be advised to approach a door or wheelchair head-on and position themselves straight in front while they take stock of their immediate environment. Once they have processed the visual information correctly, they can then proceed more accurately and safely.

SPATIAL PROCESSING

Neuropsychological tests of spatial processing

For people to move and act successfully, they must make a myriad of spatial judgements. They must know where every part of their body is and where every part of their immediate environment is. Any action requires sophisticated computations to determine the precise movement which will, for example, bring a foot to a ball or a hand to a cup. Some spatial judgements are very broad, for example taking to the back streets to avoid a traffic jam and managing to drive in the right direction. Other spatial judgements are very fine, for example threading a needle.

The VOSP (Warrington & James 1991) includes four tests which are widely used in the clinical evaluation of spatial perception. They require no manual manipulation of test material by the patient and are, therefore, free of any effects of praxic difficulties. The tests are to:

- count random scatters of dots
- decide which of two dots is exactly centred in its square
- identify the position of a dot in a square by selecting a number in the identical position in a second square
- calculate how many cubes would be required to build a pile of cubes, represented in a two-dimensional line drawing.

The VSOP provides a stringent, diagnostic screen of the spatial localisation of small visual stimuli. More complex deficits of spatial processing can result in a disregard of parts of space, which is termed a 'neglect'. The Behavioural Inattention Test (BIT; Wilson et al 1987) evaluates a patient's performance on both conventional, table-top tests of neglect and tests of neglect in everyday life. The conventional tests include line bisection, figure and shape copying and cancelling specified shapes presented among distracter shapes. The everyday tests include telephone dialling, telling the time and address copying. The BIT gives a wide-ranging assessment of the patient's spatial neglect.

Clinical observations of patients with spatial impairments

A good review of spatial perception and processing can be found in De Renzi (1982). Patients with spatial processing deficits will often move inappropriately; for example, they may be seen to fumble as they reach for the brake on a wheel-

chair. If distance judgement is poor, transfers may be unsafe and wheelchair mobility may be inefficient. The transfers are compromised because positioning the wheelchair correctly alongside the bed, and moving the body an appropriate distance, may require a great deal of effort and checking in order to overcome poor distance judgement. Where mid-air corrections are required that place heavy demands on balance, patients may tend to overshoot or undershoot when transferring. Wheelchair mobility may bring special problems when doors have to be negotiated. To propel a wheelchair through a doorway requires precise spatial awareness and calculation.

A unilateral neglect results in patients disregarding up to half of their body or disregarding up to half of the space that surrounds them. This syndrome can occur independently of hemiparesis and hemianopia. An example of the result of a patient with unilateral neglect attempting to copy a symmetrical stack of blocks is given in Figure 4.2. An overview of clinical and research findings in unilateral neglect is given in Robertson & Marshall (1993). In clinical settings, patients may be observed to knock into the left side of door frames, because they have failed to allow enough space for the left side of their body to pass through the door frame. They may arrive for therapy with the left side of their body undressed, because they have failed to put their left arm into the left sleeve of a garment. In therapy, the neglected part of the body may be

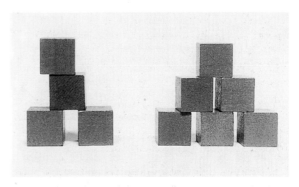

Figure 4.2 The result of a patient with unilateral neglect attempting to copy a symmetrical stack of blocks.

ignored, and the hand and arm may be left to dangle and risk injury. Patients usually have no insight into the nature or presence of their difficulty.

Sometimes it can be difficult to determine whether a patient is disabled by a unilateral neglect syndrome or a disturbance of midline perception; for example, a patient who regularly bangs his left arm into the door frame as he walks through the door. The difference may be identified if minimal contact is maintained to keep the patient in an upright stance, but not to influence his walking direction, as he walks through a doorway. If he negotiates the door successfully when walking in an upright position, then it is unlikely that a unilateral neglect is the impairment. A patient with unilateral neglect would probably neglect his left side, or the left side of space, whatever the angle of his body. If, therefore, the patient bangs into the left side of the door frame even when her body is correctly positioned, then unilateral neglect is more likely to explain her poor negotiation of doorways.

Treatment strategies for patients with spatial impairments

Sometimes making patients aware of the pattern of their difficulties, and advising them to take their time and check during activities when spatial judgements are crucial will be enough to overcome the problem. In cases where the patient's awareness of her own body positioning is good, she can usefully employ techniques where she positions a hand or foot as a guide before transferring her weight. Another approach is to identify a target for the patient through a doorway, for example a picture hung on the wall opposite the doorway, and establishing that if the patient looks at the picture and aims for it as she wheels herself through a doorway, then she will pass centrally through the door frame.

There have been some recent interesting developments in techniques for treating patients with unilateral neglect. Robertson et al (1992) used a combination of two techniques when treating three patients with severe left neglect. First, the patients were trained to use their left arm as a spatial marker by positioning it at the left border of any activity. They were also trained to look at it frequently. Secondly, they moved the affected limb. One patient was only told to activate the affected limb. All three patients demonstrated improvements in either table-top neglect tasks or everyday mobility. It appears that by 'activating' the neglected side with simple, repetitive activity, the patient is 'alerted' to the previously neglected hemispace.

Both of these approaches can be adopted, but they require a great deal of prompting and monitoring while patients are trained to position and monitor their left hand and then activate it during walking. Clenching and unclenching the left hand is the activation usually employed, but any kind of congenial, sustainable movement would probably suffice. There can be some problems with patient acceptance and compliance because, typically, insight is low and patients may be unwilling to embark on a lengthy retraining programme if they cannot comprehend the need for it.

PRAXIS
Neuropsychological tests of praxis

Strictly speaking, apraxia is a disorder of voluntary action that can neither be explained by any peripheral sensory or motor dysfunction nor by any generalised cognitive impairment, such as dementia. The unsatisfactory basis of defining apraxia, by exclusion of alternative explanations, has been noted (Tate & McDonald 1995). However, pure cases without additional physical or cognitive impairment are exceedingly rare and, in general clinical practice, one is more likely to be dealing with a person whose voluntary actions are less skilled than would be predicted by their other physical and cognitive impairments. These problems of definition have contributed to the dearth of reliable and valid tests of apraxia for the clinical context.

Clinical observation of praxis

The classical signs of apraxia are failures to perform simple motor routines such as making a cup of coffee, or using a tin opener. Errors might consist of putting the coffee in the kettle instead of the cup, or banging the tin opener on the side of the tin. Apraxias are not confined to the upper limbs. Oral apraxia and gait apraxia are both well described in the literature. Quick tests require patients to mime everyday activities, blow out a lighted match or draw a figure of eight with their feet. In the context of other physical and cognitive deficits, apraxia can be very hard to discern in a clinical situation.

Treatment strategies for patients with apraxia

Verbal guidance of motor activities, either from a therapist or carer, or by the patient from a rote-learnt spoken script or a generalised internal speech prompt might all improve voluntary action. A very simple strategy of slowing down might be all that is required. But if the patient requires fine motor dexterity at a fixed rate, for example a musician or an assembly line worker, then prospects are probably poor for a good recovery. There is evidence that interacting with objects requires several skills that can fractionate. For example, a therapy trial for activities of daily living (ADL) found stability of gains depended on continuing practice, suggesting that patients could not learn to respond appropriately to objects via first principles, but only by rote learning and then practising specific tasks (Goldenburg & Hagman 1998).

EXECUTIVE FUNCTIONS

Neuropsychological tests of executive function

The executive functions are the least well understood of the cognitive skills and the tests available to the clinician are generally less robust and reliable than those that test more focal skills. In part this may be because the executive functions are higher order, perhaps supervisory systems that tend to work through other systems, and thus are hard to test precisely and exclusively. Another feature which makes them test-shy is

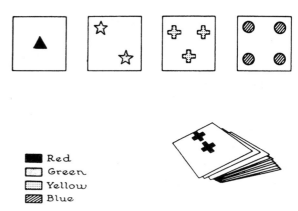

■ Red
□ Green
▤ Yellow
▨ Blue

Figure 4.3 The Wisconsin Card Sorting Test (Reproduced from Milner 1963).

that they tend to become apparent in complicated tasks with many features, which are not easy to package in a cardboard box or rehearse in a clinic setting.

The best-known test of executive function was devised by Milner (1963). It consists of four key cards, which are placed in a row before the patient (Fig. 4.3). A large pack of cards with abstract shapes in various numbers and colours is given to the patient. The patient places a card from the pack with one of the four key cards, in an attempt to determine a sorting rule. The tester says whether the placed card is right or wrong and the procedure is repeated until the patient demonstrates 10 consistently correct sorts. At this point, the sorting rule is changed. There are three rules which are applied through two cycles.

Clinical observation of dysexecutive syndrome

An overview of research in this area can be found in Perecman (1987). Patients with dysexecutive syndrome can often present as lethargic and poorly motivated. They may be passive. They will often be weak at planning and organisation. Initiation will be especially problematic. They can also be impulsive and disinhibited, the manifestation of which can range from over-jocularity, to over-familiarity, to extreme cases, where the speech can include much swearing and obscenity. Apart from affecting conversation, impulsivity can be observed during activity, when patients who are physically able to walk compromise the safety of their mobility by walking too fast. Similarly, impulsivity in transfers can also compromise safety in patients who have the basic physical ability to transfer easily.

It can be hard for these patients to generate alternative strategies if one movement or action is discovered to be wrong. For example, patients attempting to steer through a doorway can be seen to drive into the frame, hitting the left side of the frame with their left wheelchair footplate. They then reverse and repeat exactly the same trajectory that caused the previous crash. This can be repeated several times. The problem is that they cannot initiate a change of direction so that their new wheelchair trajectory will take them through the centre of the doorway without incident. They cannot use the feedback of their left footplate crashing into the door frame to make an appropriate modification to their behaviour. Instead, they repeat the identical move that led to the crash.

Sometimes there is clear evidence of poor problem solving at a more complex level. It may be hard for such patients to appreciate the nature and extent of their disease and disability, in which case their application in therapy is likely to be sporadic at best. They will often fail to grasp the implications of threats to their well-being. They may appear unconcerned about their disability. They will probably not be able to think things through and, in conversation, give the impression of not having an understanding of anything beyond the immediate and the obvious.

Treatment strategies for patients with dysexecutive syndrome

A treatment regime for helping brain-injured patients with problem-solving disorders is described by Yves von Cramon & Matthes von Cramon (1992). A combination of individual and group therapy was utilised, taking about 5 hours each week for 5 weeks. Exercises aim to improve selective encoding and comparison, selective combination, idea generation and action planning. Problem solving cannot be tackled exten-

sively as part of a physiotherapy session, but clear, concrete accounts of the implications of various courses of action and adoption of movement pattern can aid understanding and help patients to overcome their difficulty in grasping the importance of the therapy. It is probably best to start from the premise that nothing is obvious to the patient.

Apathy and poor organisation can sometimes be helped by adding structure. Calendars, diaries and charts of exercises to be performed may help. Prompting and monitoring may be necessary. If there are possible hazards or other problems at home in relation to movement, it is probably best to consider them explicitly and discuss appropriate courses of action in clear, concrete terms.

For impulsivity in movement, a verbal commentary by the therapist or patient, which may eventually be internalised, can help. This can range from a simple counting protocol to pace movement to a safe slow pace, to a list of movements and checks to be made during a specific manoeuvre. If initiation of, for example, pressure care is a problem, an electronic beeper may be a sufficient prompt to turn in bed.

If disinhibition in conversation and behaviour is a problem in therapy, then a strict behavioural approach may help. This requires that all inappropriate acts and comments are ignored and all appropriate attempts to communicate are reinforced by immediate responses. If this is not enough, then feedback about unacceptable behaviour may be necessary. A consistent approach is essential. It is unfair to patients to smile at a risqué compliment and then later turn your back on them when they tell a crude joke.

INSIGHT

Neuropsychological testing of insight

In essence, insight is determined by the comparison of two things: the first is the patient's view and the second is the clinician's. Usually, if they coincide, the patient's insight is deemed to be good. If they do not, a problem has been identified. Lack of insight has been shown to discriminate patients who have undergone brain injury from patients who have undergone surgery to other parts of their body (Andrewes et al 1998). Some researchers have attempted to quantify patients' insight, by comparing the patients' ratings of themselves with their scores on formal tests of particular cognitive skills.

McMillan (1984) developed the Subjective Memory Questionnaire (SMQ), which asks patients a number of questions about their everyday memory function, and includes collected comparison data from healthy subjects. Patients with severe head injury and their relatives completed the SMQ and both groups reported the head-injured patients' everyday function to be weaker than a matched control group (Schwartz & McMillan 1989). It appeared that both the patients with severe head injuries and their relatives had some appreciation of the patients' memory dysfunction.

In contrast, patients with MS appear to have less awareness of their memory difficulties in everyday life. Langdon & Thompson (1994) compared the reports of patients with advanced MS and their carers' reports on the SMQ, with the patients' scores on formal tests of memory function. Both patients with advanced MS and their carers reported the patients' general level of everyday memory function to be similar to that of previously reported control groups. The patients' reports were unrelated to formal tests of memory function but were related to the patients' level of emotional distress. In contrast, the carers' reports of the patients' everyday memory function were related to the patients' formal memory test performance but were not influenced by the patients' emotional distress. It seems that the carers were able to be more objective. The patients were communicating something important when they reported everyday memory dysfunction, probably that their coping skills were not up to the task of managing their day.

Clinical observation of insight

It is arguably the case that a patient's view of the situation is the most important cognitive factor in his or her recovery or rehabilitation potential. If patients do not think that they have a problem, they are unlikely to attend for therapy. If they do not think the clinician will be able to benefit them significantly, they are unlikely to attend for therapy. If they cannot see the possibility of a worthwhile improvement in their life, they are unlikely to attend for therapy. Patients with weak insight may present as difficult and non-compliant. They may appear unconcerned or off-hand to the clinician. They may be distressed and irritated by attempts at therapeutic intervention. A detailed consideration of difficulties with insight after head injury can be found in Prigatano (1991).

Treatment strategies for patients with poor insight

For some patients, careful discussion and negotiation will enable them to appreciate the need for therapy. Also the emphasis on the routine nature of the intervention can help to reassure and recruit patients. However, poor insight can be very entrenched and it may be that the patient will never explicitly agree with the therapist concerning the need, efficacy or outcome of treatment. It may still be possible, however, to engage the patient in therapy on a contractual basis. For example, progress in therapy might facilitate an earlier discharge from an inpatient ward. Although it can be hard for clinicians to endure patients constantly decrying the effectiveness of their work, the ultimate goal is the patient's physical progress, not their commendation of the clinician. Sometimes a meeting with a patient in which his or her view is explicitly acknowledged to differ from that of the clinician can be helpful, if some common ground can be found as a result to form the basis of the patient's participation in therapy.

EMOTIONAL DISTRESS
Neuropsychological tests of emotional distress

If patients experience depression, anxiety, or any affective disturbance, their view of themselves and the world is affected. This shift in outlook and judgement forms the basis of a widely used test of depression, the Beck Inventory of Depression (BDI; Beck et al 1979). It consists of 21 sets of four statements, each relating to some aspect of daily life or self-view. The first is a normal response (e.g. 'I do not feel sad') and the statements progress to a very depressed level (e.g. 'I am so sad or unhappy that I can't stand it'). Patients must select one statement from each group of four, which best describes how they have been feeling over the past week. Each statement has a numerical score and these are added together to give a degree of depression, which may fall within the normal or clinical ranges.

Another example of a widely used test of affective disturbance is the State-Trait Anxiety Inventory (STAI; Spielberger 1983). This test examines both immediate, or state, anxiety and background, or trait, anxiety. Items include 'I feel calm', 'I feel nervous'. Patients rate their degree of agreement with 20 statements for each scale.

Clinical observations of emotional distress

Gainotti (1993) has written a good review of work relating to emotional distress following head injury, and many of his observations have a wider application to other neurological conditions. Depressed patients may be tearful. They may be lethargic and find it hard to motivate themselves. They will typically be very negative, constantly producing reasons as to why there is no reason for therapy, no reason for progress and no reason for hope. They will discount the positive and predict the future negatively. They will present a poor view of themselves and their own effectiveness. They will tend to catastrophise, that is predict disastrous consequences from small setbacks.

Anxiety is usually very apparent. Patients will appear tense and worried. They may voice their worries freely, be over-concerned for their safety, perhaps be seen to delay discharge; certain sticking points may emerge that relate to previous bad experiences (e.g. a fall down stairs). In general, if physical progress is not in line with physical ability, then it might be worth considering whether some emotional factor is blocking the patient's advance.

The relation of patients' emotional status to their physical progress is not well understood. The interplay between emotional adjustment and physical disability is especially difficult to determine in an unpredictable condition of varying course, such as MS. Some group studies have examined the relation between emotional distress and the disease process of MS (see Knight 1992, Ch. 5, for a review). The fine detail and temporal dynamics of this relation can only be properly appreciated at the single case level.

A 16-year-old girl experienced her second MS relapse in 8 months. She had suddenly lost a great deal of physical function and had become dependent on a wheelchair for mobility. On admission to the rehabilitation unit, she was clearly distressed by her current situation and the possibility of permanent physical disability. She had planned to commence a 2-year course of study at her local sixth form college in September. On admission she was adamant that she would not attend the college using a wheelchair, or any other aid to mobility. She maintained this view throughout her 7-week stay on the unit.

Assessments were made of the girl's emotional status at fortnightly intervals. The measures used were the BDI (Beck et al 1979), the STAI (Spielberger 1983) and the Spielberger State-Trait Anger Inventory (STAXI; Spielberger 1988). She was also asked to rate how uncomfortable she thought that she would feel in each of 15 everyday situations, on a scale ranging from 0, which represented 'not at all uncomfortable', to 100, which represented 'the most uncomfortable I've ever been'. During her admission, she progressed from using a wheelchair, to a rollator, to walking with two sticks by the time of her discharge. The details of her scores are given in Table 4.2.

Although her score on the BDI never reached the clinically depressed range, there were more negative thoughts reported at the start of the admission, when she scored 9, than by discharge, when she scored 1. In contrast, an abnormal level of anxiety was reported on admission, but this,

Table 4.2   Changes in measures of emotion and social discomfort across a 7-week neurorehabilitation programme

	15.07.94		27.07.94		09.08.94		16.08.94		25.08.94	
Mobility	Wheelchair		Wheelchair		Wheelchair		Rollator		Two sticks	
Depression BDI (not depressed <10)	9		4		2		0		1	
Anxiety STAI										
State (immediate) %	97		45		42		17		3	
Trait (background) %	72		31		10		6		0	
Anger STAXI										
State (immediate) %	81		68		56		56		56	
Trait (background) %	50		10		5		0		2	
Social discomfort	A	F	A	F	A	F	A	F	A	F
Park	61	83	2	14	0	2	0	0	0	2
Supermarket	55	81	2	17	2	2	0	0	0	0
Bus stop	62	82	2	12	0	0	0	0	0	0
Fast food	46	78	1	4	1	1	0	0	0	0
Disco	86	87	–	24	4	5	0	0	0	0
Coffee shop	50	83	–	15	1	1	0	0	0	0
Cinema	50	86	4	–	1	3	0	0	0	0
Home	19	26	1	–	0	0	0	0	0	0
Hospital	20	22	2	4	0	0	0	0	0	0
Cosmetic shop	62	80	2	14	0	2	0	0	0	0
College	83	87	–	54	7	8	0	0	0	0
Corner shop	84	84	3	5	0	0	0	0	0	0
Party	69	94	17	30	2	7	0	0	0	0
Theatre	78	87	2	25	0	3	0	0	0	0
Restaurant	41	93	3	22	0	7	0	0	0	0

A = alone; **F** = with friends; – = not assessed

along with trait anxiety and trait anger, had reduced to very low levels by the time of her discharge. Although state anger also reduced over the same period, a significant level was still recorded at discharge. Her ratings of predicted discomfort in the everyday situations also reduced, ahead of a full physical recovery. It appears that her anticipation of a full physical recovery led her to predict levels of discomfort in line with physical independence from mobility aids, before her physical progress had reached that point. It is interesting to note that her predicted level of discomfort in situations with her friends does not reduce as quickly as her discomfort ratings of her being in situations alone. The ratings for 27 July show this discrepancy. This is probably reflecting her anxieties about her friends' attitudes towards her.

Clearly, the relation between physical progress, fears about disability and emotion is complex. Emotional responses to neurological disease cannot be directly predicted by level of physical disability. They have their own rhythm and rationale, which can only be brought to light by careful discussion and observation.

Treatment strategies for emotionally distressed patients

A significant level of emotional distress will probably require specialist help and certainly any expressions of suicidal intent or other self-harm should be brought to the attention of a psychologist or psychiatrist. But a large number of patients with some degree of emotional distress can be helped through a therapy programme and neither need nor want a consultation with a specialist in abnormal behaviour or mental illness. The basis of formulating a therapy programme is to assess what is the nature of the patient's distress. Are they tense and nervous about their illness or recovery? Then the programme probably needs to take account of their anxiety. Are there problems at home that are overwhelming them? Then they probably need a counselling referral. Are they very negative and pessimistic about everything and everyone? Then the programme needs to be formulated to reduce their negativity.

If patients are very anxious about their illness or recovery, it may help to arrange a consultation with a member of the medical staff to provide them with information. Some anxieties are not so easily allayed and in most cases it is not a good idea to spend large amounts of physiotherapy time discussing the anxieties. Try to arrange for patients to have specific counselling sessions and agree with them to concentrate on physiotherapy when they are with you. In most instances, an anxious patient is likely to proceed slowly and a paced approach is often most productive, where small agreed increases in physical activity that are well within the patient's capabilities are made each day. Slow, steady progress is the aim and setbacks should be avoided wherever possible.

If the anxiety relates to a past incident, for example a recent fall on stairs resulting in a patient being loath to try stairs again, despite an obvious physical capability, then a brief discussion of the previous event, which includes how the future experience differs (supervision, physical recovery, more effective movement) may help. Sometimes it may be necessary to talk through the feared event. In the current example, discuss what would happen if the patient did fall on the stairs (minimal contact assistance would be maintained, she would not be allowed to injure or hurt herself). It is a characteristic of emotional judgements that the facts often do not speak for themselves. Facts which are apparently obvious may not have gained full acceptance in the patient's mind and may thus fail to influence their perception of risk. By discussing their specific fear, and even what would happen if there was a repeat of the feared event during therapy, patients mentally rehearse the feared event and perceive a happier outcome than they would have imagined without the discussion. Patients may only feel able to tackle a few stairs at first, but this may be an important and positive learning experience. Feedback and reassurance will be required constantly, with special emphasis on the safe completion of each activity.

Reassurance and discussion may not be as effective with depressed patients who are very negative. If they are told that everything is all right, they may well feel alienated or irritated, because their established view of the world is likely to be bleak and hopeless. For an introduction to psychological techniques used to treat depression, see Beck et al (1979). One approach that is often successful in this situation is a very tight focus of conversation and action towards the specific functional gains identified for the therapy session.

Any negative statements that relate directly to therapy, therapeutic outcome or attendance at therapy should be challenged; a neutral, low-key tone is probably best. Rather than being drawn into an argument about whose view is right, it is best to rely on concrete evidence. If possible, try things out with the patient to demonstrate benefits. Failing that, draw on evidence of previous cases, especially previous cases who started out from the same negative stance. It may be necessary to explicitly acknowledge that patients can see no possible benefit, in which case compliance in therapy can be promoted to patients on the basis that they cannot be harmed by the process, or that it might help to take their minds off things. By attending and working in therapy they are at least giving themselves a chance of progress. Once they are involved in therapy, a diary or chart recording their progress in concrete terms can be helpful in providing evidence for the benefits of the treatment programme.

CONCLUSIONS

Neuropsychological tests

Only a handful of neuropsychological tests have been introduced in this chapter. They have been used to give a brief impression of the kinds of tools that tease out the aspects of a patient's cognitive and emotional skills that have been affected by neurological disease. They are a useful starting point in the design of a treatment programme, but their relation to a patient's physical recovery or rehabilitation needs to be carefully examined. Most patients with cortical involvement of their disease will have widespread cognitive and emotional difficulties. The most striking features of a psychological assessment may not be the most salient in treatment. For any treatment programme, the interaction between all current impairments must be considered and the most appropriate way to achieve necessary functional gains identified.

Clinical observation

There is no substitute for observing a patient's physical activity, if the aim is to understand the nature of their difficulties. It is necessary to monitor constantly for the effects of cognitive and emotional dysfunction. A patient's neurological status can change, affecting the pattern of cognitive impairment. Emotional status can change for a whole host of reasons, many independent of the disease process. Patients who first come to therapy with a high level of physical disability may not demonstrate any cognitive deficits. For example, a patient recovering from a severe head injury may learn to turn in bed without difficulty. Turning in bed makes relatively low cognitive demands on the patient, with little precision, timing or spatial calculation required. However, as the patient's recovery progresses and his physical activity progresses to more complex tasks, the confounding effects of cognitive dysfunction may become obvious.

Treatment strategies

Some patients may have suffered sensory or motor deficits that are relatively peripheral and in addition there is a possibility of cognitive dysfunction. In these cases it may be hard to clarify the pattern of impairment that is causing an observed movement problem. One approach is to try either the most likely or the simplest treatment strategy. If this is sufficiently effective, then there is no need to consider the other option in therapy. If the trial has very disappointing results, it may be best to try a strategy designed to help the other impairment and abandon the first approach. A careful trial of alternative treatment strategies, although initially cumbersome, can eventually be the most efficient intervention, because it avoids spending time on ineffective or inappropriate interventions later. However, many patients suffer from a mixture of peripheral and central impairments. For them, a combined approach may be necessary.

Textbooks can be disappointing in that they invariably fail to describe the particular constellation of impairment and disability that one's patients demonstrate. But in fairness to textbooks, the neurological patients for whom a 'prêt-à-porter' treatment package can unhesitatingly be adopted are few. It is the absorbing challenge of neurology to fuse the variety of observed clinical features into a platform on which to build an effective treatment programme. It was the aim of this chapter to help you to add a few planks to that platform.

REFERENCES

Andrewes D G, Hordern C, Kaye A 1998 The everyday functioning questionnaire: a new measure of cognitive and emotional status for neurosurgical outpatients Neuropsychological Rehabilitation 8: 377–392

Beck A T, Rush A J, Shaw B F, Emery G 1979 Cognitive therapy of depression. Guildford, New York

De Renzi E 1982 Disorders of space exploration and cognition. John Wiley, Chichester

Ellis A W, Young A W 1988 Human cognitive neuropsychology. Lawrence Erlbaum, Hove

Gainotti G 1993 Emotional and psychosocial problems after brain injury. Neuropsychological Rehabilitation 3: 259–277

Goldenburg G, Hagman S 1998 Therapy of activities of daily living in patients with apraxia. Neuropsychological Rehabilitation 8: 123–141

Gray J M, Robertson I H, Pentland B, Anderson S 1992 Microcomputer-based attentional retraining after brain damage: a randomised group controlled trial. Neuropsychological Rehabilitation 2: 97–115

Gronwall D M A 1977 Paced auditory serial addition task: a measure of recovery from concussion. Perceptual and Motor Skills 44: 367–373

Holden U, Woods R 1995 Positive approaches to dementia care. Churchill Livingstone, Edinburgh

Howard D, Hatfield F M 1987 Aphasia therapy: historical and contemporary issues. Lawrence Erlbaum, Hove

Kapur N 1988 Memory disorders in clinical practice. Butterworths, London

Kay J, Lesser R, Coltheart M 1992 Psycholinguistic assessments of language processing in aphasia. Lawrence Erlbaum, Hove

Kinsella G J 1998 Assessment of attention following traumatic brain injury: a review. Neuropsychological Rehabilitation 8: 351–375

Knight R G 1992 The neuropsychology of degenerative brain disease. Lawrence Erlbaum, Hillsdale

Langdon D W, Thompson A J 1994 Relationship of objective and self-report measures of memory in multiple sclerosis. Journal of Neurology 241: S150

Langdon D W, Thompson A J 1999 A preliminary study of selected variables affecting rehabilitation outcome. Multiple Sclerosis 5: 94–100

Langdon D W, Thompson A J 2000 Relation of impairment to everyday competence in visual disorientation syndrome: evidence from a single case study. Archives of Physical Medicine and Rehabilitation 81: 689–691

Langdon D W, Warrington E K 1995 The VESPAR: a verbal and spatial reasoning test. Lawrence Erlbaum, Hove

McCarthy R A, Warrington E K 1990 Cognitive neuropsychology: a clinical introduction. Academic Press, San Diego

McKenna P, Warrington E K 1983 Graded naming test. NFER, Windsor

McMillan T M 1984 Investigation of everyday memory in normal subjects using the subjective memory questionnaire (SMQ). Cortex 20: 333–347

Marr D 1982 Vision. Freeman, San Francisco

Milner B 1963 Effects of different lesions on card sorting. Archives of Neurology 9: 90–100

Nelson H E, McKenna P 1975 The use of current reading ability in the assessment of dementia. British Journal of Social and Clinical Psychology 14: 259–267

Nelson H E, O'Connell A 1978 Dementia: the estimation of premorbid intelligence levels using the new adult reading test. Cortex 14: 234–244

Nelson H E, Willison J 1992 Restandardisation of the NART against the WAIS-R. NFER, Windsor

Obrzut 1986 Child neuropsychology. Academic Press, San Diego

Perecman E (ed) 1987 The frontal lobes revisited. IRBN, New York

Prigatano G P 1991 Awareness of deficit after brain injury. Oxford University Press, New York

Robertson I H, Marshall J C 1993 Unilateral neglect: clinical and experimental studies. Lawrence Erlbaum, Hove

Robertson I H, North N, Geggie C 1992 Spatio-motor cueing in unilateral neglect: three single case studies of its therapeutic effects. Journal of Neurology, Neurosurgery and Psychiatry 55: 799–805

Robertson I H, Ward T, Ridgeway V, Nimmo-Smith I 1994 The test of everyday attention. Thames Valley, Bury St Edmunds

Schwartz A F, McMillan T M 1989 Assessment of everyday memory after severe head injury. Cortex 25: 665–671

Spielberger C D 1983 Manual for the state-trait anxiety inventory. Consulting Psychologists, Palo Alto

Spielberger C D 1988 The state-trait anger expression inventory. Psychological Assessment Resources, Odessa

Tate R L, McDonald S 1995 What is apraxia? The clinician's dilemma. Neuropsychological Rehabilitation 5: 273–297

von Cramon Y D, von Cramon M G 1992 Reflection on the treatment of brain-injured patients suffering from problem-solving disorders. Neuropsychological Rehabilitation 2: 207–229

Warrington E K 1984 Recognition memory test. NFER, Windsor

Warrington E K 1986 Visual deficits associated with occipital lobe lesions in man. Experimental Brain Research Supplement 11: 247–261

Warrington E K, James M 1991 The visual object and space perception battery. Thames Valley, Bury St Edmunds

Wechsler D 1997 WAIS-III administration and scoring manual. The Psychological Corporation, San Antonio

Wilson B A 1987 Rehabilitation of memory. Guildford, New York

Wilson B A, Moffat N (eds) 1984 Clinical management of memory problems. Croom Helm, London

Wilson C, Robertson I H 1992 A home-based intervention for attentional slips during reading following a head injury: a single case study. Neuropsychological Rehabilitation 2: 193–205

Wilson B, Cockburn J, Baddeley A 1985 The Rivermead behavioural memory test. Thames Valley, Bury St Edmunds

Wilson B A, Cockburn J, Halligan P 1987 The behavioural inattention test. Thames Valley Test Company, Bury St Edmunds

Wilson B A, Baddeley A, Evans J, Shiel A 1994 Errorless learning in the rehabilitation of memory impaired people. Neuropsychological Rehabilitation 4: 307–326

5

Abnormal tone and movement as a result of neurological impairment: considerations for treatment

Susan Edwards

INTRODUCTION

Impaired movement and abnormal muscle tone is a common sequel following central (cerebral or spinal) or peripheral lesions of the nervous system. The severity of the movement impairment and the quality and type of the prevailing tone is dependent upon the site and extent of the damage. Damage to the central nervous system (CNS) often leads to increased tone whereas lower motor neurone damage leads to hypotonia or flaccidity.

Tone is the resistance offered by muscles to continuous passive stretch (Brooks 1986). The two mechanisms which contribute to this resistance are the inherent viscoelastic properties of the muscle itself and the tension set up in the muscle by reflex contraction caused by muscle stretch (Rothwell 1994). In a relaxed human subject with no neurological deficit, the resistance to passive movement is due to mechanical factors such as the compliance of muscles, tendons, ligaments and joints rather than neural mechanisms (Burke 1988, Sheean 1998). The relative contribution of neural and non-neural mechanisms which contribute to the quality of tone in individuals with neurological damage is constantly being challenged and continues to stimulate much debate (Dietz 1992, Given et al 1995, O'Dwyer et al 1996, Carr & Shepherd 1998).

Investigations such as computed tomography (CT), magnetic resonance imaging (MRI), functional MRI, positron emission tomography (PET) and transcranial magnetic stimulation (TMS) have revolutionised diagnosis in neurology. Prior to the introduction of this new technology, the site and extent of the lesion was mainly determined by the clinical signs and symptoms. In a sense, the focus of physiotherapy is still at this stage where treatment is determined by the clinical presentation and effects of, for example, weakness, abnormal tone, sensory impairment and perceptual problems. The exact cause and extent of damage is considered of secondary importance to the clinical distribution and severity of impairments. There may be little correlation between the lesion and the disability: even with sophisticated assessment and monitoring, exact physical disabilities cannot be predicted from the type and extent of the lesion.

This section will discuss the pathophysiology and physical treatment and management of the more common types of motor impairments resulting from damage to the nervous system.

SPASTICITY AND THE UPPER MOTOR NEURONE SYNDROME

The comment made by Young (1994) that 'although spasticity is difficult to define, neurologists recognise spasticity when they see it – at least they think they do' may equally apply to physiotherapists.

Definition

There appears to be a general lack of consensus in the use of the word 'spasticity' in that it is often used to describe diverse clinical features observed in patients with neurological damage (Carr & Shepherd 1998, Sheean 1998). There is clearly a difference, both pathophysiologically and clinically, between hypertonus of cerebral as opposed to spinal origin and also between the severe hypertonus emerging in the immediate aftermath of head injury and the slowly evolving hypertonus following a more focal lesion such as stroke. However, in spite of these obvious differences, the term 'spasticity' is used synonymously by medical and therapy staff alike.

The physiological definition, that spasticity is 'a motor disorder characterised by a velocity-dependent increase in tonic stretch reflexes (muscle tone) with exaggerated tendon jerks, resulting from hyper-excitability of the stretch reflex as one component of the upper motor neurone (UMN) syndrome' (Lance 1980), is widely accepted and is invariably included in the introduction to all medical and therapy literature relating to spasticity. However, almost without exception, this definition is expanded within the text to encompass all features associated with the UMN syndrome.

The UMN syndrome is a more general term used to describe patients with abnormal motor function which may result from cerebral or spinal cord lesions (Katz & Rymer 1989). The clinical features of the UMN syndrome are broadly divided into negative and positive phenomena. The negative features or performance deficits include weakness and loss of dexterity, whereas the positive features or abnormal behaviours are characterised by excessive or inappropriate motor activity (Katz & Rymer 1989). Spasticity, as defined by Lance (1980), is but one component of this syndrome.

Unlike spasticity, which is velocity dependent and is apparent when the relaxed spastic muscle is stretched (Rothwell 1994), other types of muscle hypertonia may give rise to abnormal postures as a consequence of increased tonic muscle contraction which continues in the absence of movement. This latter abnormality of tone is referred to as spastic dystonia (Burke 1988, Young 1994). It is proposed that the abnormal posture and the sustained chronic contraction of affected muscle groups associated with hemiplegia, flexion of the upper limb and extension of the lower limb, should be considered to be a form of spastic dystonia (Young 1994). Whereas 'true spasticity' is dependent upon afferent information from feedback following movement of the stretched muscle, spastic dystonia is considered to be a form of sustained efferent muscular hyperactivity, dependent upon continuous supraspinal drive to the alpha motoneurones (Burke 1988, Sheean 1998).

For ease of purpose, the term hypertonia as opposed to spasticity will be used throughout this section.

Neural components

Descending pathways

The role of the motoneurone pool is to translate the varied and complex information from afferent and descending fibres and from interneurones into an output that will precisely control the contraction of muscle fibres to develop a particular force or pattern of movement (Davidoff 1992). If the information received is inappropriate or of insufficient neural drive at this spinal segmental level, the quality and control of movement will be impaired which may lead to changes in the characteristic properties of muscle (Jones & Round 1990, Cameron & Calancie 1995).

UMNs are neurones of any long descending tract that have an influence upon the excitability of the lower motor neurone either through direct synapse or via interneurones. They modulate segmental motor reflex activity in the spinal cord. Therefore, while a UMN lesion can occur anywhere along its pathway, the pathophysiological derangement responsible for most of the positive features of the UMN syndrome occurs at the level of spinal segments and therefore may be considered a 'spinal' phenomenon (Sheean 1998).

Although the UMN syndrome is often referred to as pyramidal tract injury, a discrete lesion of the pyramidal/corticospinal tract does not give rise to 'spasticity' (Burke 1988, Brown 1994, Rothwell 1994, Young 1994). The main symptoms resulting from damage to the corticospinal tract are those of weakness and loss of dexterity which is greater in distal than in proximal muscles (Kuypers 1981).

The supraspinal control of muscle tone is primarily dependent upon the balanced interaction between parapyramidal tracts which arise in the brain stem. The key tracts are the dorsal reticulospinal tract (DRT), the medial reticulospinal tract (MRT) and the vestibulospinal tract (VST). These descending pathways synapse upon interneuronal networks within the spinal cord. The DRT has an inhibitory influence and the MRT and VST have a facilitatory effect on extensor tone. All three systems are thought to inhibit flexor reflex afferents responsible for flexor spasms (Brown 1994, Sheean 1998).

Unlike the MRT and VST, the DRT is under direct cortical control from the pre-motor and supplementary motor areas via corticoreticular neurones that descend through the internal capsule. Damage to this cortical drive, such as may occur with a lesion in the internal capsule will reduce the activity of the DRT, leaving the facilitatory effects of the MRT and VST relatively unopposed, producing hypertonus (Sheean 1998).

Damage to the DRT in the lateral funiculus of the spinal cord, with sparing of the facilitatory tracts, will give rise to paraplegia in extension. This is frequently observed in patients with multiple sclerosis. The demyelinating lesions have a predilection for the lateral funiculi and this pathology may explain why extensor hypertonus is often more pronounced in the legs in the early course of multiple sclerosis (Brown 1994).

In severe or complete cord lesions there is a loss of all supraspinal control, which leads to abnormalities in spinal cord function and integration. Patients with hypertonia show reduced reciprocal inhibition between agonist and antagonist muscles and reduced recurrent inhibition mediated via the Renshaw cell (Katz & Pierrot-Deseilligny 1982). Hypertonia is not as marked as in some patients with incomplete cord lesions because the excitatory systems are no longer acting unopposed. However, flexor spasms are very prominent as flexor reflexes are released from the inhibitory influences of the DRT, MRT and the VST (Brown 1994).

Evolution of hypertonia

Depending on the site and extent of the CNS damage, patients with either cerebral or spinal lesions may demonstrate flaccidity or hypotonia for a variable period of time post-lesion before the emergence of hypertonia and exaggerated reflex activity. This is referred to as the period of shock during which time the muscles may be toneless and areflexic (Brown 1994, Rothwell 1994). Shock is rarely apparent in more slowly evolving lesions (Burke 1988). It is suggested that the delayed appearance of hypertonus may involve some functional or structural rearrangement within the CNS. Collateral sprouting and increased receptor sensitivity have been implicated in these plastic changes (Katz & Rymer 1989, Sheean 1998).

Non-neural components

The intrinsic stiffness of the muscle is a significant contributor to muscle tone and, given that muscle normally exhibits spring-like behaviour, it has been suggested that an increase in the intrinsic mechanical stiffness of the muscle is responsible for spastic hypertonia (Dietz 1992, Brown 1994, Ada et al 1998). This stiffness may be mediated by permanent structural changes in the mechanical properties of muscle or connective tissues, or be variable in character (Katz & Rymer 1989, Carey & Burghardt 1993).

The contribution of mechanical factors to the clinical impression of hypertonus is controversial but is considered by many to be the major cause of residual disability (Thilmann et al 1991, Dietz 1992, Given et al 1995, O'Dwyer et al 1996, Ada et al 1998, Carr & Shepherd 1998). In particular, in patients with more long-standing hypertonia, the continued contribution of neural activity has been questioned (Hufschmidt & Mauritz 1985, Thilmann et al 1991, Given et al 1995).

The contribution of mechanical factors to hypertonus may vary in different muscle groups. For example, Given et al (1995) demonstrated that there was increased passive stiffness of the ankle plantar flexors in comparison to the elbow flexors on the paretic side of patients following stroke. It was suggested that the greater cross-sectional area of the triceps surae was associated with increased amounts of intramuscular connective tissue, which may be responsible in part for the higher stiffness at the ankle joint. In agreement with this, Thilmann et al (1991) found that hypertonus at the elbow was always associated with velocity-dependent electromyographic (EMG) activity, whereas this was not the case with the ankle plantar flexors where again a significant contribution to raised tone arises due to changes in the passive properties of these muscles.

However, despite the importance of mechanical factors to the genesis of hypertonus, it must be appreciated that the mechanical contribution to hypertonia would not arise without the damage to the CNS producing the reduced activity and/or stereotypical postures associated with UMN lesions. The influence of neural and mechanical factors on tone and function change over time but the relative contribution of neural and non-neural components at any point in time remains unclear (Brown 1994).

Changes in muscle fibre property

Following neurological damage, changes in muscle fibre type distribution can occur and a relative increase in both the proportion of either fast or slow fibres has been described. An increase in the proportion of fast fibres may be caused by atrophy, resulting from a decreased drive on to the motoneuronal pool. In contrast, abnormal continuous muscle activity resulting from abnormal descending drives to the muscle and the compensatory movement strategies that ensue, may cause a change from fast to slow fibre types.

Atrophy

In spite of the sustained muscle activity apparent in many patients with hypertonus, atrophy of affected muscle groups is a notable feature. Disruption to the central and segmental synaptic drive onto spinal interneurones such as occurs in UMN lesions results in disuse atrophy (Gordon & Mao 1994, Rothwell 1994).

On the basis that muscle activity and stretch are prerequisites for the maintenance of slow-twitch muscle fibre properties, in the absence of activity fast fibres will predominate (Goldspink et al 1992). Patients with acquired neurological disability who have a movement impairment which interferes with their ability to maintain postural control against gravity, and in maintaining stretch and muscle activity, will demonstrate a change in proportion of fibre type from slow to fast (Martin et al 1992, Vrbova et al 1995).

It seems logical, that those patients who are unable to sustain muscle activity against gravity will be unable to maintain the muscle characteristics associated with postural control. The slow-twitch fibres responsible for this function will readily atrophy, tipping the balance towards an increased dominance of fast-twitch fibres. The development of postural control during recovery from a UMN lesion may then be dependent upon activity of fast-twitch muscle fibres which are not suited to this task as they cannot sustain force.

Changes in fibre type resulting from altered muscle activity

Conversely, it has been demonstrated following stroke and in the presence of hypertonia that there can be a gradual change in fibre type composition with increased numbers of slow muscle fibres (Dietz 1992). This may be the result of a muscle fibre transformation following continuous activity in hypertonus (Dattola et al 1993). Further, the altered muscle activity accompanying compensatory movement strategies may lead to a change in fibre type. For example, a predominance of type 1 with a deficiency of type II fibre type was found following biopsy of the gastrocnemius muscle of children with spastic cerebral palsy (Ito et al 1996). The author feels that this may be due to the sustained activity of gastrocnemius, in conjunction with soleus, to generate extensor activity to overcome the predominantly flexor gait pattern.

Functional consequence of fibre type change

A change in fibre type can have important functional consequences. As stated in Chapter 3, slow-twitch muscle fibres develop larger forces at lower firing rates and are recruited first. Therefore, an increase in their proportion may contribute to a gradual increase in hypertonia (Edstrom 1970, Vrbova et al 1995). It has also been suggested that the selective atrophy of fast-twitch muscle fibres may contribute to the reduction in voluntary power in hemiparesis, paraparesis and Parkinson's disease (Edstrom 1970).

Summary

The development of hypertonia is dependent not only on the extent and severity of the neuro-logical impairment but also on the resultant non-neural factors, which include weakness and changes in the properties of muscle. The dominant, overactive muscles will be held in a shortened position while the antagonists will be held in a lengthened position. These length changes imposed by this sustained posturing may lead to structural and physiological changes within the muscles (Goldspink & Williams 1990).

Although many emphasise the non-neural components of hypertonia as being the major contributory factor in the level of disability (Dietz 1992, Young 1994, Carr & Shepherd 1998), it is impossible to consider the supraspinal damage which leads to abnormal tone and changes in muscle property as separate entities in the management of people with hypertonia (Nash et al 1989).

Despite the controversial nature of hypertonia, the nature of the movement disorder is clear: abnormal movement synergies, weakness and incoordination all contribute to the level of disability.

Specific pathological activity associated with patients with hypertonus

Positive support reaction

The positive support reaction was first described by Magnus (1926; as cited by Bobath 1990) as a process by which the leg changes into a stiff pillar. It is a term used to describe a pattern of plantar flexion which occurs on attempted weight bearing through the foot. It affects agonists and antagonists simultaneously, producing a rigidly extended leg and a subsequent inability to balance with normal alignment of the trunk and pelvis. Bobath (1990) describes a dual stimulus:

- a proprioceptive stimulus evoked by stretch of the intrinsic muscles of the foot, and
- an exteroceptive stimulus evoked by the contact of the pads of the foot with the ground.

The positive support reaction is considered to be of distal origin, arising from hypersensitivity, which leads to the inability of the foot to adapt

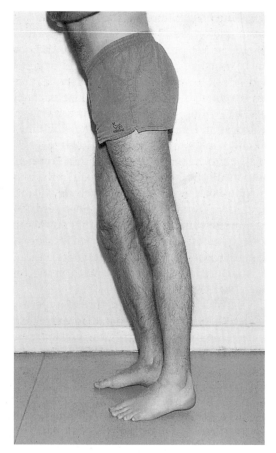

Figure 5.1 Positive support reaction.

and accept the base of support (Fig. 5.1). Compensatory strategies arise proximally in an attempt to maintain balance. This reaction is associated with extensor hypertonus in the first instance, although a modification of this response, whereby flexion may dominate, has been observed in clinical practice.

The term 'positive support reaction' would appear to be one used predominantly by physiotherapists. There is little in the literature to clarify this terminology. Massion & Woollacott (1996) refer to the positive supporting reaction, originating from distal cutaneous or proprioceptive receptors, as regulating the level of co-contraction of the limb muscles as a function of weight bearing. Schomburg (1990) commented that pressure on the plantar skin of the foot leads normally to what he terms an 'extensor thrust' and this is felt to stabilise the foot in standing and during the stance phase of gait. Certainly, pressure sensors in the sole of the foot are vital for balance and in the control of movement (Rothwell 1994). The integration of afferent information from these receptors may be impaired following cerebral or spinal cord damage, which may give rise to the response described above.

Clinical features. Plantar flexor hypertonia is a primary and obvious feature of this reaction and is frequently associated with inversion of the foot. Secondary involvement includes shortening of the intrinsic foot musculature due to the inability to transfer weight across the full surface of the foot and loss of range in the plantar fascia. The triceps surae may become shortened due to the inability to attain a plantigrade position during the stance phase of walking; this further exacerbates the inability to transfer weight or to adapt to irregularities in ground surface (Dietz 1992).

One consequence of this reaction is compensatory hip flexion in an attempt to maintain balance. The pelvis is retracted as the weight is displaced backwards by the pressure from the ball of the foot against the supporting surface, the patient being unable to transfer the weight over the full support and thus achieve extension at the hip.

Although the knee is maintained in a position of extension, this is not achieved on the basis of appropriate quadriceps activity and it is not uncommon to observe wasting of this muscle group. In many instances the knee becomes hyperextended as a result of the inability to attain normal alignment of the pelvis over the foot, impaired interaction between the hamstrings and quadriceps muscle groups and shortening of gastrocnemius. The flexed, retracted position of the hip and pelvis may lead to shortening of the hip flexors, adductors and medial rotators, producing a mechanical obstruction to correct alignment of the hip during stance phase.

The pressure exerted by the foot pushing into plantar flexion prevents release of the knee. Attempts by the patient to move the foot away from the floor result in compensatory strategies whereby the extended leg is hitched forwards in order to step through (Dietz 1992). This action demands greater activity from, in particular, latissimus dorsi with a resultant shortening of the trunk side flexors. The insertion of latissimus dorsi at the humerus produces medial rotation of the upper limb and each time the patient attempts to hitch the leg forwards, the trunk side flexors and the upper limb demonstrate an increase in pathological flexor activity, through the action of latissimus dorsi. The hypertonus of the upper limb appears to be influenced by the amount of effort expended by the patient to step forwards with the affected leg. This seemingly proportional response, of increased hypertonus in the upper limb being determined by the effort necessary to accomplish a step, is an example of what is referred to as an associated reaction (see p. 97).

The positive support reaction will also affect the ability to stand up from sitting and sit down from standing. The resistance from the hypertonic plantar flexors prevents the transference of weight forwards over the foot as the individual prepares to stand. The leg becomes stiff in extension and the patient is pushed back into the chair. The situation is reversed when attempting to sit down. The leg is unable to flex and the patient falls back into the chair. Patients with hemiplegia will tend to stand up and sit down predominantly on their sound leg because of this inability to take weight through the affected limb.

More recently, a flexor component of the positive support reaction has been observed in clinical practice. As the patient attempts to bring the leg forwards there is a notable increase in flexor activity. In this situation, the sensitivity of the foot remains the primary problem, but the weight-bearing mechanics are altered. The foot is maintained in a position of inversion and the ball of the foot does not make contact with the ground, leading to adaptive shortening of affected muscle groups. Weight is taken over the lateral border of the foot with an almost instant withdrawal into flexion as an attempt is made to step through.

Treatment of the positive support reaction should be directed towards mobilisation of the foot, the triceps surae and the Achilles the first instance, in an attempt to desensitise against both the intrinsic and extrinsic stimuli (Lynch & Grisogono 1991). Therapists are often advised not to stimulate the ball of the foot but in this instance appropriate handling and facilitation of transference of weight over the foot are important to reduce the effects of this reaction.

Botulinum toxin is increasingly being used to weaken the dominant muscle groups responsible for the positive support reaction (Dengler et al 1992, Hesse et al 1994, Dunne et al 1995, Richardson et al 2000) (see Chapter 7). Used in conjunction with physiotherapy and in some cases splinting (Scrutton et al 1996), this has shown promising results.

Flexor withdrawal response of the leg

Flexor withdrawal is a response which occurs in normal subjects and is well illustrated by withdrawal of the hand from a hot stove, or the foot when stepping on a drawing pin. It is associated with the crossed extensor reflex (Magnus 1926 as cited by Bobath 1990, Schomburg 1990). The withdrawal response is determined by the direction of the noxious stimulus and therefore may not necessarily be into flexion (Rothwell 1994).

Patients with neurological impairment may demonstrate this response in a more stereotyped and consistent pattern. A minimal stimulus, not necessarily noxious – for example, removing the bedclothes from a patient following spinal cord injury – may be enough to elicit this response

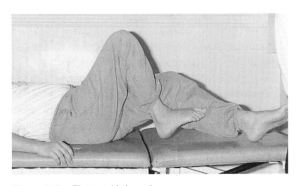

Figure 5.2 Flexor withdrawal.

(Edwards 1998). The response in the lower limbs is that of flexion, abduction and lateral rotation at the hip, flexion at the knee and inversion of the foot in conjunction with dorsiflexion or plantar flexion of the ankle (Fig. 5.2).

The problem is often exacerbated by shortening of the dominant muscle groups, particularly the hip and knee flexors which may lead to subsequent shortening of the erector spinae. This response may be stimulated by stretch of these muscles, which prevents the patient from standing up effectively (Lynch & Grisogono 1991) and from placing the foot on the floor.

In clinical practice this response may be seen in patients with severe neurological damage such as may occur following complete spinal cord transection (Brown 1994). It may also be observed in patients with neurological impairment following painful trauma such as a fracture of the neck of femur. Pressure sores, or other painful stimuli of the foot in particular, may also give rise to a flexor response (Schomburg 1990).

Removal of the noxious stimulus and/or management of the primary trauma are of immediate concern in treating the manifestations of this response. The short-term influence of such a stimulus may prove to be readily reversible, whereas prolonged exposure, particularly to pain, will have more residual effects, such as the establishment of contractures.

Treatment by physiotherapy will be determined by the extent and severity of structural changes which may have occurred. Attempts to stand a patient on a leg which is mechanically altered due to contracture will further aggravate the situation, not least by imposing an additional painful stimulus. It is essential first to regain the required range of movement at the hip and pelvis, thereby allowing the leg to be released sufficiently to attain its normal length.

'Normal' standing can only be achieved on the basis of mechanical and structural alignment of the pelvis and lower limbs. In their absence compensation, particularly at the trunk and pelvis, is inevitable. Mobilisation of shortened muscles and soft tissues may cause some discomfort, but it is important to distinguish between pain resulting from muscle stretch and joint pain which

may occur through forcing a malaligned joint. As a general rule, any intervention should be pain-free, it being impossible to inhibit pathological or, indeed, normal protective muscle spasm in the presence of pain.

Davies (1985) advocates the use of a back slab to maintain the leg in extension and thereby facilitate weight bearing. This procedure may be of benefit in the early stages of counteracting increasing flexor activity of the leg but should be used with caution in patients with more long-standing problems, particularly where there is loss of range. Attempts to force the leg into a back slab may cause pain and thereby nullify any positive effects.

More recently, intrathecal baclofen has been used to good effect in carefully selected patients with severe flexor hypertonus (Porter 1997). Details of this treatment intervention are to be found in Chapter 7.

Grasp reflex

The grasp reflex is a normal phenomenon in human infants which disappears within a few months of birth. In the adult it is always pathological (Rothwell 1994). The stimulus for initiating this response is to the hand and fingers, particularly the palm. Desensitisation of this reflex must therefore incorporate mobilisation and appropriate tactile stimulation to the hand within the patient's tolerance. This must involve all personnel involved in the management of such patients, not least the patients themselves and their carers. Movements of the hand should also include an appropriate response from the whole of the upper limb and, wherever possible, produce a functional outcome.

The use of splinting to prevent contracture in the presence of a severe grasp reflex remains a controversial issue and is discussed in Chapter 10.

Extensor response

This response may be observed following severe head injury and in people with multiple sclerosis or dystonic/athetoid cerebral palsy. Extreme cases will include extension of all four limbs with arching of the spine (see Rigidity, p. 105). It is initiated and perpetuated by stimulation and contact between the back of the head and the supporting surface and is exacerbated in extensor positions such as supine lying.

Patients described as displaying the 'out of line' or 'pusher' syndrome (Davies 1985) may also demonstrate an extensor thrust of the head and upper trunk but this is often in conjunction with flexor hypertonus of the affected lower leg.

There are differing degrees of severity but it is important to recognise the influence of positions of extension and the susceptibility of a stimulus – for example, the head support of a wheelchair – in triggering this response. It may be an extensor thrust which is responsible for preventing the patient from accepting the support of a chair, with the result that he is constantly pushing himself out (see Ch. 9). If this is the case, it is important to desensitise this response rather than merely attempting to restrain the patient in the chair.

The extensor response is indicative of gross cerebral pathology, and it may be questioned whether any physiotherapeutic intervention can have an effect on outcome. It is difficult to prevent the development of contractures if the patient is constantly held in this extreme position of extension. Physiotherapy is based on the principle that changes in the environment will influence potential for change in the CNS. Modification of the extended position to introduce an element of flexion will create a temporary release from what can only be assumed to be a painful maintenance of extensor hypertonus. This may be achieved not only by modifying the supporting surface of the bed, as described in Chapter 6, but also by the use of the gymnastic ball whereby the patient is mobilised into flexion over an adaptable as opposed to a rigid surface (Fig. 5.3).

The patient may also be facilitated into standing, preferably with a therapist in front to support the knees and another behind to provide a mobile support in an attempt to prevent stimulation of the thrust into extension. A tilt table is often used for this purpose and in some instances this may be the only practicable way of the

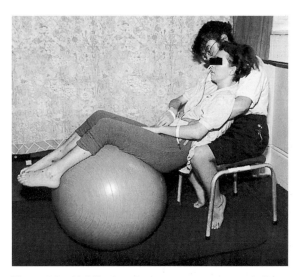

Figure 5.3   Mobilisation of extensor response over ball.

patient attaining the standing position. Difficulties may arise using this method as the table provides a rigid support against which the patient can push and, at the same time, minimises the opportunity of mobilising the patient while upright against gravity (see Ch. 6).

The extensor response is invariably accompanied by plantar flexor hypertonus. Treatment as advocated above may have some influence on this particular aspect of management. Unfortunately, contracture of the triceps surae is a well-documented complication of extensor hypertonus (Booth et al 1983, Yarkony & Sahgal 1987, Kent et al 1990, Davidson & Waters 1999). Application of below-knee inhibitory casts as a prophylactic measure has been recommended as a means of preventing or minimising this disabling complication (Conine et al 1990, Moseley 1993, 1997) and is discussed in Chapter 10.

Associated reactions

Associated reactions (ARs) were originally described as 'released postural reactions in muscles deprived of voluntary control' (Riddoch & Buzzard 1921, Walshe 1923) and appear as involuntary stereotyped abnormal patterns of movement at a body segment of the affected side, which coincide with or follow effort exerted at another body site (Davies 1985, Dickstein et al 1996). They are thought to be pathological movements which are indicative of the potential for development of hypertonus or an accentuation of the prevailing spastic synergy (Bobath 1990).

ARs may occur throughout the body but are most apparent distally, such as in the arm and hand and the leg and foot. They may be initiated not only as a result of attempted movement but also at the preparatory stage of movement (Dickstein et al 1995) and they may also be observed with involuntary actions such as yawning, coughing and sneezing (Mulley 1982). Attempts to communicate by patients with dysphasia or cognitive problems may also produce this response.

Following damage to the central nervous system, it is generally believed that the severity of the ARs is directly related to the degree of hypertonus: the more severe the hypertonus, the more forceful and longer lasting the associated reaction and the larger the magnitude of the limb excursion (Davies 1990, Cornall 1991, Dvir & Panturin 1993, Dvir et al 1996). However, Dickstein et al (1996) suggest that this relationship is not so clearly defined. When examining the displacement of the paretic elbow into flexion of hemiplegic patients during walking, they identified two distinct movement stages. The first abrupt increase in elbow flexion, which occurred during the first four steps, appeared to be reflexive in nature, whereas they suggest that the preservation of elbow flexion during walking may be an expression of stiffening of the elbow flexor muscle fibres.

Stephenson et al (1998) highlighted the confusion in terminology between ARs and associated movements. Bobath (1985) makes a clear distinction between ARs, which are always pathological, and associated movements, which are normally coordinated movements occurring as a result of reinforcement of movements initiated and performed with effort, such as when learning a new skill. In contrast, Carr & Shepherd (1980) and Shepherd (1998) refer to associated movements in the context of both normal and pathological response to concentrated or effortful movement, and Brunnstrom (1970) uses this term

to describe involuntary limb movement. In addition to the terms ARs and associated movements, motor overflow has also been used to describe this phenomenon (Lazarus 1992).

ARs have been described previously in relation to compensation for the positive support reaction (see p. 95). The extensor hypertonus in the lower limb necessitates increased effort in taking the leg forwards during the swing phase of gait. This effort is reflected in an increase of tonus throughout the affected side, producing, in many instances, a stereotyped response of flexor hypertonus in the arm and side flexion of the trunk. It is suggested that this pathological response is indicative of the severity of the hypertonus (Dvir et al 1996). Dickstein et al (1995) also reported an increase in EMG activity of the biceps muscle of the paretic upper limb in stroke patients, which was associated with foot lifting, and in many instances this EMG activity started before the foot was lifted. However, this response also occurred, although to a lesser degree, in the non-paretic limb and in healthy controls.

The use of ARs has been advocated to describe and grade the severity of hypertonus, to evaluate and direct therapeutic intervention and as a prognostic indicator (Davies 1985, 1990, Bobath 1990, Lynch & Grisogono 1991). Dvir & Panturin (1993) found that improvement in effort-related ARs mirrored a decrease in hypertonus and, in a study by Cornall (1991), ARs were used to assess the effects on hypertonus when self-propelling a wheelchair.

In a recent small-scale survey of physiotherapy departments in the Yorkshire region of England, the use of ARs to grade hypertonus and to guide therapeutic intervention was found to be the most common means of assessing hypertonus in the clinical setting (Stephenson 1996). The use of this assessment scale, referred to as a 'Bobath' assessment, as a clinically relevant measure, was supported by Lynch-Ellerington (1998) on the basis that 'the facilitation of the control of associated reactions by the patient produces the rewards of recovery of sensation, proprioception, posture and selective movement and hence function'. However, although it may appear logical that ARs are a positive feature of the UMN syndrome, there is no conclusive evidence with regard to reliability, validity or responsiveness that this is the case (Stephenson et al 1998). Furthermore, they are variable, their magnitude and duration differing drastically on repeated trials (Dvir et al 1996) and, therefore, it has been suggested that they may not be the most appropriate means of measuring hypertonus (Haas 1994).

Clinical implications. It is suggested that sustained ARs, may give rise to a deteriorating level of function in that movement. Repeated movements, for example of the arm into flexion, may lead to a gradual loss of range and ultimately contracture (Davies 1990, Dvir & Panturin 1993). Movement requiring excessive effort is cited as causing this pathological response, and assistance from the therapist to reduce the amount of effort required is recommended (Davies 1994).

Although ARs are generally associated with hypertonus, their appearance and severity may be due to underlying low tone. Patients with hypotonia may demonstrate marked ARs due to lack of stability at the trunk and proximal key points. Unless this true cause is identified and addressed in treatment, 'inhibition' of ARs will have no functional carry-over. While mobilising and stretching the upper limb may be effective in maintaining range of movement, there will be no lasting change without improved proximal stability and without the patient being able to actively use the affected limb.

Aims of physiotherapy intervention in the management of hypertonus

There are many assumptions and beliefs regarding the treatment of hypertonus, many of which are unsubstantiated. One major issue is whether weakness is apparent or real. Bobath (1990) attributes the 'weakness' of hypertonic muscles to exaggerated co-contraction of opposing muscle groups and hypothesises that resisted exercise and effort will further increase the hypertonus. However, as discussed above, there is now conclusive evidence that weakness is a very real and disabling feature following UMN lesions.

Secondary effects include muscle atrophy and the potential for development of contractures.

Specific interventions such as mobilisation, stretch of affected muscle groups and possibly splinting are clearly indicated to prevent muscle shortening and to enable muscles to be activated more efficiently, but to what extent should the patient be encouraged to use graded resisted exercises? The theory that resisted exercise causes a marked loss of coordination and an increase in co-contraction was refuted in a recent study by Miller & Light (1997), who concluded that strength training with paretic muscles could benefit individuals post-stroke. Furthermore, aerobic exercise has also been shown to be related to improvement of overall sensorimotor function after stroke (Potempa et al 1996).

Tone reduction is clearly indicated for patients with pathological overactivity in dominant muscle groups. However, if functional tasks produce an increase in tone, for example an associated reaction, should this activity be discouraged? Walking is an oft-cited example of function versus quality of movement and many therapists recommend that patients avoid this activity until they are deemed (by the physiotherapist) to be 'ready to walk' (Davidson & Waters 2000). However, as suggested in this study, if delay in walking is advocated on the grounds of quality issues, the benefits and effectiveness of treatment need to be substantiated.

Physiotherapy intervention to assess and treat the patient with hypertonus is determined by assumptions about its nature and cause. If the neural components of hypertonus are the perceived problem, the purpose of therapy will be to 'inhibit' the stereotyped response and to facilitate more normal postures and movement patterns. However, while reducing or eliminating hypertonus may increase range of movement, this may reveal underlying weakness rather than underlying control (Giuliani 1992, Nielsen & Sinkjaer 2000). The main influence of tone reduction would appear to be on the non-neural components. Maintaining or increasing the length of muscle gives a better biomechanical advantage for optimal force production, more efficient activation of muscle and the potential for carry-over into functional tasks.

Conventional clinical practice in the UK is based on the Bobath approach. This approach emphasises the facilitation of normal muscle tone and movement; activities which perpetuate or increase abnormal tone are strongly discouraged (Bobath 1990). However, research evidence for the effectiveness of interventions indicates that resisted exercise training and using equipment such as the treadmill, splints and walking aids enhance performance of movement (Pomeroy & Tallis 2000).

The primary goal of physiotherapy is to change functional performance, and one aspect of treatment to achieve this goal is the reduction of hypertonus. However, merely to reduce hypertonus is not the answer. The patient must be active in order for there to be any influence on the neural components of tone because, without this, no carry-over is possible.

ATAXIA

Ataxia is a general term meaning a decomposition of movement (Holmes 1939). Morgan (1980) describes three main types of ataxia: sensory, labyrinthine (vestibular) and cerebellar.

Sensory ataxia

This results from lesions affecting peripheral sensory nerves conveying proprioceptive and cutaneous information or in conditions affecting the dorsal columns or the primary sensory cortex (Morgan 1980). Symptoms vary depending on the pattern of sensory loss. For example, proprioceptive input from both the distal legs and the lumbar spine and pelvis are essential for initiating and modulating postural adjustments in standing (Ingilis et al 1994, Allum et al 1995, Allum 1996). Patients with sensory loss of the lower limbs have a wide-based gait with eyes fixed to the ground for visual feedback (Lajoie et al 1996). The amplitude of postural sway when standing with feet together is greatly increased with the eyes closed (Notermans et al 1994).

Patients with loss of proprioception of the upper limb are unable to plan for or compensate for the biomechanical variations that naturally occur with multi-joint movements such as reaching (Sainburg et al 1993, 1995). When assessing the impact of sensory loss on upper limb function, the importance of cutaneous input from the palmar aspect of the hand and fingers must be recognised (Johansson 1996). These patients often compensate for poor grip control by applying excessive force (Carey 1995).

Vestibular ataxia

This may occur with peripheral vestibular disorders or central disorders which affect the vestibular nuclei and/or their afferent/efferent connections, for example with medullary strokes (Brandt & Dieterich 2000). Peripheral lesions may be either bilateral or, more commonly, unilateral (Fetter 2000).

The vestibular apparatus comprises the semicircular canals and otoliths that detect angular and linear acceleration of the head, respectively. The otoliths also detect the position of the head with respect to gravity, thus contributing to the person's orientation to gravity and the midline (Hain et al 2000). The vestibular apparatus is involved in the initiation and modulation of postural adjustments and in stabilising the head against gravity (Allum et al 1997, Horak & Shupert 2000). The patient with vestibular ataxia may have poor righting reactions and abnormalities in postural strategies in both sitting and standing.

Patients with bilateral peripheral lesions often lean backwards in standing while those with a unilateral lesion tend to lean towards the side of the lesion. They tend to stagger and have a wide-based gait. To maintain standing balance, patients are often over-reliant on one of the remaining sensations, such as vision, often to the exclusion of other potentially useful sensations such as somatosensory information or any remaining vestibular information. This inappropriate reliance may lead to disequilibrium when these sensory cues are absent, reduced or inappropriate (Shumway-Cook et al 1996, Herdman & Whitney 2000). Head, trunk and subsequently upper limb movements are often decreased and disequilibrium is increased by head movement while walking (Gill-Body & Krebs 1994, Herdman & Whitney 2000).

Vestibular ataxia may be accompanied by poor perception of the midline, vertigo, blurred vision and nystagmus due to the vestibular system's role in sensing and perceiving self-motion and in stabilising gaze (Horak & Shupert 2000). It is important to determine the factors that precipitate these distressing but potentially treatable symptoms as they may greatly limit functional recovery. Patients may limit head movements to avoid precipitating vertigo, leading not only to neck stiffness but also to inadequate use of somatosensory or remaining vestibular information which is important for the recovery of gaze control and balance (Herdman & Whitney 2000).

Cerebellar ataxia

This results from lesions affecting the cerebellum or its afferent or efferent connections. The cerebellum may be divided into specific functional areas (Thompson & Day 1993). Lesions of the midline structures, the vermis and flocculonodular lobe produce bilateral symptoms affecting axial parts of the body, which manifest as truncal ataxia and titubation and abnormalities of gait and equilibrium. Occulomotor abnormalities and dysarthria may also be associated with this pathology (Lewis & Zee 1993). Lesions affecting the hemispheres give rise to ipsilateral limb symptoms (Ghez 1991).

Symptoms associated with cerebellar ataxia

Dysmetria. This refers to inaccuracy in achieving a final end position (hypermetria equals overshoot; hypometria equals undershoot). This is clearly demonstrated by the patient attempting the finger–nose test. The movement may overshoot or undershoot the target, with overcorrection resulting in additional movements.

Tremor

- Kinetic tremor, which is the oscillation that occurs during the course of the movement.
- Intention tremor, which is the increase in tremor towards the end of the movement.

- Postural tremor, which occurs when holding a limb in a given position.
- Titubation, which is tremor affecting the head and upper trunk, typically occurs after lesions of the vermis.
- Postural truncal tremor, which affects the legs and lower trunk, is typically seen in anterior cerebellar lobe lesions as often results from chronic alcoholism (Thompson & Day 1993).

Dyssynergia and visuomotor incoordination. Dyssynergia is the incoordination of movement involving multiple joints. The cerebellum is involved in programming, initiation and ongoing control of multi-joint movements towards visual targets (Stein 1986, Thach et al 1992, Haggard et al 1994). The influence of the cerebellum in the initiation of a movement can be seen in the increased reaction time to a given task after cerebellar dysfunction (Diener & Dichgans 1992).

The cerebellum is also vitally important for the control of eye movements and eye–hand coordination (Dichgans 1984, van Donkelaar & Lee 1994). During reaching, coordination of the eye and hand is essential for accuracy (Jeannerod 1988). Abnormalities in multi-joint movements, eye movement and their coordination all occur in cerebellar ataxia and therefore all contribute to the inaccuracy of reaching seen after a cerebellar lesion (van Donkelaar & Lee 1994).

Dysdiadochokinesia. This is the inability to perform rapidly alternating movements such as alternately tapping with palm up and palm down. The rhythm is poor and the force of each tap is variable (Diener & Dichgans 1992, Rothwell 1994).

Posture and gait. Patients with anterior lobe lesions show an increased postural sway in an anteroposterior direction, which is increased with eye closure. Patients with lesions of the vestibulocerebellum (flocculonodular lobe) show an increased postural sway in all directions. The effect of eye closure on postural sway in these patients is minimal (Mauritz et al 1979, Diener et al 1984).

Following cerebellar lesions, postural adjustments may be impaired. Patients with anterior lobe damage show poorly scaled, hypermetric responses to a sudden unexpected movement that leads to instability (Horak & Diener 1994, Timman & Horak 1998). The abnormalities in predictive and reactive postural adjustments and the presence of dysynergic leg movements may contribute to the staggering gait, with poor precision of foot placement seen in these patients (Diener & Dichgans 1996).

Other symptoms associated with cerebellar dysfunction

Hypotonia. This occurs with acute cerebellar lesions (Holmes 1922) but it is rarely seen in chronic lesions (Gilman 1969, Diener & Dichgans 1992, Rothwell 1994). Physiotherapists often view hypotonia as a symptom of ataxia (Atkinson 1986, Davies 1994). However, although hypotonia is a symptom of cerebellar dysfunction it is not a causative factor of ataxia and usually disappears within a few weeks following acute lesions (Diener & Dichgans 1992).

Weakness and fatigue. Holmes (1922, 1939) describes a generalised non-specific weakness as a feature of cerebellar dysfunction. This occurs more often with extensive and deep lesions and is most apparent in the proximal musculature. The weakness decreases over months; the maximal voluntary contraction of a patient with a chronic cerebellar disorder is similar to that of a normal subject (Mai et al 1988). However, on clinical observation, it would seem that patients with long-term ataxia do show signs of weakness. This may result from their lack of spontaneous movement and the adoption of compensatory movement strategies. Frustration may lead to the patient with chronic ataxia becoming increasingly inactive and dependent and, therefore, merely preventing disuse may be helpful (Hardie 1993). Fatigue has also been noted as a common feature of cerebellar dysfunction (Holmes 1922).

Motor learning. It is generally agreed that motor learning is a process which involves the whole nervous system (Halsband & Freund 1993). However, some researchers feel the cerebellum to be a major site of motor learning in that it is specialised to combine simple movements into more complex synergies. These synergies or motor patterns are then stored in the cerebellum

(Thach et al 1992). This theory remains somewhat controversial (Cordo et al 1997). Patients with cerebellar cortical atrophy have recently been shown to be deficient in learning a conditioned reflex (Topka et al 1993) and more complex motor skills (Sanes et al 1990, Thach et al 1992), which may have implications for the effectiveness of physiotherapy intervention (Hardie 1993).

Cognition. A cognitive affective syndrome has been described in subjects with specific cerebellar lesions (Schmahmann 1997, 1998). Symptoms include executive deficits, such as difficulties with planning, working memory and poor visuospatial memory, as well as abnormalities of personality and behaviour. These cognitive deficits may further affect both the patient's function and the treatment strategies that the clinician may adopt (Chafetz et al 1996).

Treatment strategies

Cerebellar ataxia. Many strategies have been advocated in the treatment of cerebellar-type ataxia. They include the use of weights (Morgan et al 1975), manual guidance/resistance (DeSouza 1990), rhythmic stabilisations (Gardiner 1976), horse riding (Saywell 1975) and the gymnastic ball (Hasler 1981). Factors that increase the weight of a limb or its resistance to movement, such as the application of weights, decrease tremor (Morgan et al 1975). However, tremor will return after removal of a weight, often greater than before, and can cause fatigue, particularly in patients with multiple sclerosis (DeSouza 1990). The use of weights to reduce truncal tremor has shown variable results (Lucy & Hayes 1985). More recently, there has been renewed interest in thalamotomies and thalamic stimulation as treatments for the symptomatic relief of tremor (Nguyen et al 1996, see Ch. 7).

Ataxia is primarily a disorder affecting postural control and the coordination of multi-joint movements (DeSouza 1990). The patient is aware of the movement disorder and adopts compensatory strategies to effect function (Gordon 1990). An example of this is the use of excessive fixation when using gait aids to improve stability (Balliet et al 1987).

There is a greater deficit in multi-joint as opposed to single-joint movement (Goodkin et al 1993) and Bastian (1997) has suggested that the use of single-joint, as opposed to multi-joint movements, should be encouraged to improve function. However, although some fixation may be inevitable and possibly even useful, it does limit the potential for improving proximal control and multi-joint movements. Specific mobilisation, particularly of the head and trunk, in conjunction with goal-directed, multi-joint movements have been recommended (DeSouza 1990).

Vestibular ataxia

Unilateral vestibular lesions. Improvement of symptoms following a unilateral vestibular lesion requires the active participation of the patient, although some spontaneous recovery may occur (Zee 2000). Treatment approaches vary: with habituation exercises, symptoms decrease with repeated exposure to the provocative stimulus (Herdman & Whitney 2000). The mechanisms of this action are unclear but it is this principle that underlies treatments for vertigo and impaired balance (Cawthorne 1944, Cooksey 1946, Norre & DeWeerdt 1980). Although specific regimes differ, positioning and movements that provoke symptoms are performed two to three times a day. As the symptoms improve, the position may be changed or the speed of movement increased.

Other exercises have been developed that utilise the vestibular system's ability to increase the size (or gain) of an eye movement or postural response to a given stimulus induced by head motion or position. When the patient moves, an error signal is produced that the vestibular system is not functioning optimally. The CNS then attempts to reduce this error signal by increasing the response of the vestibular system (Curthoys & Halmagyi 1995). Such an error signal must be produced by active movement of the patient, such as when moving the head while attempting to visually fixate a target. If gaze stability is poor, the image will move, producing an erroneous retinal slip. With repeated movements over time the vestibular system adapts, the eye movements increase in amplitude and this retinal slip is decreased (Herdman & Whitney 2000).

This need to facilitate vestibular adaptation by stressing the relevant system may also have important implications for the improvement of balance control. As Brandt et al (1981) state, a therapist should:

> expose the patient increasingly to unstable body positions in order to facilitate rearrangement and recruitment of control capacities. Stance and gait aids will alleviate only transiently patients' balance problems, but when used continuously, they will worsen the symptoms.

This may be because incorrect use of a gait aid does not allow the patient to generate an error signal that is required to improve their balance. However, in clinical practice it has been observed

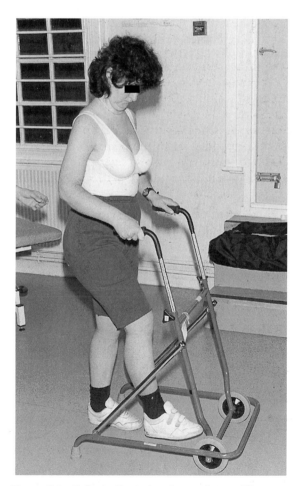

Figure 5.4 Patient with ataxia using a rollator walking frame.

that use of a rollator walking frame often serves to provide the patient with a means of more independent control. Used selectively, with emphasis on it being an aid to balance as opposed to a point of fixation, patients may use this aid as a means of progression to an independent gait (Jeka 1997; Fig. 5.4). Eventually, the majority of patients with unilateral lesions should be able to walk without an aid.

Importantly, the vestibular system demonstrates context specificity; that is, improvement will only be seen in those movements and positions performed by the patient. Any treatment regime must therefore address those movements that precipitate, for example, disequilibrium in the environment that they are normally experiencing (Curthoys & Halmagyi 1995).

Finally, improvement in symptoms may occur through substitution of absent vestibular input with other sensory inputs. For example, patients should be encouraged to learn to use all available sensations to balance. If they are over-reliant on one sensation, such as vision, they should be taught to balance in situations where visual cues are absent or reduced. Although useful, visual and somatosensory information cannot perfectly replace the lost vestibular function. Even following a unilateral lesion, some gaze control and balance symptoms may still be experienced, especially with fast movements (Herdman & Whitney 2000).

In summary there are many ways in which vestibular function may be improved. The exercises recommended are similar despite different underlying principles. The accumulation of experimental studies of individually prescribed exercises, performed under supervision or at home, highlights the effectiveness of this approach (Strupp et al 1998, Yardley et al 1998, Blakely 1999, Herdman et al 2000).

Bilateral vestibular lesions. With a complete bilateral vestibular lesion, improvement in ataxia can only occur by substitution of visual and, more importantly, somatosensory cues. Recovery after a bilateral vestibular lesion often takes longer and is more incomplete than after a unilateral lesion. Even so, physical exercise has been demonstrated to affect the rate of recovery (Igarashi et al 1988, Krebs et al 1993) and compensatory strategies, such as turning on the light before getting out of bed, are recommended (Herdman & Clendaniel 2000).

Central lesions also demonstrate more variable recovery as the areas damaged – the brain stem, cerebellum and vestibular nuclei – are implicated in the process of recovery (Igarashi 1984). This is of particular relevance in the treatment of traumatic head injury where vestibular disorders are thought to occur in 30–65% of patients (Shumway-Cook 1994).

Sensory ataxia. Compensation with remaining senses is encouraged, such as that of vision as advocated by Frenkel's exercises (Hollis 1989). However, the over-reliance on conscious effort with these exercises detracts from the desired automatic response.

Studies have demonstrated that the sensory cortex can display some capacity for reorganisation and recovery following discrete lesions (Dannenbaum & Dykes 1988, Dannenbaum & Jones 1993, Xerri et al 1998) and, in these cases, sensory re-education may be beneficial. However, recovery in the sensibility of the hand will only occur if the area of sensory loss is small and if the patient has the required mobility and strength to use the arm functionally (Carey 1995).

Finally, if sensory loss is accompanied by a loss of thermal sensibility, care must be taken to avoid injury and maintain skin integrity (Carey 1995).

MOVEMENT DISORDERS ASSOCIATED WITH BASAL GANGLIA DISEASE

The movement disorders that result from basal ganglia damage or disease are often dramatic, and depending on the site of the lesion, can cause extreme slowness of movement and rigidity, or uncontrollable involuntary postures and movements. There also appears to be some defect of attention that is important in diseases of the basal ganglia. This may be observed in patients with Parkinson's disease who are so akinetic that they can barely move and yet may deftly sidestep an oncoming car or flee from a fire (Brown & Marsden 1998) and in dystonia, where in spite of grossly distorted postures, the patient may accomplish surprisingly skilled tasks (Marsden 1984, Britton 1998).

Mink (1996) hypothesised that the basal ganglia do not generate movements, but that the tonically active inhibitory output of the basal ganglia acts as a 'brake' on motor pattern generators (MPGs) in the cerebral cortex (via the thalamus) and brain stem. When a movement is initiated by a particular MPG, basal ganglia output neurones projecting to competing MPGs increase their firing output, thereby increasing inhibition and applying a 'brake' on those generators. Other basal ganglia output neurones projecting to the MPGs involved in the desired movement decrease their discharge, thereby removing tonic inhibition and releasing the 'brake' from those desired generators. In this way, selected movements are enabled and competing postures and movements are prevented from interfering with the one selected.

The example cited in this review is that of reaching to pick an apple off a tree. While the most obvious feature is that of reaching, multiple other motor mechanisms act together to maintain the upright posture of the body. Prior to the reach, these mechanisms are also active in the reaching arm to maintain its posture. However, as the arm reaches towards the apple, the postural mechanisms must be turned off selectively in the arm while they maintain activity in the rest of the body. When the reach is completed, the reaching MPGs must be turned off and the postural mechanisms turned back on. If the competing posture-holding and reaching mechanisms were inappropriately active at the same time, the result may be instability of posture or slowing of movement or both (Mink 1996).

When the balance of inhibition and excitation in the basal ganglia and motor cortex is upset, the symptoms and signs of rigidity and involuntary movements supervene along with abnormalities of posture and associated movement, and slowness of movement (Jones & Godwin-Austen 1998).

RIGIDITY

Rigidity is clinically defined as increased resistance to stretch and the inability to achieve complete muscle relaxation (Wichmann & DeLong 1993). The stiffness or involuntary muscle contraction is maintained throughout the range of movement, relatively independent of the velocity of stretch and for as long as the stretch is maintained (Burke 1987). In parkinsonian rigidity, tendon jerks are usually normal (Marsden 1982, Messina 1990, Rothwell 1994).

Several factors may contribute to the increase in resistance during passive movement of the limbs. These include (a) inability of the patient to relax and completely eliminate activity in the muscles; (b) increased stiffness due to altered viscoelastic properties of the muscles; (c) abnormal co-activation of agonist–antagonist muscle groups; and (d) increased stretch reflexes (Lee 1989). Enhancement of long-latency stretch reflexes and a reduction in inhibition of interneuronal circuits have been implicated in parkinsonian rigidity (Hallett 1993) and it is suggested that there may be an inability to suppress unwanted reflex activity generally (Mink 1996).

Rigidity may occur in different forms. It is one of the cardinal features of Parkinson's disease and may also occur with midbrain and brainstem lesions. However, decerebrate and decorticate rigidity are abnormal postures associated with coma rather than a specific type of hypertonus, and Britton (1998) suggests that the terms decorticate and decerebrate posturing would be more appropriate. Burke (1987) supports this view in that, with 'decerebrate rigidity', the patient is usually flaccid at rest and transiently assumes the rigid posture when stimulated. Rigidity also occurs with stiff man or stiff limb syndrome (Barker et al 1998).

Marsden (1982) identified excessive and uncontrollable supraspinal drive to alpha motoneurones as the most important cause of rigidity in Parkinson's disease. He concluded that rigidity

represents a positive symptom resulting from release of other brain structures that are normally inhibited by basal ganglia function. Rigidity indicates the operation of remaining intact motor systems and tells little of the normal function of the basal ganglia.

The clinical presentation of rigidity and possible treatment strategies will be discussed in the context of Parkinson's disease, as opposed to rigidity as an independent movement disorder.

Clinical presentation of Parkinson's disease

Features which are associated with rigidity in patients with Parkinson's disease include akinesia and bradykinesia. However, neither is caused by restraint of active movement since both conditions can be present when rigidity is absent (Gordon 1990).

Akinesia. This term describes the paucity of movement and 'freezing' and has been attributed to an impairment in the initiation of movement or delay in the reaction time. In patients with Parkinson's disease this is most prominent for movements which are internally generated rather than those which occur in response to sensory stimuli (Miller & DeLong 1988, Lee 1989). Other features of akinesia in relation to Parkinson's disease are:

- lack of spontaneous movements
- lack of associated movements, such as arm swinging during walking
- abnormally small amplitude movements, such as very small steps during walking or micrographia
- a tendency for repetitive movements to show a decrease in amplitude and eventually fade out
- difficulty performing two simultaneous movements (Lee 1989).

Bradykinesia. Bradykinesia is a term which should be used exclusively to refer to slowness in the execution of the movement (Lee 1989). This has been associated with both reduced magnitude of agonist muscle activity (Hallett & Khoshbin 1980) and excessive co-contraction of the antagonist during movement (Hayashi et al 1988), with the inability to 'turn off' the antagonist being more impaired than the ability to 'turn on' the agonist (Corcos et al 1996). Bradykinesia appears as a disorder in voluntary movement in daily life and is considered to be partly responsible for disorders in posture and locomotion (Yanagisawa et al 1989).

Although these different definitions are used, they would appear to be of academic rather than practical value. Marsden (1986) and Hallett (1993) provide a more global definition in referring to akinesia as an inability to move and bradykinesia as slowness of movement. In Parkinson's disease, rigidity is considered to be a positive symptom resulting from release of other brain structures that are normally inhibited by basal ganglia function, whereas akinesia or bradykinesia are the key negative features of loss of normal basal ganglia function (Marsden 1982).

The delay in initiation of movement in Parkinson's disease is more evident with internally generated or self-initiated movements than with movements occurring in response to sensory stimuli (Lee 1989). Various types of sensory input may partially compensate for akinesia. Brooks (1986) suggests the use of visual, auditory and vestibular cues, such as bouncing a ball, rocking the patient's shoulders back and forth or tilting them forwards to facilitate movement. It is well recognised that patients with Parkinson's disease may 'freeze' at a doorway and yet have no problem passing through if, for example, a stick is placed on the floor for them to step over. They may be unable to reach forwards with their arm on command but may be able to pick up a glass.

Parkinson's disease is characterised by an inability to perform two separate motor actions at the same time. For example, the patient may be able to stand up and shake hands as two individual motor acts but he is unable to perform these two actions simultaneously (Marsden 1982, Rothwell 1994).

Aims of physiotherapy

Normal movement is dependent upon an intact CNS providing for an adaptable and integrated level of tonus. Patients with Parkinson's disease become more flexed as the condition deteriorates (Gordon 1990). Rotation is dependent upon balanced activity between flexor and extensor muscle groups and, as previously described in Chapter 3, a dominance of either muscle group will impair rotation. The lack of rotation with reduced or loss of arm swing is a notable feature of Parkinson's disease (Marsden 1984, Lee 1989, Pentland 1993).

In the past, the emphasis of physiotherapy treatment was to improve rotation. To that effect, walking sticks were placed in the patient's hands with which the therapist would initiate arm swing. In normal subjects, arm swing, a relatively passive action, occurs as a result of interaction between the pelvis and shoulder girdles on the basis of an extended, upright posture. The ageing process clearly supports this analysis, in that, as the elderly adopt a more flexed posture, the arm swing is reduced (Elble et al 1991).

Patients with Parkinson's disease may become more flexed both through the CNS pathology and the ageing process. Attempts to superimpose arm swing as described above, with this predominantly flexed posture, will inevitably be doomed to failure. Analysis of the primary move-

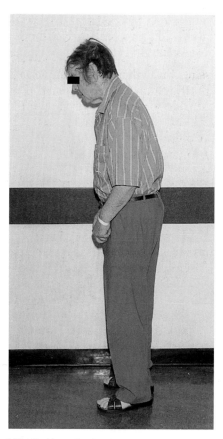

Figure 5.5 Parkinson's posture.

ment disorder will identify the lack of extension as a significant factor. Although the increased tone is equally distributed on passive manipulation of the joints, the evidence of increasing flexion is evident (Fig. 5.5).

Turnbull (1992) proposed a 'progressive' model of management for patients with Parkinson's disease which includes early and ongoing intervention by physiotherapy. This model was designed to prevent secondary complications and maintain function, instead of waiting until the disability is advanced before initiating a therapy programme.

Assessment is essential to identify treatment priorities and to monitor progress with early implementation of an exercise programme and targeted intervention, focusing on areas of deterioration (Jones & Godwin-Austen 1998). Awareness on the part of the patient of the expected progression of the disease in terms of the impairment of movement and an appropriate home exercise programme to reduce the insidious onset of flexion and maintain extension may go some way to maintaining function.

The administration of dopamine agonists often has a dramatic effect for patients with Parkinson's disease and in many cases determines the functional options (Marsden 1986). In severe cases, physiotherapy may only be possible after administration of these drugs. In providing the experience of more normal movement and the maintenance of an upright posture, physiotherapy as an adjunct to medication is appropriate and beneficial in the management of this patient group. Equally, advice and management of specific problems which arise in the more disabled population, such as the inability to turn over in bed, will be of tremendous benefit to patients and their carers. They will direct therapy in that they identify a problem, and then the therapist determines the causative factors and instigates appropriate treatment or coping strategies to enable a greater degree of function.

DYSTONIA

Dystonia is a syndrome dominated by muscle contraction frequently causing twisting and repetitive movements, or abnormal posture that may be sustained or intermittent (Fahn et al 1987).

Classification and prevalence

The current classification of dystonia describes each patient with dystonia in three separate categories: age at onset, distribution and aetiology (Fahn et al 1987). The distribution of dystonia may be either focal, affecting a single body part; segmental, affecting adjacent body parts or a segment of the body; hemidystonia, involving one side of the body; or generalised dystonia, affecting two or more body segments (Berardelli et al 1998). Dystonia can affect virtually any area of the body and there are familiar names for dystonia at different sites (Table 5.1).

The aetiological classification of dystonia has recently been subdivided in the light of genetic, pathological and biochemical advances (Fahn et al 1998):

(a) Primary dystonia is the most common form of dystonia and has been found to be associated with several different gene abnormalities. Primary dystonia shows no consistent pathological change and appears to be neurochemical in origin, rather than a neurodegenerative disorder with neuronal loss.

(b) Dystonia-plus is also a neurochemical disorder that includes neurological features such as parkinsonism and myoclonus. The dystonic-parkinsonian syndrome is also referred to as dopa-responsive dystonia.

(c) Secondary dystonia is a disorder that develops mainly as a result of an insult to the brain. This includes dystonias associated with cerebral palsy, cerebral hypoxia and following stroke.

(d) Heredodegenerative dystonia occurs when there is underlying brain degeneration: for example, in Wilson's disease and multiple system atrophy (Fahn et al 1998).

Dystonia is estimated to be more common than other well known neurological diseases such as Huntington's disease, motor neurone disease and myasthenia gravis (Marsden & Quinn 1990), with a prevalence of 108 per million, of which 40 per million have cervical dystonia (Warner 1999). These figures are based on those patients with primary dystonia who have been diagnosed by a neurologist. However, many general practitioners are unfamiliar with the signs and symptoms and referral to a neurologist may be delayed or not occur (Dystonia Society 1999).

Table 5.1 Common names used to describe dystonia affecting specific parts of the body (Marsden & Quinn 1990)

Name	Muscles contracting involuntarily
Blepharospasm	Orbicularis oculi and neighbouring facial muscles
Oromandibular dystonia	Jaw and mouth
Lingual dystonia	Tongue
Spasmodic dysphonia	Laryngeal, causing cord adduction and a strangulated speech, or cord abduction and whispering dysphonia
Dystonic dysphagia	Pharyngeal
Spasmodic torticollis	Sternocleidomastoid and posterior neck
Writer's cramp and other occupational cramps	Hand, forearm and arm
Axial dystonia	Back and trunk, causing scoliosis, lordosis, kyphosis or tortipelvis
Leg dystonia	Foot, leg and thigh

A combination of blepharospasm and oromandibular and lingual dystonia is known as cranial dystonia, Meige's or Brueghel's syndrome.
A combination of cranial dystonia and torticollis is known as craniocervical dystonia.

Pathophysiology

Dystonia is the least well understood, in terms of the underlying pathophysiology, of all movement disorders associated with basal ganglia dysfunction (Crossman & Brotchie 1998). Evidence suggests that primary dystonia results from a functional disturbance of the basal ganglia which causes altered thalamic control of cortical motor planning and executive areas and abnormal regulation of brain stem and spinal cord inhibitory interneuronal mechanisms (Berardelli et al 1998). Reciprocal inhibition, for example, is reduced in patients with both generalised and focal dystonia (Rothwell et al 1983, Panizza et al

1990) and this may be abnormal even in asymptomatic limbs, in people with blepharospasm (Hallett 1998).

The involuntary movements are often exacerbated during voluntary movements and are characterised by an abnormal pattern of EMG activity with co-contraction of agonists and antagonists and overflow into inappropriate muscles (Berardelli et al 1998).

Hallett (1995) has proposed that dystonia could be primarily a sensory disorder in that sensory symptoms or trauma may precede the onset of dystonia. Voluntary repetitive movements, to relieve the sensory symptom, have been reported by patients to have become uncontrolled (Ghika et al 1993) and it has been suggested that repeated use of a body part may be a precedent for dystonia of that body part (Byl et al 1996, Hallett 1998). Interestingly, it has been reported that there is abnormal perception of movement, but not of position, in dystonic subjects (Grunewald et al 1997).

It is only recently that dystonia has become a recognised, organic condition as opposed to a hysterical disorder (Hallett 1995). However, Rondot et al (1991) found that no fewer than 61% of 220 patients suggested different events which they held responsible for the onset of cervical dystonia (spasmodic torticollis), and the authors concluded that 'in the complex of factors leading to spasmodic torticollis, psychological aspects do indeed play a role'.

Clinical presentation

Dystonia can be present at rest but, in general, is more likely to appear during voluntary activity (Hallett 1993). These dystonic spasms are characterised by co-contraction of agonist and antagonist muscles rather than the more usual reciprocal pattern seen in normal voluntary movement (Hallett 1993, Rothwell 1994). There is a loss of selectivity when attempting to perform discrete independent movements which results in an overflow of activity to remote muscle groups that are not normally activated in the movement and the time taken to switch between components of a complex movement is prolonged (Berardelli et al 1998).

Although there have been no studies yet on change in the biomechanical properties of muscle, Hallett (1993) suggests that such changes are as likely to occur in dystonia as in any other long-standing disease where there have been fixed postures.

The spasms may contort the body into grotesque postures which may severely limit activities of daily living with considerable socio-economic implications (Crossman & Brotchie 1998). While this is more apparent in those with generalised dystonia, problems also arise for those with focal dystonia. For example, a person with cervical dystonia may be unable to drink from a glass and one with blepharospasm may be unable to drive.

Dystonia exhibits a variability under different conditions such as stress and fatigue and in the performance of certain motor acts such as walking (Lorentz et al 1991). In many instances, people develop their own strategies to control their movements: those with cervical dystonia may touch the side of the chin (the 'geste antagoniste'); people with blepharospasm may apply pressure on the eyelids; and a toothpick in the mouth may relieve tongue dystonia.

Treatment

Symptomatic treatment, particularly of the focal dystonias, has been revolutionised with the advent of botulinum toxin (see Ch. 7). Its use has proved so successful that, as recommended by Marsden & Quinn (1990), the majority of regional neuroscience centres in the United Kingdom now provide this treatment. Botulinum toxin is administered by injection to the primarily affected muscles. This is now the treatment of choice for most focal dystonias, particularly blepharospasm (Britton 1998) and cervical dystonia (Anderson et al 1992). The injections are usually repeated, on average, at 3- to 4-monthly intervals. The use of botulinum toxin is thought to be less effective in the treatment of cervical dystonia than in blepharospasm, possibly because there are more and often deeper-sited muscles affected (Berardelli et al 1993).

Surgical treatment has been advocated in the past, such as facial nerve sectioning or myomectomy for patients with blepharospasm and various procedures for cervical dystonia. These include selective peripheral denervation and stereotactic thalamotomy (Bertrand et al 1987, Bertrand 1993). Surgery may still be indicated for some patients who do not respond to botulinum toxin.

There is little documented on physiotherapy for patients with dystonia. Marsden & Quinn (1990) consider that physiotherapy is of great benefit in preventing contractures but cannot teach the brain to deliver normal motor programmes. Braces and other forms of restraint are thought to be ineffective (Marsden & Quinn 1990).

Electromyography has revealed complete inhibition of antagonist muscles in cervical dystonia (Bertrand 1993), and retraining of these muscles is recommended (Dykstra et al 1993). On the basis of this evidence, providing patients with an individual exercise programme following injection of botulinum toxin might enable more effective activity of the antagonist muscles and thereby improve postural control of the head and neck for a longer period of time between injections. Indeed, specific exercises for people with cervical dystonia have been developed and are reported to be effective in improving postural control of the head and neck (Bleton 1994). However, while the beneficial effect of specific exercises seems plausible theoretically, few carefully planned studies have been undertaken and little objective evidence exists to support this. Similarly, other approaches such as increasing proprioceptive input by compression or stretch and using 'mobile weight bearing through the hands and feet' to allow the patient to feel postural adaptation, as recommended by Thornton & Kilbride (1998), require further evaluation.

Basic science and clinical research can and should be used to validate the efficacy of physiotherapy (Byl & Topp 1998). Repetitive, highly stereotyped movements applied in a learning context have been shown to actively degrade cortical representations of sensory information guiding fine motor hand movements in monkeys. It has been hypothesised that this cortical plasticity/learning-based degradation of sensory feedback information from the hand contributes to the genesis of occupationally derived repetitive strain injuries and focal dystonia of the hand (Byl et al 1996). In a single case study of a patient with a focal hand dystonia that developed after excessive use of a computer keyboard, Byl & Topp (1998) reported improvement in cortical sensory processing, motor control, physical performance and independent function, including work status. This followed an intensive programme lasting 1 year, which included sensory discriminative therapy and keyboard retraining. Although the amount of repetition necessary for sensory retraining required a high level of patient compliance, restoration of sensory function was associated with improved motor control.

In addition to the sensory retraining of patients with occupational focal dystonias, this may also prove effective in the management of the more generalised dystonias. The term 'torsion dystonia' is frequently used with these patients. This aptly describes the effect of the dystonic movements pulling the patient into distorted asymmetrical postures which may lead to further deformity and degradation of cortical sensory information. Advice on posture and seating for people with generalised dystonia is of paramount importance. Patients requiring wheelchairs must have a detailed assessment of their particular needs with appropriate adaptations as indicated (see Ch. 9).

As with all people with disability, it is important to recognise that the individuals with the disability are often more knowledgeable about the management of their condition than the majority of health care workers involved in their management. This is particularly so for people with dystonia.

CHOREA AND ATHETOSIS

Chorea and athetosis are common symptoms of basal ganglia disease or damage and describe involuntary, writhing movements of the body. The term chorea is usually applied to movements at proximal or axial joints, while athetosis is used more frequently to describe movements of the distal parts of the limbs (Rothwell 1994). Mink (1996) defines the sudden, random twitch-like movements that involve any body part as chorea and, if they are accompanied by slower writhing voluntary movements, as choreoathetosis.

All muscle groups tend to be affected, including those of the eyes and tongue, with the movements moving randomly from one part of the body to another. Writhing of the head and limbs, grimacing and twitching often occur unpredictably. Speech is invariably affected. Hallett (1993) comments that the most appropriate adjective to describe chorea is 'random'. Random muscles throughout the body are affected at random times and make movements of random duration. Chorea occurs at rest, on posture and on movement whether it be fast or slow (Marsden 1984).

It is difficult to distinguish between chorea and athetosis as they display similar characteristics. Athetosis is the term most frequently used to describe this dyskinesia in children with cerebral palsy whereas chorea is used to describe the movement disorder in, for example, Huntington's disease. In most cases there is involvement of both proximal and distal musculature and for the purpose of discussion regarding treatment the two will be considered as one.

The motor plan involves the selection, sequencing and delivery of the correct collection of motor programmes required to achieve the desired motor behaviour. In chorea, the correct attempt to move is made by the patient but its success is disrupted by the abnormal co-contraction of synergists, antagonists and postural fixators, so the details of the motor programme are abnormally specified (Marsden 1984). The initiation and execution of movement are disturbed but chorea tends to increase on attempted movement and this movement-related increase in chorea occurs in both the moving and non-moving body parts (Mink 1996). However, in spite of this, function may be achieved, often in a somewhat contorted manner, in spite of the severity of the dyskinesia (Marsden 1984).

Clinical presentation

The general features of athetosis are those of fluctuating abnormal tone with poor grading of posture and movement associated with involuntary movements that are accentuated by volitional activity and stimulation. The resting tonus is generally low but attempts at volitional activity reinforce the involuntary movement due to insufficient and unstable postural tone. In the majority of patients, the whole body is involved, with the upper part more affected than the legs.

Course notes from the Bobath Centre (1997) describe three different types of involuntary movements:

- *Mobile spasms.* These are alternating writhing limb movements and are often rhythmical in nature.
- *Fleeting irregular, localised contractions.* These affect muscle groups throughout the body and, if severe, may produce exaggerated postures and movements such as facial grimacing and bizarre distal movements (Fig 5.6). More localised or weaker contractions may be observed as minor twitches.
- *Intermittent tonic spasms, so-called 'dystonic'.* These are predictable in pattern but not in timing and are often dependent on changes in head position. The individual may be temporarily fixed in extreme patterns which may involve the whole body, proximal body parts or only a limb. These extreme postures are more commonly seen in children but their influence may persist throughout life.

Problems associated with communication and eating

People with athetosis often have the additional problem of impaired communication. In some cases, the involuntary movements affecting the face may preclude intelligible speech. The autobiography, *My Left Foot* (Brown 1989), gives great insight into the frustration arising from this inability to communicate. Computers are now widely used to provide a means of both communication and education. Although communication may be considered primarily the remit

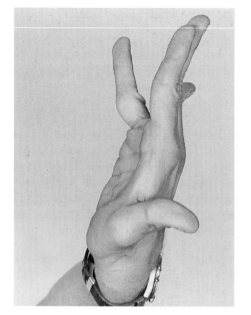

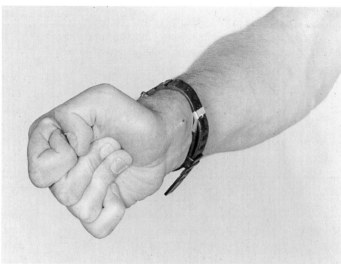

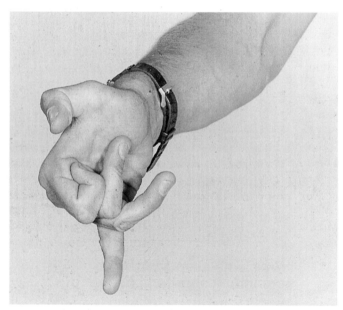

Figure 5.6   Athetoid hands.

of the speech and language therapist, control of posture and respiration are essential prerequisites and will also be addressed by the physiotherapist in collaboration with the speech and language therapist.

Similarly, eating is a problem both in terms of the uncontrolled orofacial movements and the mechanical difficulty of taking the food to the mouth. Very few people with athetosis are overweight, which may be a combination of the eating difficulties and the constant involuntary movement throughout the body. Advice and treatment to address this problem should include:

● Desensitisation of the mouth including the lips, tongue, gums and, where present, the bite reflex. Instruction should be sought from an experienced speech and language therapist or physiotherapist.

- Supported sitting, with the arms resting forwards supported on a table. This will reduce the tendency to push back into extension as the food approaches the mouth.
- Maintenance of elongation of the cervical spine to facilitate movement of the head towards the food.

Communication and eating difficulties are two of the most distressing aspects of athetosis and, for this reason, treatment techniques or strategies which prove to be of benefit must be constantly reinforced by the patient and/or his assistant.

Problems arising with posture and gait

Inevitably there are many patients with athetosis who will become, or remain, wheelchair dependent. Determining the appropriate chair and adaptations is complex and requires detailed assessment and continual reappraisal.

Those born with athetosis initially present with very low tone and may be referred to as 'floppy children'. Depending on the severity of symptoms, it may take several years for children to develop sufficient tone to maintain themselves upright against gravity. The constant fluctuations of tone throughout the body severely hamper grading of all movement. Facilitation and constant repetition of a more controlled movement is essential for the child to develop adequate stability. Positioning to improve symmetry and alignment and use of bilateral grasp is also recommended (Bobath Centre 1997).

People with athetosis who are ambulant often demonstrate a somewhat bizarre gait pattern characterised by marked retraction of the head, trunk and hips. On clinical observation it would seem that the shoulder girdles are retracted with the arms in either flexion or extension depending on the stability afforded at the pelvis. This stability may be provided by adequate tone in the less severely affected legs or by mechanical factors, as in the patient with lower tone, who may sta-

bilise the hip in extension by 'hanging' on the iliofemoral ligament.

The swing-through phase differs depending on the fluctuations and degree of increased tone. For example:

- Those people with greater fluctuations in tone tend to initiate a step using a total pattern of flexion to break up the prevailing extensor tone required to maintain them upright against gravity. In this instance the impression is one of utilisation of alternate flexor and extensor synergies, affecting the whole body.
- People with predominantly low tone, using the iliofemoral ligament to provide stability, demonstrate increased extensor activity in the head and trunk in their attempt to step forwards.

Similarly the stance phase differs:

- People with marked fluctuations in tone demonstrate a more rigidly extended leg in the extensor synergy, often with flexion of the hip due to the overall increase in flexion as the opposite leg steps through.
- Those with lower tone use the more mechanical stability of extension of the hip and hyperextension of the knee counteracted by increased extension of the trunk.

Pure athetosis is rare, particularly in the cerebral palsy population. Those with predominant hypotonia may also have what are described as dystonic spasms, whereas others with higher tone may also demonstrate symptoms associated with the positive features of an upper motor neurone lesion (Fig. 5.7).

While people with pure athetosis are unlikely to develop contractures due to the prevailing low tone and constant movements, those with asymmetrical dystonic spasms may develop severe deformity, even joint displacement, depending on the severity of these spasms. Dislocation of the hip in children with cerebral palsy is a not infrequent complication with repeated spasms of the leg into adduction and medial rotation. Those with a combination of athetosis and hypertonus are more susceptible to the development of more general contractures because there is less variety

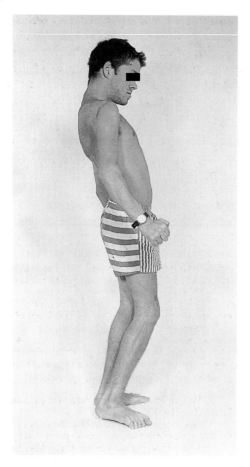

Figure 5.7 Athetoid standing position.

of movement and the basic tone is higher and in more stereotyped patterns.

Management

People with long-standing choreoathetosis develop strategies, often unique to each individual, to compensate for their unstable tone and involuntary movement. These strategies are essential for them to function. In most instances physiotherapy intervention is required for complications arising from the disability, such as pain or contracture, as opposed to treatment of the movement disorder itself. Invariably it is the abnormal movement which causes the problem for which the person seeks treatment, but mutually agreed goals must be established to deter-

mine appropriate treatment. For example, many people with athetosis defy the laws of balance in their means of ambulation, and physiotherapists must recognise that this is successful and functional for them. Attempts to improve their gait pattern, unless this is established to be the cause of the complication, will generally be met with a distinct lack of enthusiasm.

SUMMARY

Physical disability is often characterised by abnormal tone and movement which contribute to the functional deficit. Some of the different types of movement disorders have been described, with emphasis on the clinical presentation and examples of physiotherapy intervention which may prove of benefit.

Although the neurological impairment in many instances is non-progressive, the disability arising from the pathology may increase over time. This deterioration may occur as a result of enforced immobility or dominance of stereotyped movement patterns. Any individual who is restricted to a limited or inappropriate repertoire of movement is in danger of developing structural changes of affected muscle groups, which may further decrease functional capability.

Physiotherapists should have an understanding of the pathophysiology of the different types of movement disorder to formulate effective treatment interventions. Many patients, particularly those with severe symptoms, develop compensatory strategies which are appropriate to their functional needs. The physiotherapist must recognise that restoration of 'normal movement' is often an inappropriate and unattainable goal and work with the patient to ensure the optimal functional outcome. In the majority of cases, there should be a balance between re-education of more normal movement patterns and acceptance and promotion of necessary and desirable compensation to attain optimal function. While in many instances it is necessary to work for component parts of movement patterns, the patient must appreciate that the outcome of this improved activity will have functional significance, otherwise motivation and cooperation will be diminished (Carr & Shepherd 1987, 1998, Ada et al 1990).

At the present time there is no evidence to suggest that physiotherapy can influence the disease processes or pathology in conditions such as muscular dystrophy or stroke. The main aim of physiotherapy is to retrain motor skills to enable people with neurological disability to move and function more effectively. However, the physiotherapist cannot work in isolation. With the increasing time and financial con-straints imposed on health services throughout the world, treatment plans must be devised in consultation with the patient, other health care workers and family and friends to ensure the continued and ongoing effectiveness of inter-vention. One hour of physiotherapy a day may be totally inadequate in maintaining any lasting effects unless this is supported by appropriate positioning, handling and practice of tasks in addition to altering the environment to facilitate this process.

REFERENCES

Ada L, Canning C, Westwood P 1990 The patient as an active learner. In: Ada L, Canning C (eds) Key issues in neurological physiotherapy. Heinemann Medical, Oxford

Ada L, Vattanasilp W, O'Dwyer N J, Crosbie J 1998 Does spasticity contribute to walking dysfunction after stroke. Journal of Neurology, Neurosurgery and Psychiatry 64: 628–635

Allum J H J 1996 Vestibulospinal and proprioceptive reflex assessment of balance control. In: Bronstein A M, Brandt T H, Woollacott M (eds) Clinical disorders of balance, posture and gait. Arnold, London

Allum J H J, Honegger F, Acuna H 1995 Differential control of leg and trunk muscle activity by vestibulo-spinal and proprioceptive signals during human balance corrections. Acta Otolaryngology 115: 124–129

Allum J H J, Gresty M, Keshner E, Shupert C 1997 The control of head movements during balance corrections. Journal of Vestibular Research 7: 189–218

Anderson T J, Rivest J, Stell R et al 1992 Botulinum toxin treatment of spasmodic torticollis. Journal of the Royal Society of Medicine 85: 524–529

Atkinson H W 1986 Aspects of neuro anatomy and physiology. In: Downie P A (ed) Cash's textbook of neurology for physiotherapists. Faber & Faber, London

Balliet R, Harbst K B, Kim D, Stewart R V 1987 Retraining of functional gait through the reduction of upper extremity weight-bearing in chronic cerebellar ataxia. International Rehabilitation Medicine 8: 148–153

Barker R A, Reeves T, Thom M, Marsden C D, Brown P 1998 Review of 23 patients affected by the stiff man syndrome: clinical subdivision into stiff trunk (man) syndrome, stiff limb syndrome and progressive encephalomyelitis with rigidity. Journal of Neurology, Neurosurgery and Psychiatry 65: 633–640

Bastian A J 1997 Mechanisms of ataxia. Physical Therapy 77: 1112–1113

Berardelli A, Formica A, Mercuri B et al 1993 Botulinum toxin treatment in patients with focal dystonia and hemifacial spasm. A multicentre study of the Italian movement disorder group. Italian Journal of Neurology 14: 361–367

Berardelli A, Rothwell J C, Thompson P D, Manfredi M, Marsden C D 1998 The pathophysiology of primary dystonia. Brain 121: 1195–1212

Bertrand C, Molina-Negro P, Bouvier G, Gorczyca W 1987 Observations and analysis of results in 131 cases of spasmodic torticollis after selective denervation. Applied Neurophysiology 50: 319–323

Bertrand C M 1993 Selective peripheral denervation for spasmodic torticollis: surgical techniques, results and observations in 260 cases. Surgical Neurology 14: 96–103

Blakely 1999 Vestibular rehabilitation on a budget. Journal of Otolaryngology 28: 205–210

Bleton J-P 1994 Spasmodic torticollis. Handbook of rehabilitative physiotherapy. Editions Frison-Roche, Paris

Bobath B 1985 Abnormal postural reflex activity caused by brain lesions, 3rd edn. Heinemann Physiotherapy, London

Bobath B 1990 Adult hemiplegia: evaluation and treatment, 3rd edn. Heinemann Medical Books, London

Bobath Centre 1997 Course notes to accompany the 8 week course in cerebral palsy. The Bobath Centre, London

Booth B, Doyle M, Montgomery J 1983 Serial casting for the management of spasticity in the head-injured adult. Physical Therapy 63(12): 1960–1966

Brandt T H, Dieterich M 2000 Assessment and management of central vestibular disorders. In: Herdman S (ed) Vestibular rehabilitation, 2nd edn. F A Davis, Philadelphia

Brandt T H, Krafczyk S, Malsbenden I 1981 Postural imbalance with head extension: improvement by training as a model for ataxia therapy. Annals of the New York Academy of Sciences 374: 636–649

Britton T C 1998 Abnormalities of muscle tone and movement. In: Stokes M (ed) Neurological physiotherapy. Mosby, London

Brooks V 1986 The neural basis of motor control. Oxford University Press, Oxford

Brown C 1989 My left foot. Mandarin Paperbacks, London

Brown P 1994 Pathophysiology of spasticity. Journal of Neurology, Neurosurgery and Psychiatry 57: 773–777

Brown P, Marsden C D 1998 What do the basal ganglia do? Lancet 351: 1801–1804

Brunnstrom S 1970 Movement therapy in hemiplegia. Harper & Row, New York

Burke D 1987 Pathophysiological aspects of rigidity and dystonia. Advances in Neurology 47: 87–100

Burke D 1988 Spasticity as an adaptation to pyramidal tract injury. Advances in Neurology 47: 401–423

Byl N N, Topp K S 1998 Focal hand dystonia. Physical Therapy Case Reports 1: 39–52

Byl N N, Merzenich M M, Jenkins W M 1996 A primate genesis model of focal dystonia and repetitive strain injury: 1. Learning-induced dedifferentiation of the representation of the hand in the primary somatosensory cortex in adult monkeys. Neurology 47: 508–520

Cameron T, Calancie B 1995 Mechanical and fatigue properties of wrist flexor muscles during repetitive contractions after cervical spinal cord injury. Archives of Physical Medicine and Rehabilitation 76: 929–933

Carey J, Burghardt T 1993 Movement dysfunction following central nervous system lesions: a problem of neurologic or muscular impairment? Physical Therapy 73: 538–547

Carey L M 1995 Somatosensory loss after stroke. Critical Reviews in Physical and Rehabilitation Medicine 7: 51–91

Carr J H, Shepherd R B 1980 Physiotherapy in disorders of the brain. Heinemann Medical Books, London

Carr J H, Shepherd R B 1987 A motor relearning programme for stroke, 2nd edn. Heinemann Medical, Oxford

Carr J H, Shepherd R B 1998 Neurological rehabilitation: optimising motor performance. Butterworth-Heinemann, Oxford

Cawthorne T 1944 The physiological basis for head exercises. Journal of the Chartered Society of Physiotherapy 30: 106–107

Chafetz M D, Freidman A L, Kevorkian G, Levy J K 1996 The cerebellum and cognitive function: implications for rehabilitation. Archives of Physical Medicine and Rehabilitation 77: 1303–1308

Conine T, Sullivan T, Mackie T, Goodman M 1990 Effects of serial casting for the prevention of equinus in patients with acute head injury. Archives of Physical Medicine and Rehabilitation 71: 310–312

Cooksey F S 1946 Rehabilitation in vestibular injuries. Proceedings of the Royal Society of Medicine 39: 273–275

Corcos D M, Chen C-M, Quinn N P, McAuley J, Rothwell J C 1996 Strength in Parkinson's disease: relationship to rate of force generation and clinical status. Annals of Neurology 39: 79–88

Cordo P, Bell C, Harnad S 1997 Motor learning and synaptic plasticity in the cerebellum. Cambridge University Press, Cambridge

Cornall C 1991 Self propelling wheelchairs: the effect on spasticity in hemiplegic patients. Physiotherapy Theory and Practice 7: 13–21

Crossman A R, Brotchie J M 1998 Pathophysiology of dystonia. Dystonia 3: Advances in Neurology 78: 19–25

Curthoys I S, Halmagyi E S 1995 Vestibular compensation: a review of the oculomotor, neural and clinical consequences of unilateral vestibular loss. Journal of Vestibular Research 5: 67–107

Dannenbaum R M, Dykes R 1988 Sensory loss in the hand after sensory stroke: therapeutic rationale. Archives of Physical Medicine and Rehabilitation 69: 833–839

Dannenbaum R M, Jones L A 1993 The assessment and treatment of patients who have sensory loss following cortical lesions. Journal of Hand Therapy 130–138

Dattola R, Girlanda P, Vita G et al 1993 Muscle rearrangement in patients with hemiparesis after stroke: an electrophysiological and morphological study. European Neurology 33: 109–114

Davidoff R A 1992 Skeletal muscle tone and the misunderstood stretch reflex. Neurology 42: 951–963

Davidson I, Waters K 2000 Physiotherapists working with stroke patients. A national survey. Physiotherapy 86: 69–80

Davies P M 1985 Steps to follow: a guide to the treatment of hemiplegia. Springer-Verlag, Berlin

Davies P M 1990 Right in the middle. Springer-Verlag, Berlin

Davies P M 1994 Starting again: early rehabilitation after traumatic brain injury or other severe brain lesions. Springer-Verlag, Berlin

Dengler R, Neyer U, Wohlfarth K, Bettig U, Janzik H H 1992 Local botulinum toxin in the treatment of spastic drop foot. Journal of Neurology 239: 375–378

DeSouza L 1990 Multiple sclerosis: approaches to management. Chapman & Hall, London

Dichgans J 1984 Clinical significance of cerebellar dysfunction and their topo-diagnostical significance. Human Neurobiology 2: 269–279

Dickstein R, Pillar T, Abulaffio N 1995 Electromyographic activity of the biceps brachii muscles and elbow flexion during associated reactions in hemiparetic patients. American Journal of Physical Medicine and Rehabilitation 74: 427–431

Dickstein R, Heffes Y, Abulaffio N 1996 Electromyographic and positional changes in the elbows of spastic hemiplegic patients during walking. Electroencephalography and Clinical Neurophysiology 101: 491–496

Diener H-C, Dichgans J 1992 Pathophysiology of cerebellar ataxia. Movement Disorders 7: 95–109

Diener H-C, Dichgans J 1996 Cerebellar and spinocerebellar gait disorders. In: Bronstein A M, Brandt T H, Woollacott M (eds) Clinical disorders of balance, posture and gait. Arnold, London

Diener H-C, Dichgans J, Bacher M, Gompf B 1984 Quantification of postural sway in normals and patients with cerebellar diseases. Electroencephalography and Clinical Neurophysiology 57: 134–142

Dietz V 1992 Human neuronal control of automatic functional movements: interaction between central programs and afferent input. Physiological Reviews 72(1): 33–69

Dunne J W, Heye N, Dunne S L 1995 Treatment of chronic limb spasticity with botulinum toxin A. Journal of Neurology, Neurosurgery and Psychiatry 58: 232–235

Dvir Z, Panturin E 1993 Measurement of spasticity and associated reactions in stroke patients before and after physiotherapeutic intervention. Clinical Rehabilitation 7: 15–21

Dvir Z, Panturin E, Prop I 1996 The effect of graded effort on the severity of associated reactions in hemiplegic patients. Clinical Rehabilitation 10: 155–158

Dykstra D, Elleringham C, Belfie A, Baxter T, Lee M, Voelker A 1993 Quantitative measurement of cervical range of motion in patients with torticollis treated with botulinum A toxin. Movement Disorders 8: 38–42

Dystonia Society Newsletter 1999 Winter: 3–4

Edstrom L 1970 Selective changes in the sizes of red and white muscle fibres in upper motor lesions and parkinsonism. Journal of Neurological Science 11: 537–550

Edwards S 1998 The incomplete spinal lesion. In: Bromley I (ed) Tetraplegia and paraplegia: a guide for physiotherapists, 5th edn. Churchill Livingstone, London

Elble R J, Sienko Thomas S, Higgins C, Colliver J 1991 Stride-dependent changes in gait of older people. Journal of Neurology 238: 1–5

Fahn S, Marsden C D, Calne D B 1987 Classification and investigation of dystonia. In: Marsden C D, Fahn S (eds) Movement disorders 2. Butterworths, London

Fahn S, Bressman S B, Marsden C D 1998 Classification of dystonia. Dystonia 3: Advances in Neurology 78: 1–10

Fetter M 2000 Vestibular system disorders. In: Herdman S (ed) Vestibular rehabilitation, 2nd edn. F A Davis, Philadelphia

Gardiner M D 1976 The principles of exercise therapy. G Bell, London

Ghez C 1991 The cerebellum. In: Kandel E R, Schwartz J H, Jessell T M (eds) Principles of neural science, 3rd edn. Appleton & Lange, London

Ghika J, Regli F, Growdon J H 1993 Sensory symptoms in cranial dystonia: a potential role in the etiology? Journal of Neurological Science 116: 142–147

Gill-Body K M, Krebs D E 1994 Locomotor stability problems associated with vestibulopathy. Assessment and treatment. Physical Therapy Theory and Practice 3: 232–245

Gilman S 1969 The mechanism of cerebellar hypotonia: an experimental study in the monkey. Brain 92: 621–638

Giuliani C A 1992 Dorsal rhizotomy as a treatment for improving function in children with cerebral palsy. In: Forssberg H, Hirschfeld H (eds) Movement disorders in children. Karger, Basel

Given J D, Dewald J P A, Rymer W Z 1995 Joint dependent passive stiffness in paretic and contralateral limbs of spastic patients with hemiparetic stroke. Journal of Neurology, Neurosurgery and Psychiatry 59: 271–279

Goldspink G, Williams P 1990 Muscle fibre and connective tissue changes associated with use and disuse. In: Ada L, Canning C (eds) Key issues in neurological physiotherapy. Butterworth-Heinemann, Oxford

Goldspink G, Scutt A, Loughna P T, Wells D J, Jaenicke T, Gerlach G F 1992 Gene expression in skeletal muscle in response to stretch and force generation. American Journal of Physiology 262: R356–R363

Goodkin H P, Keating J G, Martin T A, Thach W T 1993 Preserved simple and impaired compound movement after infarction in the territory of the superior cerebellar artery. Canadian Journal of Neurosciences 20: S93–104

Gordon J 1990 Disorders of motor control. In: Ada L, Canning C (eds) Key issues in neurological physiotherapy. Butterworth-Heinemann, London

Gordon T, Mao J 1994 Muscle atrophy and procedures for training after spinal cord injury. Physical Therapy 74: 50–60

Grunewald R A, Yoneda Y, Shipman J M, Sagar H J 1997 Idiopathic focal dystonia: a disorder of muscle spindle afferent processing? Brain 120: 2170–2185

Haas B 1994 Measuring spasticity: a survey of current practice among health-care professionals. British Journal of Therapy and Rehabilitation 1: 90–95

Haggard P, Jenner J, Wing A 1994 Co-ordination of aimed movements in a case of unilateral cerebellar damage. Neuropsychologia 32: 827–846

Hain T C, Ramaswamy T S, Hillman M A 2000 Anatomy and physiology of the normal vestibular system. In: Herdman S (ed) Vestibular rehabilitation, 2nd edn. F A Davis, Philadelphia

Hallett M 1993 Physiology of basal ganglia disorders: an overview. Canadian Journal of Neurological Sciences 20: 177–183

Hallett M 1995 Is dystonia a sensory disorder? Annals of Neurology 38: 139–140

Hallett M 1998 Physiology of dystonia. Dystonia 3: Advances in Neurology 78: 11–18

Hallett M, Khoshbin S 1980 A physiological mechanism of bradykinesia. Brain 103: 301–314

Halsband U, Freund H-J 1993 Motor learning. Current Opinion in Neurobiology 3: 940–949

Hardie R 1993 Tremor and ataxia. In: Greenwood R, Barnes M P, McMillan T M, Ward C D (eds) Neurological rehabilitation. Churchill Livingstone, London

Hasler D 1981 Developing a sense of symmetry. Therapy Aug 27: 3

Hayashi A, Kagamihara Y, Nakajima Y, Narabayashi H, Okuma Y, Tanaka R 1988 Disorder in reciprocal innervation upon initiation of voluntary movement in patients with Parkinson's disease. Exploratory Brain Research 70: 437–440

Herdman S J, Clendaniel R A 2000 Assessment and treatment of complete vestibular loss. In: Herdman S (ed) Vestibular rehabilitation, 2nd edn. F A Davis, Philadelphia

Herdman S J, Whitney S L 2000 Assessment and management of central vestibular disorders. In: Herdman S (ed) Vestibular rehabilitation, 2nd edn. F A Davis, Philadelphia

Herdman S J, Blatt P J, Shupert M C 2000 Vestibular rehabilitation of patients with vestibular hypofunction or with benign paroxysmal positional vertigo. Current Opinion in Neurology 13: 39–43

Hesse S, Lucke D, Malezic M et al 1994 Botulinum toxin treatment for lower limb extensor spasticity in chronic hemiplegic patients. Journal of Neurology, Neurosurgery and Psychiatry 57: 1321–1324

Hollis M 1989 Special regimes. In: Hollis M (ed) Practical exercise therapy, 3rd edn. Blackwell Scientific Publications, London

Holmes G 1922 On the clinical symptoms of cerebellar disease and their interpretation. Lancet 1: 1177–1182

Holmes G 1939 The cerebellum of man. Brain 62: 1–30

Horak F B, Diener H-C 1994 Cerebellar control of postural scaling and central set in stance. Journal of Neurophysiology 72: 479–493

Horak F B, Shupert C L 2000 Role of the vestibular system in postural control. In: Herdman S (ed) Vestibular rehabilitation, 2nd edn. F A Davis, Philadelphia

Hufschmidt A, Mauritz K-H 1985 Chronic transformation of muscle in spasticity: a peripheral contribution to increased tone. Journal of Neurology, Neurosurgery and Psychiatry 48: 676–685

Igarashi M 1984 Vestibular compensation. An overview. Acta Otolaryngol (Stockholm) Suppl 406: 78–82

Igarashi M, Ishikawa K, Ishii M, Yamane H 1988 Physical exercise and balance compensation after total ablation of vestibular organs. Progress in Brain Research 76: 395–401

Ingilis J T, Horak F B, Shupert C L, Jones-Rycewicz C 1994 The importance of somatosensory information in triggering and scaling automatic postural responses in humans. Experimental Brain Research 100: 93–106

Ito J, Araki A, Tanaka H, Tasaki T, Cho K, Yamazaki R 1996 Muscle histopathology in spastic cerebral palsy. Brain and Development 18: 299–303

Jeannerod M 1988 The neural and behavioural organisation of goal-directed movements. Oxford Science Publications, Oxford

Jeka J J 1997 Light touch contact as a balance aid. Physical Therapy 77: 476–487

Johansson R S 1996 Sensory control of dextrous manipulation in humans. In: Wing A M, Haggard P, Flanagan J R (eds) Hand and brain. The neurophysiology and psychology of hand movements. Academic Press, London

Jones D, Godwin-Austen R B 1998 Parkinson's disease. In: Stokes M (ed) Neurological physiotherapy. Mosby, London

Jones D A, Round J M 1990 Histochemistry, contractile properties and motor control. In: Jones D A, Round J M (eds) Skeletal muscle in health and disease: a textbook of muscle physiology. Manchester University Press, Manchester

Katz R, Pierrot-Deseilligny E 1982 Recurrent inhibition of α-motoneurones in patients with upper motor neurone lesions. Brain 105: 103–124

Katz R T, Rymer W Z 1989 Spastic hypertonia: mechanisms and measurement. Archives of Physical Medicine and Rehabilitation 70: 144–155

Kent H, Hershler C, Conine T, Hershler R 1990 Case control study of lower limb extremity serial casting in adult patients with head injury. Physiotherapy Canada 42(4): 189–191

Krebs D E, Gill-Body K M, Riley P O, Parker S W 1993 Double-blind, placebo-controlled trial of rehabilitation for bilateral vestibular hypofunction: preliminary report. Otolaryngology, Head and Neck Surgery 109: 735–741

Kuypers H G J M 1981 Anatomy of the descending pathways. In: Brookhart J M, Mountcastle V B (eds) Handbook of physiology, section 1, The nervous system, vol II, Motor control, part 1, pp 597–666

Lajoie Y, Teasdale N, Cole J D et al 1996 Gait of a different subject without large myelinated sensory fibres below the neck. Annals of Neurology 47: 109–115

Lance J W 1980 Symposium synopsis. In: Feldman R G, Young R R, Koella W P (eds) Spasticity: disordered motor control. Year book, Chicago

Lazarus J-A 1992 Associated movement in hemiplegia: the effect of force exerted, limb usage and inhibitory training. Archives of Physical Medicine and Rehabilitation 73: 1044–1049

Lee R G 1989 Pathophysiology of rigidity and akinesia in Parkinson's disease. European Neurology 29 (Suppl 1): 13–18

Lewis R S, Zee D S 1993 Ocular motor disorders associated with cerebellar lesions: pathophysiology and topical localisation. Revue Neurologique 149: 665–677

Lorentz I T, Shanthi Subramaniam S, Yiannikas C 1991 Treatment of idiopathic spasmodic torticollis with botulinum toxin A: a double-blind study on twenty-three patients. Movement Disorders 6: 145–150

Lucy S D, Hayes K C 1985 Postural sway profiles: normal subjects and subjects with cerebellar ataxia. Physiotherapy Canada 37(3): 140–148

Lynch M, Grisogono V 1991 Strokes and head injuries. John Murray, London

Lynch-Ellerington 1998 Letter. Physiotherapy Research International 3: 76–78

Mai N, Bolsinger P, Avarello M, Diener H-C, Dichgans J 1988 Control of isometric finger force in patients with cerebellar disease. Brain 111: 973–998

Marsden C D 1982 The mysterious motor function of the basal ganglia. The Robert Wartenburg Lecture. Neurology 32: 514–539

Marsden C D 1984 Motor disorders in basal ganglia disease. Human Neurobiology 2: 245–250

Marsden C D 1986 Movement disorders and the basal ganglia. Trends in Neuroscience 512–515

Marsden C D, Quinn N 1990 The dystonias. British Medical Journal 300: 139–144

Martin T P, Stein R B, Hoeppner P H, Reid D C 1992 Influence of electrical stimulation on the morphological and metabolic properties of paralysed muscle. Journal of Applied Physiology 72: 1401–1406

Massion J, Woollacott M 1996 Posture and equilibrium. In: Bronstein A M, Brandt T, Woollacott M (eds) Clinical disorders of balance posture and gait. Arnold, London

Mauritz K-H, Dichgans J, Hufschmidt A 1979 Quantitative analysis of stance in late cortical cerebellar atrophy of the anterior lobe and other forms of cerebellar ataxia. Brain 102: 461–482

Messina C 1990 Pathophysiology of muscle tone. Functional Neurology 5: 217–223

Miller G J T, Light K E 1997 Strength training in spastic hemiparesis: should it be avoided? NeuroRehabilitation 9: 17–28

Miller W, DeLong M R 1988 Parkinsonian symptomatology: an anatomical and physiological analysis. Annals of the New York Academy of Sciences 515: 287–302

Mink J W 1996 The basal ganglia: focused selection and inhibition of competing motor programmes. Progress in Neurobiology 50: 381–425

Morgan M H 1980 Ataxia: its causes, measurement and management. International Rehabilitation Medicine 2: 126–132

Morgan M H, Langton Hewer R, Cooper R 1975 Application of an objective method of assessing intention tremor: a further study on the use of weights to reduce intention tremor. Journal of Neurology, Neurosurgery and Psychiatry 38: 259–264

Moseley A M 1993 The effect of a regimen of casting and prolonged stretching on passive ankle dorsiflexion in traumatic head-injured adults. Physiotherapy Theory and Practice 9: 215–221

Moseley A M 1997 The effect of casting combined with stretching on passive ankle dorsiflexion in adults with traumatic head injuries. Physical Therapy 77: 240–247

Mulley G 1982 Associated reactions in the hemiplegic arm. Scandinavian Journal of Rehabilitative Medicine 14: 117–120

Nash J, Neilson P D, O'Dwyer N J 1989 Reducing spasticity to control muscle contracture of children with cerebral palsy. Developmental Medicine and Child Neurology 31: 471–480

Nguyen J P, Feve A, Keravel Y 1996 Is electrostimulation preferable to surgery for upper limb ataxia? Current Opinion in Neurology 9: 445–450

Nielsen I F, Sinkjaer T 2000 Peripheral and central effect of baclofen on ankle joint stiffness in multiple sclerosis. Muscle Nerve 23: 98–105

Norré M E, DeWeerdt W 1980 Treatment of vertigo based on habituation. Journal of Laryngology and Otology 94: 689

Notermans N C, van Dijk E W, van der Groaf Y, van Gijh J, Wokke J H J 1994 Measuring ataxia: quantification based on the standard neurological examination. Journal of Neurology, Neurosurgery and Psychiatry 57: 22–26

O'Dwyer N J, Ada L, Neilson P D 1996 Spasticity and muscle contracture following stroke. Brain 119: 1737–1749

Panizza M, Lelli S, Nilsson J, Hallett 1990 H-reflex recovery curve and reciprocal inhibition of H-reflexes in different kinds of dystonia. Neurology 40: 824–828

Pentland B 1993 Parkinsonism and dystonia. In: Greenwood R, Barnes M, McMillan T, Ward C (eds) Neurological rehabilitation. Churchill Livingstone, London

Pomeroy V M, Tallis R C 2000 Physical therapy to improve movement performance and functional ability post-stroke. Part 1. Existing evidence. Reviews in Clinical Gerontology 10: 261–290

Porter B 1997 A review of intrathecal baclofen in the management of spasticity. British Journal of Nursing 6: 253–262

Potempa K, Braun L T, Tinknell T, Popovich J 1996 Benefits of aerobic exercise after stroke. Sports Medicine 21: 337–346

Richardson D, Greenwood R, Sheean G, Thompson A, Edwards S 2000 Treatment of focal spasticity with botulinum toxin: effect on 'positive support reaction'. Physiotherapy Research International 5: 62–71

Riddoch G, Buzzard E 1921 Reflex movements and postural reactions in quadriplegia and hemiplegia, with especial reference to those of the upper limb. Brain 44: 397–489

Rondot P, Marchand M P, Dellatolas G 1991 Spasmodic torticollis – review of 220 patients. Canadian Journal of Neurological Sciences 18: 143–151

Rothwell J 1994 Control of human voluntary movement, 2nd edn. Chapman & Hall, London

Rothwell J C, Obeso J A, Bay B L, Marsden C D 1983 Pathophysiology of dystonias. Advances in Neurology 39: 851–863

Sainburg R L, Poizner H, Ghez C 1993 Loss of proprioception produces deficits in interjoint co-ordination. Journal of Neurophysiology 70: 2136–2147

Sainburg R L, Ghilardi M F, Poizner H, Ghez C 1995 Control of limb dynamics in normal subjects and patients without proprioception. Journal of Neurophysiology 73: 820–835

Sanes J N, Dimitrov B, Hallett M 1990 Motor learning in patients with cerebellar dysfunction. Brain 113: 103–120

Saywell S Y 1975 Riding and ataxia. Physiotherapy 61: 334–335

Schmahmann J D 1997 The cerebellum and cognition. Academic Press, London

Schmahmann J D 1998 The cerebellar cognitive affective syndrome. Brain 121: 561–579

Schomburg E D 1990 Spinal sensorimotor systems and their supraspinal control. Neuroscience Research 7: 265–340

Scrutton J, Edwards S, Sheean G, Thompson A 1996 A little bit of toxin does you good? Physiotherapy Research International 3: 141–147

Sheean G L 1998 Pathophysiology of spasticity. In: Sheean G (ed) Spasticity rehabilitation. Churchill Communications, Europe Ltd., London

Shepherd R 1998 Stephenson et al – a response. Letter, Physiotherapy Research International 3: 78–80

Shumway-Cook A 1994 Vestibular rehabilitation in traumatic brain injury. In: Herdman S J (ed) Vestibular rehabilitation. F A Davis, Philadelphia

Shumway-Cook A, Horak F B, Yardley L, Bronstein A M 1996 Rehabilitation of balance disorders in the patient with vestibular pathology. In: Bronstein A M, Brandt T H, Woollacott M (eds) Clinical disorders of balance, posture and gait. Arnold, London

Stein J F 1986 Role of the cerebellum in the visual guidance of movement. Nature 323: 217–221

Stephenson R 1996 A survey of the assessment and grading of spasticity by physiotherapists in the Yorkshire region. Synapse pp 2–6

Stephenson R, Edwards S, Freeman J 1998 Associated reactions: their value in clinical practice? Physiotherapy Research International 3: 69–78

Strupp M, Arbusow V, Maag K P, Gall C, Brandt T H 1998 Vestibular exercises improve central vestibular compensation after vestibular neuritis. Neurology 51: 838–844

Thach W T, Goodkin H P, Keating J G 1992 The cerebellum and the adaptive coordination of movement. Annual Review of Neuroscience 15: 403–442

Thilmann A F, Fellows S J, Ross H F 1991 Biomechanical changes at the ankle after stroke. Journal of Neurology, Neurosurgery and Psychiatry 54: 134–139

Thompson P D, Day B L 1993 The anatomy and physiology of cerebellar disease. Advances in Neurology 61: 15–31

Thornton H, Kilbride C 1998 Physical management of abnormal tone and movement. In: Stokes M (ed) Neurological physiotherapy. Mosby, London

Timman D, Horak F B 1998 Perturbed step initiation in cerebellar subjects 1 Modification of postural responses. Experimental Brain Research 119: 73–84

Topka H, Valls-Sole J, Massaquoi S E, Hallett M 1993 Deficit in classical conditioning in patients with cerebellar degeneration. Brain 116: 961–969

Turnbull G I 1992 Physical therapy management of Parkinson's disease. Churchill Livingstone, London

van Donkelaar P, Lee R G 1994 Interactions between the eye and hand motor systems: disruptions due to cerebellar dysfunction. Journal of Neurophysiology 72(4): 1674–1685

Vrbova G, Gordon T, Jones R 1995 Nerve–muscle interaction. Chapman & Hall, London

Walshe F 1923 On certain tonic or postural reflexes in hemiplegia, with special reference to the so-called 'Associated Movements'. Brain 46: 1–37

Warner T T on behalf of the Epidemiological Study of Dystonia in Europe (ESDE) collaborative group 1999 Sex related influences on the frequency and age of onset of primary dystonia. Neurology 53: 1871–1873

Wichmann T, DeLong M R 1993 Pathophysiology of parkinsonian motor abnormalities. Advances in Neurology 60: 53–61

Xerri C, Merzenich M M, Peterson B E, Jenkins W 1998 Plasticity of primary somatosensory cortex paralleling sensorimotor skill recovery from stroke in adult monkeys. Journal of Neurophysiology 79: 2119–2148

Yanagisawa N, Fujimoto S, Tamaru F 1989 Bradykinesia in Parkinson's disease: disorders of onset and execution of fast movement. European Neurology 29 (suppl 1): 19–28

Yardley L, Beech S, Zander L, Evans T, Weinman J 1998 A randomised controlled trial of exercise therapy for dizziness and vertigo in primary care. British General Practice 48: 1136–1140

Yarkony G M, Sahgal V 1987 Contractures: a major complication of craniocerebral trauma. Clinical Orthopaedics and Related Research 219: 93–96

Young R R 1994 Spasticity: a review. Neurology 44 (suppl 9): S12–S20

Zee D 2000 Vestibular adaptation. In: Herdman S (ed) Vestibular rehabilitation, 2nd edn. F A Davis, Philadelphia

6

General principles of treatment

Philippa Carter
Susan Edwards

The purpose of this chapter is to describe principles of treatment which apply to all stages of management of patients with neurological disability. This includes acute and chronic disorders. The emphasis is on early physiotherapy intervention when patients are usually hospitalised and includes management of respiratory and neurological dysfunction.

Some sections of this chapter are well referenced whereas in others there is no literature to support current practice. The description of physiotherapy management is based on the authors' clinical experience and should not be considered as definitive. It is hoped that many research questions will be raised to either substantiate or disprove this treatment approach.

TREATMENT AND MANAGEMENT OF RESPIRATORY DYSFUNCTION

This section concentrates on how the neurological status of a patient may affect the respiratory management rather than examining the more detailed aspects of respiratory care. The management of patients with traumatic brain injury (TBI) and patients with respiratory muscle impairment following spinal cord injury (SCI) and neuromuscular disease is discussed.

TRAUMATIC BRAIN INJURY

Brain injury can be divided into primary and secondary brain damage. Primary damage is caused at the time of insult and is irreversible. Secondary damage occurs later and is caused by several factors, including raised intracranial pressure (ICP) and decreased cerebral perfusion pressure (CPP) which may follow hypotension, haemorrhage, hypoxia and hypercapnia. Recovery from any type of brain injury depends on the extent of the initial injury and the secondary damage (Reilly & Lewis 1997, Arbour 1998).

Medical intervention is directed at maintaining adequate cerebral blood flow (CBF) and minimising secondary damage which can have devastating effects on the overall outcome (Snyder 1983, March et al 1990). In order to plan appropriate physiotherapy intervention one must understand intracranial dynamics and the physiology of intracranial hypertension.

Intracranial dynamics

The skull forms a rigid box containing brain tissue (80% of the total volume), cerebrospinal fluid (CSF) (10%) and blood, which is the final 10% (Andrus 1991). These components are in dynamic equilibrium: if the volume of one component increases, there must be a relative decrease in other components to keep the overall volume constant (Odell 1996, Arbour 1998).

Intracranial pressure

Intracranial pressure (ICP) is defined as the pressure exerted within the skull and meninges by the brain tissue, CSF and cerebral blood volume (CBV) (Andrus 1991) and can be measured by a variety of monitoring devices (German 1998, Chitnavis & Polkey 1988).

The normal range of values for ICP is between 0 and 15 mmHg (Garradd & Bullock 1986, Chudley 1994). Intracranial hypertension occurs when the ICP exceeds 15 mmHg, and treatment is normally required above 20 mmHg. A persistently high ICP may be associated with a poor prognosis and uncontrollable ICP is often fatal (Tobin 1989).

Intracranial compliance

Intracranial compliance is the ability of the brain to tolerate increases in volume without a cor-

responding increase in ICP (Arbour 1998). With an expanding intracranial lesion, compensatory mechanisms include:

- displacement of CSF from the cranial to the spinal subarachnoid space
- decreased CSF production
- decreased CBV.

When compliance is normal, increases in volume of brain tissue, blood or CSF do not initially produce increases in ICP (Fig. 6.1 A–B). When compliance is poor, a small increase in volume may cause a dramatic increase in ICP (Fig. 6.1 B–C) demonstrated by the intracranial pressure volume curve (Lindsay & Bone 1997).

Cerebral perfusion pressure

Cerebral perfusion pressure is the pressure at which the brain tissue is perfused with blood and is a measure of the adequacy of the cerebral circulation (March et al 1990). It is the difference between the mean arterial pressure (MAP) and the ICP. The normal range for CPP is 70–100 mmHg. A CPP less than 50–60 mmHg may adversely affect prognosis (Leurssen & Marshall 1990, Rosner et al 1995).

At present, ICP and CPP monitoring remain the most commonly used clinical parameters for assessing intracranial dynamics. By continuous observation and regulation of the ICP and the MAP, the CPP can be maintained (Brucia & Rudy 1996, Imle et al 1997).

Cerebral blood flow

Cerebral oxygen delivery is the product of cerebral blood flow (CBF) and arterial oxygen content. The CBF is closely coupled to the energy requirements of brain tissue; if the cerebral metabolic rate (CMR) is high then the oxygen consumption is high and oxygen demand is great (Kerr et al 1995).

The average CBF is 50–55 ml/100 g/min and is calculated as

$$CBF = \frac{CPP}{CVR}$$

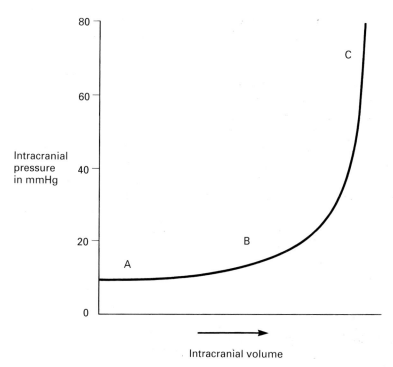

Figure 6.1 Intracranial pressure-volume curve.

where CPP = MAP – ICP and CVR is the cerebral vascular resistance (the pressure across the cerebrovascular circulation from the arteries to the jugular veins). It may be altered by oedema, vasospasm and pre-existing hypertension (Johnson et al 1989).

In many neuroscience units new methods such as jugular bulb oximetry, transcranial Doppler ultrasonography and radioactive zenon are used to measure CBF, brain tissue metabolism and its need for oxygen (Kerr et al 1995, Reilly & Lewis 1997, Berré et al 1998, Cruz 1998).

Factors affecting the cerebral vasculature

Autoregulation

Autoregulation is the ability of the brain to maintain a constant CBF, by regulating the CVR despite wide variations in systemic arterial blood pressure (SABP) and metabolic demands. Autoregulation is effective between a MAP of 60 and 130 mmHg. Within these limits if there is a

drop in SABP the cerebral vessels vasodilate to maintain CBF and vasoconstrict if there is a rise in SABP. Above a MAP of 130 mmHg, the vessels are unable to compensate and an increase in ICP occurs. If the MAP falls to below 60 mmHg, CBF may decrease, causing cerebral ischeamia (Arbour 1998).

Chemoregulation

The cerebral vessels are very sensitive to arterial partial pressures of carbon dioxide ($PaCO_2$) and oxygen (PaO_2), being more sensitive to changes in $PaCO_2$ than PaO_2. An increase in $PaCO_2$ or or reduction in PaO_2 causes reflex cerebral vasodilation, which increases the CBV and ICP. If the SABP remains unchanged, a reduction in the CPP and CBF will occur (Rudy et al 1986).

Intracranial hypertension

A variety of injuries and conditions may cause changes in intracranial dynamics (Arbour 1998).

Altered patterns of cerebral blood flow occur when autoregulation is lost and intracranial compliance diminished. All these factors put the patient at risk of intracranial hypertension and cerebral ischaemia which is associated with a poor neurological outcome (Dexter 1997, Kerr et al 1997).

The effect of brain injury on the respiratory system

Traumatic brain injury may impair lung function both directly and indirectly, at the time of the original trauma or later. The resulting respiratory insufficiency leads to hypoxaemia and hypercapnia, both of which may compromise cerebral oxygenation (Warren 1983). Pneumonia ranks second to intracranial hypertension as the leading cause of death in patients with TBI (Imle et al 1997).

Direct damage to the chest wall, respiratory muscles, pleura or lungs may produce ineffective respiratory mechanics and hypoventilation (Prasad & Tasker 1990, Parataz & Burns 1993, Arbour 1998).

Indirect respiratory insufficiency may be due to:

- Depressed level of consciousness, resulting in an inability to maintain the airway and hypoxia (Warren 1983).
- Compromise of the respiratory centre in the brainstem, leading to altered respiratory patterns, hypoventilation and increased $PaCO_2$. Concurrent suppression of the cough and gag reflex will result in poor airway protection and increase the risk of aspiration (Warren 1983, Prasad & Tasker 1990).
- Neurogenic pulmonary oedema, the exact cause of which is unknown but which in most cases develops within 24 hours after the initial injury. The symptoms are similar to those seen in acute respiratory distress syndrome (ARDS) (Warren 1983).
- Immobility or tonal changes resulting in reduced tidal volumes, small airway closure and atelectasis (Warren 1983, Arbour 1998).

Medical management of intracranial hypertension

Patients with severe neurological injuries who are at risk of hypoxia require early aggressive airway management to prevent secondary complications by maintaining CBF (Brucia & Rudy 1996, Dexter 1997). Sedation and occasionally paralysing agents are used in the first 48–72 h and then withdrawn to assess the patient's state of consciousness (Garradd & Bullock 1986). If the patient becomes agitated or has severely elevated ICP, it may be necessary to resedate and paralyse the patient.

A venticular drain may be used to measure ICP and drain CSF as a means of reducing ICP. The drain is clamped when the patient is moved during physiotherapy and unclamped and realigned afterwards.

Hyperventilation

Hyperventilation has been the cornerstone in treating patients with intracranial hypertension, but its use has become increasingly controversial (Dexter 1997, Arbour 1998). Hyperventilation decreases the $PaCO_2$ to between 4 and 4.5 kPa, producing cerebral vasoconstriction and a decrease in CBF and ICP. The effect is short lived. What is not clear is whether the resulting decrease in CBF places patients with TBI at risk of regional cerebral ischaemia (Dexter 1997). Extreme hyperventilation, where the $PaCO_2$ falls below 3 kPa, may cause profound cerebral vasoconstriction, resulting in cerebral ischaemia (Kerr & Brucia 1993, Dexter 1997).

Positive end-expiratory pressure

Positive end-expiratory pressure (PEEP) is often used in ventilated patients to maintain the patency of airways at the end of expiration and improve oxygenation. However, it must be used with caution, as PEEP in excess of 7.5 cmH$_2$O may decrease intracranial compliance by increasing intrathoracic pressure (ITP), CBV and ICP (Feldman et al 1997).

Drug therapies

Propofol is often used for sedation, decreasing cerebral metabolic rate, CBF and ICP. However, it will reduce the SABP, which may compromise the CPP. Paralysing agents immobilise the patient and reduce the systemic consumption of oxygen. Inotropic support may be necessary to maintain an adequate MAP and CPP. Bolus doses of mannitol, an osmotic diuretic, are used to reduce ICP by establishing an osmotic gradient between the plasma and brain tissue, thereby reducing cerebral oedema. High-dose barbiturates, for example thiopentone, reduce the cerebral metabolic rate of oxygen and stabilise or reduce the cerebral blood flow (Lindsay & Bone 1997, Arbour 1998).

Physiotherapy intervention

The physiotherapist must understand intracranial dynamics and the effect of physiotherapy in order to assess accurately and treat effectively. The following factors should be considered:

- conscious level, as measured on the Glasgow Coma Scale (GCS)
- pupil response before and after intervention
- vital signs including ICP, SABP and CPP and how these are influenced by turning, pressure relief and oral hygiene procedures.

Prior to physiotherapy, sedation or painkillers may be given. The timing of the drug administration is vital and close liaison with the nursing staff is essential.

Suctioning

Suction is a necessary adjunct to ventilator therapy. It ensures airway patency, removes pulmonary secretions and promotes ventilatory exchange (Brucia & Rudy 1996, Kerr et al 1997). Suction causes a progressive increase in ICP with each insertion of the suction catheter. In most patients, elevations in ICP are transient and return to baseline level within minutes (Kerr et al 1998). Induced hypercapnia and hypoxia may cause ICP to rise during suction (Chudley 1994).

While coughing assists with removal of secretions, increased intrathoracic pressure reduces cerebral venous return and increases CBV and ICP (Wainwright & Gould 1996, Kerr et al 1998).

Findings from several studies show that increased ICP during suctioning occurs due to direct tracheal stimulation (Brucia & Rudy 1996, Fisher et al 1982). Transient increases in ICP result from direct carina stimulation but a sustained rise in ICP is due to the increase in ITP associated with coughing. Patients with reduced intracranial compliance have the most pronounced elevations in ICP on suctioning and are less able to tolerate these elevations. Care must be taken when suctioning patients with an ICP above 20 mmHg (Kerr et al 1998).

Considerations when suctioning

- Hyperoxygenation, for example, 100% O_2 for 2 minutes prior to suctioning, minimises transient periods of hypoxia and hypercapnia (Rudy et al 1986, Chudley 1994, Kerr et al 1997).
- Crosby & Parsons (1992) recommend at least 60 seconds of manual hyperventilation between each suction with 2 minutes undisturbed rest to allow ICP, MAP and CPP to return to baseline.
- Disconnection from the ventilator during suctioning causes a rapid drop in ITP and sudden loss of PEEP. A reduction in ICP, due to an increase in cerebral venous return, or an increase in ICP, due to abrupt elevations of the SABP, may result. Disconnection may also cause hypoxia, resulting in cerebral vasodilation (Kerr et al 1993, Imle et al 1997). Suctioning via a port adaptor on the catheter mount, or using a closed suction circuit is therefore recommended. Suction should not exceed 10–15 seconds (Kerr et al 1993).
- The catheter should pass beyond the endotracheal tube (ETT) but not contact the carina to minimise irritant receptor stimulation. The ETT must be stabilised to avoid any unnecessary tracheal stimulation (Kerr et al 1993, Brucia & Rudy 1996)
- Suction passes should be limited to a maximum of 2–3 (Garradd & Bullock 1986, Rudy et al 1991, Kerr et al 1993, Arbour 1998).

- Suction pressure should be high enough to remove secretions but not reduce functional residual capacity or cause tracheal mucosal trauma: 120 mmHg pressure is recommended (Kerr et al 1993).
- The external diameter of the catheter should not exceed half the internal diameter of the ETT to minimise the changes in airway resistance and negative pressure (George 1983, Young 1984).
- Intratracheal or intravenous lignocaine may be used to blunt ICP responses to suctioning (Rudy et al 1986).
- Neuromuscular blocking agents suppress the cough reflex and induce paralysis of the intercostal muscles and diaphragm, increasing chest wall compliance. This may be responsible for the attenuation of expected increases in ICP occurring during suction (Kerr et al 1998).

Suctioning usually increases ICP but the MAP may also increase. It therefore follows that what may be a dangerous increase in ICP may be offset by a rise in MAP maintaining an adequate CPP. Suctioning should only be performed when clinically indicated (Wainwright & Gould 1996, Imle et al 1997).

Manual hyperinflation

Manual hyperinflation (MH) provides artificial ventilation by means of a rebreathing (Water's) or non-rebreathing (Ambu) bag attached to an oxygen source. The aim is to mobilise and assist the clearance of excess bronchial secretions, to increase lung volumes and re-expand areas of lung collapse (Pryor & Webber 1998).

A larger tidal volume is delivered, producing an increase in ITP, which leads to a reduction in cerebral venous return and increase in CBV and ICP (Snyder 1983, Imle et al 1997). If the SABP is low, the induced increase in ITP reduces systemic venous return, lowering the cardiac output, further lowering the SABP and compromising the CPP (Ersson et al 1990, Prasad & Tasker 1990). If SABP is high, MH can increase it to a critical level (Ada et al 1990). The increased levels of PaO_2 induced by MH may have a slight vaso-constrictive effect on the cerebral vasculature, reducing the CBV and ICP (Rudy et al 1991, Kerr & Brucia 1993). Hyperinflation should be interspersed with short-duration hyperventilation to lower $PaCO_2$ prior to or following suction (Kerr et al 1997). Application of MH should be brief, as ICP may increase over time (Garradd & Bullock 1986, Paratz & Burns 1993).

Manual techniques

Shaking and vibrations. These are intermittent coarse or fine compressions of the chest wall during expiration, usually combined with MH. They augment the expiratory flow and facilitate large and small airway clearance by mobilising and advancing secretions (Ciesla 1989, Pryor & Webber 1998). Manual techniques with shaking may increase ICP over time; vibrations in isolation have no effect on ICP (Prasad & Tasker 1990, Imle et al 1997).

Chest clapping. These are slow rhythmical movements of the cupped hands over affected lung segments to mobilise secretions (Pryor & Webber 1998). Chest clapping does not adversely affect ICP and may even lower it (Garradd & Bullock 1986, Paratz & Burns 1993, Imle et al 1997).

Positioning

Patients with high ICP should be nursed in 30 degrees head and trunk elevation as this increases cerebral venous return and lowers ICP, without a significant decrease in CBF (Brimioulle et al 1997). Head elevations above 30 degrees may cause a decrease in SABP, which may compromise the CPP (March et al 1990, Imle et al 1997, Simmons 1997). The head and trunk should be in alignment, as neck flexion and rotation may increase ICP by compressing the internal jugular vein (Williams & Coyne 1993, Chudley 1994).

Postural drainage is a means of positioning that enables gravity to assist the clearance of bronchial secretions. Positions such as a head down tilt may cause an increase in ICP; however, they can be performed safely when strict guidelines are followed and effects of treatment carefully monitored (Lee 1989, Imle et al 1997).

Turning patients into side-lying may increase ICP, with only small changes in CPP (Mitchell et al 1981, Lee 1989, Rising 1993). If the baseline ICP is less than 15 mmHg and the CPP is greater than 50 mmHg, it is considered safe to turn the patient with TBI (Parsons & Shogan 1984). Hip flexion greater than 90 degrees limits venous drainage and will increase ICP (Arbour 1998).

In summary:

- Patients' positioning is individually determined by ICP, SABP and CPP (March et al 1990, Simmons 1997).
- Care should be taken with cervical collars and ETT ties: if too tight, these may impair cerebral venous drainage (Arbour 1998).
- Adequate time should be given to allow ICP to return to baseline (Chudley 1984). The cumulative effect of increased ICP is a major determining factor in prognosis (Shalit & Umansky 1977).

Passive movements

Passive movements to monitor range of motion and assess muscle tone are performed routinely on patients in intensive care units. They can be performed safely on patients with normal or elevated levels of ICP (Brimioulle et al 1997). Stereotyped patterns of hypertonus, producing isometric contractions with pressure of the feet against a foot board, are associated with elevations in ICP (Andrus 1991).

Conclusion

Physiotherapy usually increases ICP, but the positive benefits often outweigh the transient increase. Cerebral perfusion pressure may remain unchanged due to a corresponding increase in the SABP (Garradd & Bullock 1986, Paratz & Burns 1993). The decision whether or not to treat must be made in conjunction with the nursing and medical staff.

Physiotherapists have a role to play in the prevention of secondary brain damage, which may result from hypoxia or hypercapnia arising from respiratory dysfunction. It is essential that physiotherapists understand the relationship between brain and lung function, intracranial dynamics and how all aspects of physiotherapy are integrated with intracranial physiology.

RESPIRATORY MUSCLE IMPAIRMENT

Neuromuscular diseases often affect the respiratory muscles and may involve bulbar muscles, producing impairment of the gag reflex, laryngeal dysfunction and poor airway protection (Kelly & Luce 1991). Pulmonary complications following cervical SCI are the leading cause of death (Mansel & Norman 1990). Respiratory muscle weakness or paralysis causes hypercapnic respiratory failure associated with hypoxaemia. This results from hypoventilation, an ineffective cough and an inability to clear secretions (Kelly & Luce 1991, Roth et al 1997).

The lower motor neurone (LMN) (see Ch. 5) begins at the motoneurone and includes the peripheral nerve, neuromuscular junction and muscle. Disorders can effect the LMN anywhere along its pathway. Motoneurone disease (MND), peripheral nerve disorders, for example Guillain–Barré syndrome (GBS), neuromuscular junction disorders such as myasthenia gravis and disorders of muscle, for example muscular dystrophies, together with SCI, can have devastating effects on respiratory muscle function.

Following an acute SCI the patient may be in a state of spinal shock, with absent reflexes and flaccid paralysis lasting from days to months. For those with cervical SCI, the resultant tetraplegia may be no different from that of a patient with GBS. Similar principles of assessment and treatment therefore apply.

Physiotherapy intervention

Accurate assessment and regular review is vital to initiate preventative measures and treatment. The third to fifth days after SCI are most crucial, as increased secretions may lead to atelectasis and chest infection (Mansel & Norman 1990). The following details should be considered when assessing patients with respiratory muscle impairment:

- examination of the chest wall and upper abdomen for paradoxical movements indicating weakness of intercostal muscles or diaphragm (Brownlee & Williams 1987)
- effectiveness of the cough (Brownlee & Williams 1987, Ward 1998)
- high respiratory rate, which may indicate diaphragmatic weakness or fatigue (Ward 1998)
- repeated measurements of vital capacity: a vital capacity of less than 1 litre may indicate the need for mechanical ventilation.

Breathing exercises

Breathing exercises must be established at an early stage to encourage maximal inspiration. Patients with SCI may have absent or impaired sensation below the level of the lesion. Verbal and visual feedback, using an incentive spirometer, supplements tactile feedback (Brownlee & Williams 1987, Ward 1998).

Intermittent positive pressure breathing

Intermittent positive pressure breathing (IPPB) increases inspiratory volume and aids clearance of secretions in patients with sputum retention and lung collapse (Mansel & Norman 1990). Many neuroscience units use IPPB prophylactically in patients whose vital capacity is between 1 and 1.5 litres. Treatment should be short to avoid tiring the patient (Brownlee & Williams 1987).

Assisted coughing

Assisted coughing is vital for patients lacking sufficient intercostal and abdominal force to produce an effective cough. The therapist replaces the function of weakened or paralysed abdominal muscles by applying a compressive force upwards and inwards against the thorax as the patient attempts to cough (Fig. 6.2). Care must be taken to avoid pressure on the abdomen, particularly if paralytic ileus is suspected, and stability must be maintained at the fracture site for patients with traumatic SCI (Bromley 1998).

The patient must be encouraged to cough 3–4 times a day, and collaboration with the nursing staff is essential (Ward 1998).

Positioning

Positional changes affect respiratory function in patients with tetraplegia: for example, vital capacity may increase in supine compared with upright positions of sitting or standing (Brownlee & Williams 1987). In the supine position, paralysis of the abdominal muscles causes the abdominal contents to force the diaphragm into a higher resting position, increasing its mechanical advantage (Mansel & Norman 1990). In an upright position, the abdominal contents fall downwards and forwards, causing the diaphragm to descend lower into the abdominal cavity and thereby decreasing its effectiveness (Ward 1998).

Effects of autonomic dysfunction

Autonomic dysfunction is a vascular reflex which may occur in SCI patients with lesions above T4 or in neuromuscular disorders. There is involvement of both the sympathetic and parasympathetic systems and symptoms include sweating above the lesion, slow pulse, hypertension, headache and, in some cases, cardiac arrest (Kelly & Luce 1991). Autonomic dysreflexia may occur in response to impaired bladder and bowel function or other noxious stimulus and, although antihypertensive drugs may be given as a temporary measure (Bromley 1998), it is essential to identify and remove the cause.

Following cervical cord injury, the thoracolumbar sympathetic outflow is impaired and parasympathetic tone unopposed. Stimulation of the parasympathetic system, for example during nasopharyngeal suction, may result in bradycardia, hypotension and even cardiac arrest. Loss of vasoconstrictor tone resulting in peripheral vasodilation and diminished venous return due to paralysis of the abdominal and lower limb musculature may lead to postural hypotension (Mansel & Norman 1990). In the early stages of acute paralysis this may impact on the patient's ability to sit up in bed.

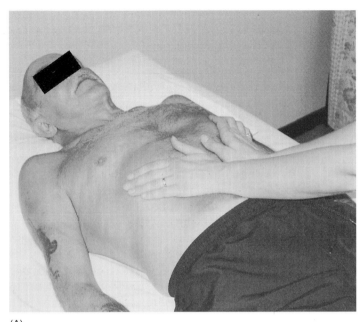

(A)

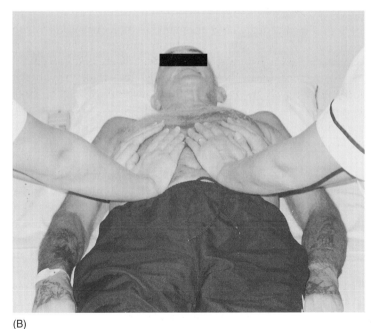

(B)

Figure 6.2   Assisted coughing.

Abdominal binders may be used to provide support to the abdominal contents, allowing the diaphragm to assume a more normal resting position in upright positions, but care must be taken that they do not restrict the movement of the lower rib cage (Brownlee & Williams 1987). They improve the vital capacity of patients with tetraplegia in sitting but not in the supine position (Goldman et al 1986) and are a useful adjunct in the early stages of mobilisation, particularly when standing the patient. Surgical stockings may also be used to good effect to control postural hypotension.

Non-invasive ventilation

Non-invasive ventilation (NIV) can improve gaseous exchange and reduce the work of breathing in patients with hypercapnic respiratory failure following respiratory muscle impairment. A nasal or full face mask is used, avoiding the problems associated with endotracheal intubation and mechanical ventilation (Simonds 1996, Pryor & Webber 1998, Parton et al 1999).

Mechanical ventilation

Depending on the extent and severity of neurological impairment, patients may require mechanical ventilatory support and early tracheostomy to avoid respiratory failure. As respiratory muscle function improves, an active weaning programme should be instigated. This may be more appropriate in the supine position for patients with cervical cord lesions, as the vital capacity is increased in this position (Mansel & Norman 1990). Patients are encouraged to breathe spontaneously for short periods several times a day and given ventilatory support at night to ensure adequate rest and the avoidance of diaphragmatic fatigue (Gardner et al 1985, Ferner et al 1987).

In patients with acute SCI, as spinal shock resolves, chest wall flaccidity may be replaced with hypertonus. In this instance, pulmonary function may improve significantly as the more rigid chest resists collapse (Kelly & Luce 1991).

Conclusion

Physiotherapists are closely involved in the assessment, treatment and management of the respiratory system of patients with SCI and neuromuscular disease. A full understanding of the function of muscles involved in respiration is essential to predict potential problems due to weakness or paralysis and to plan prophylactic measures or treatment where necessary.

MANAGEMENT OF NEUROLOGICAL DYSFUNCTION

Shumway-Cook & Wollacott (1995) propose that there are four key concepts that contribute to a comprehensive conceptual framework for clinical practice. These are:

- the clinical decision-making process, whereby essential information is gathered to develop a plan of care consistent with the problems and needs of the patient
- a hypothesis-orientated clinical practice, whereby assumptions about the nature and cause of motor control may be tested
- a model of disablement which analyses the effects of disease and enables the clinician to develop a list of problems towards which treatment may be directed
- a theory of motor control from which the assumptions about the cause and nature of normal and abnormal movement are derived.

This framework enables the therapist to make decisions about key elements to assess and treat when retraining patients with a movement disorder.

BASIC PRINCIPLES

The control of body posture includes the alignment of body segments to each other and to the supporting surface. It requires a reference point around which movement can occur. The choice of position, both for support and for the performance of movement, must be considered in respect of changes in tone, the influence of gravity, potential structural deformities and preservation of tissue viability (Dufosse & Massion 1992, Pope 1992).

Movements are regularly performed on patients who are unconscious, paralysed, or who have hypertonus, in order to maintain muscle and joint range. An understanding of normal movement as described in Chapter 3 is essential to ensure that movements are performed correctly. Emphasis should be placed on functional movements, ensuring an appropriate response throughout the whole body, rather than on purely movements of an isolated part.

Passive joint motion refers to any movement of an articulation that is produced by some external force (Frank et al 1984). By implication, the term 'passive' indicates that what is done is outside the patient's control and, as such, passive movement must be considered a powerful tool. Patients who are unconscious or who have flaccid paralysis have no resistance to any force applied, whereas those dominated by stereotyped hypertonic posturing tend to resist movements out of these patterns.

In a recent study, Nelles et al (1999) demonstrated that passive elbow movements in hemiplegic stroke patients before clinical recovery elicit some of the brain activation patterns described during active movement after substantial motor recovery (Chollet et al 1991, Weiller et al 1993). It is suggested that the recruitment of ipsilateral sensory and motor pathways early after stroke may be critical for return of voluntary control.

In the clinical setting, the term 'passive' is often inappropriate in that, irrespective of their level of consciousness, patients should be involved in the activity. Verbal instruction should be given as each movement is carried out, to inform patients of the desired response and what is expected of them, and attention given to the degree of proximal mobility and alignment to effect optimal limb movement. It is only in this way that the maintenance of muscle and joint range becomes a dynamic activity rather than a mindless, routine procedure performed on the patient.

It is impossible for the physiotherapist to replicate, for a paralysed patient, the full gamut of functional activity undertaken in everyday life. Normal movement is dependent upon the activation of appropriate agonists and antagonists, with adjustment of synergists and postural fixators (Marsden 1984). Appropriate positioning is of great importance in enabling effective movement with this concurrent response throughout the body. For example, elevation of the arm in normal subjects is influenced by the degree of thoracic excursion which complements this action. If the spine becomes stiff and immobile and is unable to accommodate to the arm movement, this movement will be performed ineffectively and may traumatise the shoulder joint and surrounding structures.

Limitation of range of movement is a common complication in patients with musculoskeletal and neurological conditions (Williams 1990, Pope 1992). Many authors stress the importance of passive movements to prevent this occurrence (Frank et al 1984, Pope 1992, Soryal et al 1992, Daud et al 1993, Davies 1994). However, Davies (1994), while advocating the use of passive movements, emphasises the need for caution, and Silver (1969) and Daud et al (1993) identified a relationship between passive movement and heterotopic bone formation in patients with spinal injury. Patients who are unable to signify pain and discomfort are at particular risk if the limb is taken to the extreme of range by a therapist intent on 'maintaining range of movement'.

The use of passive movement remains controversial. Vigorous, forceful movements carried out in the presence of severe hypertonus may cause microtears in muscle which may lead to calcification of the muscle (Ada et al 1990). Movement of a joint where there is inadequate muscular control may also lead to overstretching of tissues around the joint (Frank et al 1984). This is in part due to the lack of reciprocal activity which under normal circumstances provides proximal control and stability. Soryal et al (1992) described three patients with Guillain–Barré syndrome who had 'profound disability and social handicap over 1–3 years after acute neurological presentation primarily as a result of reduced joint mobility rather than neurogenic weakness'. This was considered to be the result of either inadequate passive movement or excessive passive movement, in the presence of hypotonia, traumatising the joints and surrounding structures.

When muscle is immobilised in a shortened position there is both a reduction in the muscle fibre length due to a loss of serial sarcomeres and a remodelling of the intramuscular connective tissue, leading to increased muscle stiffness (Goldspink & Williams 1990). Mobilisation of the muscle is therefore essential to minimise these structural changes. Periods of stretch as short as half an hour each day have been found to be effective in preventing loss of sarcomeres and reducing muscle atrophy in neurologically intact mice (Williams 1990). However, Tardieu et al (1988), in a study of the soleus muscle of children with cerebral palsy, demonstrated that it was necessary for the muscle to remain in a lengthened position for 6 hours to prevent contracture.

Passive movements of the limbs may be performed on patients once or twice a day. This is particularly so for patients in an intensive care setting where passive movements are often carried out as a routine procedure. The time taken in carrying out these movements varies, but due to other constraints, rarely exceeds 1 hour a day in total. If, for the rest of the time, the patient is dominated by stereotyped patterns which maintain the muscles in a shortened position, this intervention, on its own, is unlikely to be effective in the maintenance of muscle and joint range. Other strategies must be developed to produce a more lasting effect in the control of body posture and movement.

Early mobilisation of the patient should be encouraged as and when the medical condition allows. Movements of the limbs while the patient is confined to bed are difficult in terms of facilitating activity within the trunk. Where bed rest is unavoidable, it is important to maintain adequate movement of the trunk to maintain mobility and to stimulate postural adjustments when moving the limbs.

Of equal importance is the mobility of the nervous system itself and how it adapts to body movement (Maitland 1986, Butler 1991, Hall et al 1993, Shacklock 1995). Mobilisation of the nervous system is used extensively in the assessment and treatment of pain syndromes but it is only quite recently that its importance has been recognised in the treatment of patients with neurological disability (Davies 1994, Panturin & Stokes 1998). Patients who are unable to move or who are dominated by hypertonic stereotyped postures are in as great a danger of developing shortening of neural structures as they are of loss of range of the musculoskeletal system.

Davies (1994) advocates the use of specific tension tests for the maintenance or restoration of adaptive lengthening of the nervous system. Therapists are advised to study the techniques carefully and to practice them on normal subjects prior to using them in the treatment of patients with neurological dysfunction.

POSITIONING

Different postures and positions, and their influence on tone and movement, are discussed in Chapter 3. These should be considered in determining the most appropriate position for treatment of patients with differing types of abnormal tone. However, the optimal position is not always possible due to the patient's medical condition or the presence of contractures, and modification is necessary.

Throughout this section 'acceptance of the base of support' refers to the ability of the patient to adjust appropriately to the contours of the supporting surface.

Positioning in a variety of postures is recommended particularly for patients dominated by

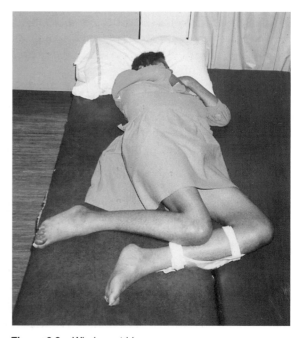

Figure 6.3 Windswept hips.

severe hypertonus. Many patients with increased tone demonstrate a degree of asymmetry which, without treatment, may lead to contracture within the stereotyped patterns. An example of this pattern of contracture is illustrated in Figure 6.3.

The pattern includes:

- rotation of the pelvis relative to the thorax
- lateral flexion of the trunk
- 'windswept' lower limbs
- unilateral hip adduction
- abduction of the opposite hip
- bilateral knee flexion (Pope et al 1991).

This pattern of contracture not only precludes sitting and standing but also adversely affects the patient's ability to accept the base of support in supine and side-lying.

Principles of positioning in bed

The patient may be confined to bed, particularly in the early stages, and is therefore able to experience only a limited variety of positions and movement. The positions are generally restricted to those of side-lying, supine, half-lying and occasionally prone. Movements are dependent upon the position and are compromised by limitations imposed by proximal inactivity or inappropriate activity as may result from hypertonus. The posi-

tions and movements must not be seen as separate entities; each is dependent on the other to ensure the optimal functional outcome.

Supine lying

Patients with hypotonia totally accept the large supportive surface and it is important to ensure that the support provided by the bed preserves the optimal alignment of muscles and joints.

Although patients are rarely placed on a totally flat surface it is important to recognise the potential complications which may arise from this positioning. With a totally flat surface, there is a tendency for the spine to adapt to the contours of the support, with the lumbar spine becoming flatter and the thoracic spine becoming more extended. The shoulder girdles tend to elevate and fall back into retraction. The feet, unless supported, become plantar flexed with the danger of contracture of the triceps surae.

Patients with extensor hypertonus may be unable to accept this large, flat base of support, pushing back against the resistance offered by the surface and thereby exacerbating this dominant posture. The patient with flexor hypertonus may be unable to release this tone to accommodate to the flat surface. In most instances, both extensor and flexor hypertonus are compounded by an element of asymmetry, making appropriate

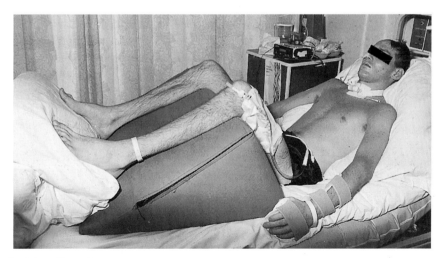

Figure 6.4 Supine lying with wedges.

placement virtually impossible. Alterations to spinal and pelvic alignment are determined by the prevailing tone.

Modification of supine lying, by the use of a wedge, T-roll or pillows, may be of value in controlling the alignment of the spine and in facilitating acceptance of this position. Wedges may be used to good effect both under the head and shoulders and under the knees (Fig. 6.4). For those with predominant extensor hypertonus, the introduction of flexion provides a point of fixation at the pelvis about which movement from lying can be facilitated. The head is in alignment with the trunk in the sagittal and coronal planes, reducing the tendency for increased extension of the cervical spine and for the shoulder girdles to pull back into retraction. The flexion introduced at the hips and knees breaks up the dominant extensor hypertonus of the legs.

Patients with predominant flexor hypertonus may be unable to release the flexor activity if the supporting surface is flat and fully extended. In cases where there is severe flexor hypertonus, a larger wedge may be required in the first instance, its size being gradually reduced as the patient becomes able to accommodate to a more extended position. If there is established shortening of the hip flexors, the graduated use of wedges can be effective in regaining range of movement. Many patients with either flexor or extensor hypertonus present with an asymmetrical posture. The use of a T-roll (Fig. 6.5) may be of value in that it promotes more equal

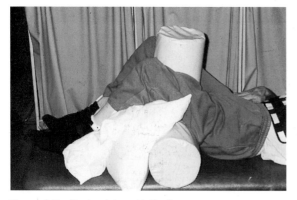

Figure 6.5 Supine lying with T-roll.

loading of tissues and can improve the alignment of body segments (Pope 1992).

This posturing is very much dependent upon the type of bed and firmness of the mattress. Many different types of mattresses are now available and air beds are frequently used in the management of people with neurological disability. Elevation of the head of the bed is often preferred to placing additional pillows or wedges to control the alignment of the head, neck and shoulder girdles. However, although elevation of the head of the bed improves the alignment of the upper body, it produces flexion at the hips, and hip flexor contractures are second only to plantar-flexor contractures as a consequence of neurological impairment (Yarkony & Sahgal 1987).

Side-lying

This position is often utilised in the management of patients with neurological dysfunction (Bobath 1990, Davies 1994). It introduces opposing influences of tone on the two sides of the body: on the supporting side, one of extension, and on the non-weight-bearing side, one of flexion. The side-lying position is similar for patients with either low tone or increased tone. The patient may be positioned with either the underneath leg extended and the uppermost leg flexed or with both legs flexed. The underneath shoulder is protracted to prevent pressure falling over the acromion process, and the pelvis is rotated slightly towards prone. Pillows are required, one or two in front of the patient to support the arm and encourage maintenance of this position towards prone, and one between the knees to stabilise the pelvis and prevent adduction of the uppermost leg. A pillow behind the patient should not be necessary, providing the pelvis is tilted slightly forwards, unless there is uncontrolled movement.

Asymmetrical posturing of the head and trunk may also be corrected or improved with the use of pillows or foam wedges. For example, pillows are used to maintain the head in alignment in the coronal plane, and positioning of a pillow under the left side, when in left side-lying, may prove effective in maintaining range within the opposing trunk side flexors.

Davies (1994) advocates the use of wedges and/or pillows to fill in the 'gaps', particularly for patients with perceptual and/or cognitive impairments. This additional support is considered to provide a feeling of greater security for these often-disorientated patients.

Prone lying

This position is recommended as a means of maintaining or correcting range into extension particularly at the hips and knees (Pope 1992, Davies 1994). However, prone lying should be used with caution in that it may exacerbate flexor hypertonus. Patients with flexor hypertonus rarely accommodate to this position without the additional support of a wedge or pillows. Davies (1994) advocates the use of pillows under the trunk or pelvis to allow acceptance of the support, gradually reducing them until the patient can lie in full extension. The feet should be positioned over the end of the bed to prevent shortening of the triceps surae muscle group.

For patients with hypotonus, prone lying may be a useful adjunct to treatment. A wedge placed under the thorax alters the contour of the spine and enables controlled weight-bearing through the forearms. The protracted position of the arms facilitates flexion at the thoracic spine, thereby overriding the tendency towards extension when the patient is positioned in supine. The extended position of the lumbar spine serves to maintain the lumbar lordosis. From this position, normal extensor activity may be recruited in the head and trunk (Fig. 6.6).

Positioning in this way may also be of benefit for patients with extensor hypertonus, as the overall influence is one of flexion. For these patients, the emphasis is more on mobilising the shoulders forwards into protraction to counteract the commonly observed retraction. Extensor activity of the cervical musculature may also be inhibited when the patient is in prone lying.

Prone lying is recommended for improving oxygenation in ventilated patients with acute respiratory failure (Wong 1998) and the presence of a tracheostomy need not be a precluding factor. The main disadvantage of this position is that there is little stimulation when lying face downwards and, in some instances, the degree of neck rotation may be limited.

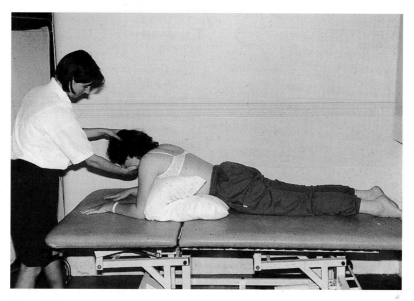

Figure 6.6 Prone lying with forearm support over pillows.

Summary

Limb movements are compromised if there is reduced spinal mobility and inadequate or inappropriate muscle tone to enable effective proximal adjustments. Where bed rest is unavoidable, it is important to maintain adequate movement within the trunk to maintain mobility and to stimulate the proximal control associated with limb movements. Although frequently less obvious than contractures affecting the limbs, loss of range and impaired coordination of the trunk musculature has a dramatic effect on function (Davies 1990).

Movement between lying positions and when coming up from lying to sitting should be carried out with care and the patient given time to adjust to the change of position, particularly when postural hypotension prevails. Turning from side to side or being hurriedly taken into sitting can also be a frightening experience, particularly if there are perceptual problems and sensory impairment.

Principles of positioning in sitting

The principles for appropriate seating are described in detail in Chapter 9.

Trunk mobilisations

In the treatment of neurological patients, trunk mobilisations refer to movements of the trunk, facilitated by the physiotherapist, which are used to modify abnormal tone and improve alignment. In this context they should not be confused with specific vertebral mobilisations as advocated by manipulative therapists.

Treatment of the patient in sitting provides an opportunity for the physiotherapist to mobilise the trunk and facilitate correct alignment with proximal control and stability. Trunk mobilisation, as used in this way, is considered by some practitioners to be a somewhat passive form of intervention. However, as with all techniques, it is dependent upon the physiotherapist's skill and expertise to elicit the desired response. Slow, rhythmical movements, providing full support from behind the patient are more effective in reducing tone and increasing mobility. Smaller range movements with less support and intermittent pressure, as required to gain a 'holding' response, are more effective in stimulating activity. Recently, Thornton & Kilbride (1998) have described handling techniques which may be used for patients with varying levels of tonus.

Patients with hemiplegia develop compensatory strategies to contend with their asymmetry. Those with hypotonus may develop excessive activity of the 'unaffected' side as they struggle to support the weight of the flaccid hemiplegic side. A general assumption among clinicians is that it is this overactivity of the sound side that precludes activity of the affected side. Mobilisation of the trunk is of particular benefit in this situation as the physiotherapist can facilitate a more appropriate response between the two sides of the body. In this situation, it is the 'unaffected' side which is in danger of becoming shortened.

However, it should be noted that in a recent study by Dickstein et al (1999) the muscles on the paretic side were not found to be activated to a lesser extent than those on the non-paretic side during symmetrical trunk movements.

Hemiplegic patients with hypertonus may develop shortening of the trunk side flexors of the affected side. Mobilisation of the trunk is again appropriate but in this instance the emphasis is on reducing the hypertonus in the affected side.

This scenario illustrates the global effects of neurological impairment. Although hemiplegia is by definition a condition affecting half of the body, the consequences of motor and sensory impairment of one side inevitably affect all aspects of movement.

Use of the gymnastic ball

The ball is made of resilient plastic and comes in various sizes. In treatment, it is used predominantly in eight directions – forwards, backwards, to each side and diagonally forwards and backwards (Lewis 1989). Carriere (1999) provides a comprehensive description of the use of the gymnastic ball.

Klein-Vogelbach (1990) gives detailed reference to specific techniques which may be used to optimise stability and/or mobility. These are active exercises performed by the patient with assistance from the therapist as required. These techniques were originally designed for the treatment of orthopaedic conditions. Hasler (1981) adapted Klein-Vogelbach's method for the treatment of patients with neurological disability and Silva & Luginbuhl (1981) and Edwards (1998) recommend its use in the treatment of patients with incomplete spinal cord injury. The gymnastic ball has also been recommended as a treatment modality for patients with hemiplegia (Lewis 1989, Davies 1990).

The ball is useful:

● to stimulate dynamic co-contraction of the trunk musculature

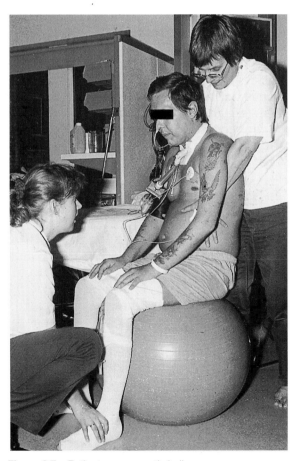

Figure 6.7 Patient on gymnastic ball.

● to mobilise the trunk and limbs
● to retrain balance reactions and coordination
● to strengthen postural muscles (Hasler 1981).

Patients may be mobilised, sitting on the ball with the physiotherapist supporting from behind. In this way the potential loss of range, especially at the thoracolumbar spine and pelvis, may be prevented or minimised. A second person may be required to control the patient's legs to prevent them falling into abduction and lateral rotation (Fig. 6.7). Slow, deliberate movements of the ball both laterally and forwards and backwards can prove most effective in inhibiting hypertonus and maintaining mobility.

Careful assessment of patients who may benefit from this intervention is essential. Great care must be taken when transferring the more disabled patients on to the ball. The ball must be stabilised by another person as the patient is moved from the chair or plinth, which should be of a similar height to that of the ball. If the patient is unable to participate in the transfer, the use of a hoist should be considered.

The gymnastic ball may be used to good effect in preserving or regaining range of movement and in stimulating postural adjustments, particularly within the trunk and lower limbs. However, it should be used with caution because such a mobile surface may provide insufficient support for the patient to effect the desired response. It should also be appreciated that, although the gymnastic ball is widely used in many neurological physiotherapy departments, there is little evidence of its effectiveness (Jackson 1998).

Principles of positioning in standing

Standing is advocated as a means of maintaining joint range and stimulating anti-gravity activity (Ada et al 1990, Pope 1992, Brown 1994). Different types of equipment are recommended to achieve this goal. The selection of the most appropriate aid is dependent upon the size and weight of the patient, the patient's medical status and the assistance available. In the light of moving and handling legislation, any type of standing aid must ensure the protection and well-being of staff and carers.

Positioning of the feet is of particular concern. Patients with low tone may be placed in standing to maintain the length of soleus and gastrocnemius and thereby prevent development of contractures (Ada et al 1990, Pope 1992). However, loss of range of the triceps surae is a recognised complication of excessive hypertonus (Yarkony & Sahgal 1987). In this situation, support must be provided under the heel to accommodate this shortening. The effect of this support is twofold:

- A foam wedge placed under the heel reduces the stress placed on shortened structures by increasing the contact area.
- This increased base of support enables more equal weight-bearing through the full surface of the foot. If there is no support under the heel, the pressure is exerted through the metatarsal heads, which may exacerbate the hypertonus. The pressure exerted by the patient's own body weight may place unacceptable strain over the medial arch and plantar fascia, and damage to these structures may ensue.

By using support in this way, the patient may gradually be able to accept a smaller wedge as the range of movement increases. Mobilisation of the plantar flexors while in standing may be effective in maintaining or regaining range of movement.

The tilt table

This is frequently used, particularly in the early stages of treatment. Patients who are unconscious and/or have hypotonus require total support to enable them to achieve an upright posture. The tilt table affords this support and is perhaps the most commonly used form of intervention. It is of particular value for patients who are excessively heavy or need a graduated means of standing while monitoring for signs of postural hypotension. The patient may be transferred on to the tilt table either by means of a hoist or by sliding them on an 'easy-slide', from their hospital bed on to the table. When using the latter technique, attention must be paid to the protection of the skin by ensuring that any rigid points are covered by a towel or other means of padding.

The tilt table is the method of choice where there is cardiovascular and/or autonomic instability with the potential danger of hypotension. In these instances, it is imperative that the patient can be restored to the horizontal position at the first sign of distress. In many cases, the blood pressure is monitored throughout the procedure to ensure there are no untoward effects.

The tilt table is perhaps the most passive means of taking the patient up into standing. The common characteristics of normal alignment in standing are dependent upon an intact neuromuscular system and have been described in Chapter 3. Where there is abnormal tone caused by neurological impairment, the patient is unable to attain this normal alignment. The use of the tilt table brings the patient up into standing but does little to facilitate the postural adjustments essential for normal standing (Cordo & Nashner 1982, Friedli et al 1984).

Patients with predominantly low tone adapt to the gravitational force, supported only by the straps securing them to the table. The pelvis tilts anteriorly, with a resultant increase in the lumbar lordosis and consequent flexion of the hips. In this position, the iliopsoas muscle is in a shortened position with the potential for development of hip flexion contractures. The knees tend to hyperextend, with the resultant loss of the plantigrade position at the feet through the shortened position of gastrocnemius. To prevent the head and shoulders falling forwards and the patient hanging on the trunk strap, the tilt table is frequently positioned a few degrees from the full vertical. The shoulder girdles retract with the head extended, precipitating shortening of the extensor muscles of the cervical spine. Clearly, if the therapist is aware of these potential complications, then adjustments can and should be made. Use of the tilt table purely to attain an upright posture is of little value to the patient in terms of regaining correct postural control.

The tilt table should be used only as an adjunct to treatment. Where possible, the straps should be removed, particularly the trunk strap. In the

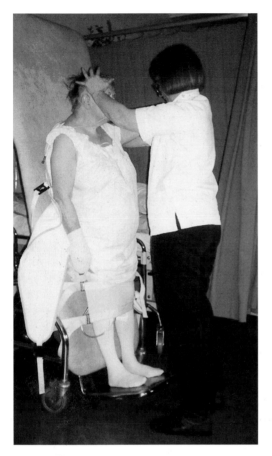

Figure 6.8 Tilt table.

majority of cases this need not be used if the therapist supports the patient from the shoulder girdles with the arms extended and thus stimulating head and trunk control (Fig. 6.8). A pillow or towel may be used behind the knee to prevent hyperextension, but it must be recognised that this in itself does not address the primary problem, that of the anterior tilt of the pelvis.

The tilt table is not generally recommended for patients with severe extensor hypertonus, primarily because it provides an extensor surface against which they may resist, thereby exacerbating their tone. For those with flexor hypertonus the tilt table may be of value in controlling the legs in a more extended position. This positioning should only be used in conjunction with mobilising techniques to first reduce the increased flexor tone. Forcing the legs into exten-

sion by means of the knee strap will not only exacerbate the hypertonus but may also cause considerable discomfort to the patient. Equally, the attainment of more extension at the knees by these means will inevitably create problems both proximally and distally. The use of force to attain improved alignment is ineffective in terms of controlling hypertonus or in the prevention of subsequent contractures.

Summary. The tilt table is a valuable tool in enabling the patient to stand. If there is any risk to staff in standing patients by more dynamic means, then the tilt table is the method of choice. Where possible, other means of standing should be considered to ensure correct alignment and to provide greater stimulation and a more dynamic response.

The Oswestry standing frame

This frame was originally designed by a paraplegic patient for paraplegic patients. These people can lift themselves up into the frame and stand independently once the straps are secured. The Oswestry standing frame has now become one of the most commonly used frames, not only in spinal injury units but also in general hospitals and certainly in the majority of neuroscience centres in the United Kingdom. It is also frequently prescribed for use in the home for physically disabled people with diverse neurological pathologies. It is durable and relatively cheap. However, its use for the more severely disabled clients is being challenged.

In the light of current moving and handling legislation, it is essential to select carefully only those patients who are able to assist bringing themselves up into standing. In the past, heavily disabled patients have been lifted up into the Oswestry standing frame by two or more therapists.

However, the possible benefit to the patient must be weighed against the difficulty for the carers in lifting the patient into the frame. In the majority of cases, certainly in the community, this is deemed to be an unacceptable risk. Alternative means of standing must therefore be considered.

The wooden frame affords tremendous stability while allowing access for the therapist from behind. Three sheepskin-covered straps attach behind the ankles, in front of the knees and behind the hips. If correctly applied, these secure the lower limbs in a position of extension and enable the therapist, standing behind the patient, to ensure correct alignment of the pelvis.

The therapist can ensure that the pelvis is in neutral or preferably in a position of slight posterior tilt. This enables full extension at the hips with mechanical lengthening of the iliofemoral ligament and the iliopsoas muscle. Maintenance of the length of these two structures prevents the compensatory lordosis of the lumbar spine and extension at the shoulder girdles. This positioning also facilitates abdominal activity.

To achieve this optimal alignment it is important that the straps are correctly applied.

- The hip strap must be taut to prevent the patient 'sitting' on it and thereby producing flexion, adduction and medial rotation at the hips.
- The knee strap must be positioned over the patella tendon, as opposed to over the patella itself, and must maintain the knees in extension. A foam wedge or towel may be placed between the knees to prevent valgus.
- The foot strap is attached behind the heels.

The Oswestry frame allows for more dynamic intervention in terms of movement. The hip strap may be removed, with the therapist standing behind and supporting the patient. In this way the therapist can allow the patient to move down towards sitting and facilitate movement back into standing, ensuring correct pelvic alignment. The therapist should have a plinth positioned behind her at the correct height to ensure that this activity is safe.

Patients may also be mobilised by use of the table. By taking the patient forwards to rest over pillows or a wedge on the table, the thoracolumbar spine may be mobilised and elongation of the cervical spine obtained. The patient may stand supported in this position to ensure extensibility of the hip extensors, knee flexors, ankle plantar flexors and of the neural structures.

Summary. The Oswestry standing frame is designed in such a way as to enable its use for:

- stimulating proximal muscle activity with correct alignment of the legs and pelvis
- mobilisation of the patient with hypertonus to prevent shortening of structures dominated by the increased tone.

It may be considered as 'an extra pair of hands' in providing proximal and lower limb stability to allow for functional use of the arms.

Manual and powered hoists have now been developed to overcome the difficulties of lifting the more heavily disabled patients up into this frame (Fig 6.9).

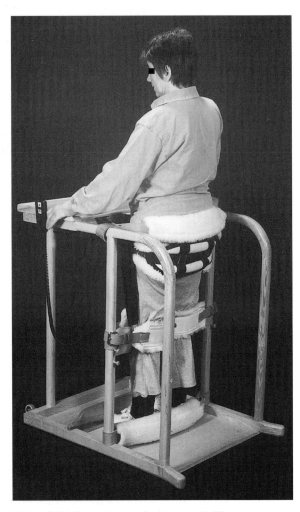

Figure 6.9 Oswestry standing frame with lifter.

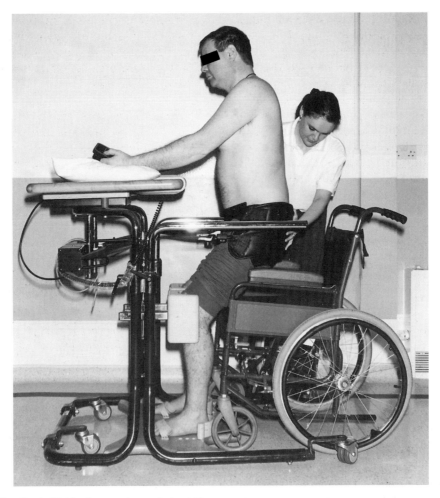

Figure 6.10   Standing in Richter frame using motorised lifter.

Standing frame with motorised lifter

Standing frames with motorised lifters are increasingly being purchased to comply with moving and handling legislation. Similar in design to the Oswestry frame, the Richter standing frame, which is but one example, enables the patient to be taken gradually from sitting, up into standing, at the touch of a button. The therapist(s) may need to support the patient as he comes up into standing, but the 'heavy work' is done by the motorised lifter (Fig 6.10).

A strap is placed under the patient's seat and attached to a mains or battery drive unit. If phys-

ically capable, the patient operates the control button himself; otherwise, the therapist takes responsibility. At any time the lift may be stopped to allow the patient time to adjust to the more upright posture. A quick release mechanism is provided in the event of an emergency, whereby the patient may be immediately restored to the sitting position.

In standing, there are a variety of accessories which may be used to support even the most severely disabled patients. These include scapulae, lateral and head supports in addition to hip, knee and foot supports which work on a similar principle to those of the Oswestry frame. However, the pads which secure the hips, knees and feet provide more control because they surround these joints, preventing medial rotation and adduction at the hip and valgus at the knee. The cup support around the foot also maintains a more stable position.

Although they are more expensive, given the moving and handling legislation, standing frames with a motorised lifter will inevitably become essential equipment in the management of people with neurological disability. Already, in the settlement of many medicolegal cases, standing frames with a motorised lifter are accepted as the norm. It is to be hoped that their provision in hospitals throughout the United Kingdom is not too far distant.

Summary. Electric standing frames enable therapists and care staff in the community to stand people with severe neurological disability in a graded and controlled fashion while minimising the risk of injury both to themselves and to the patient.

This frame is a solid, very heavy structure. It should be placed in the optimal position in the gym or in the patient's home to avoid having to move it. It is ironic that, while this frame reduces the strain on professional staff and carers in standing the patient, attempts to move the frame have been known to cause serious back injuries.

The principles of treatment underpinning its use are similar to those of the Oswestry standing frame.

Stand-up wheelchair

Wheelchairs enabling the person to stand while remaining in the chair are increasingly used in the management of children and adults with neurological disability. Details are given in Chapter 9.

Prone standing table

The prone standing table is more commonly used in the management of children with neurological disability but may also be of value for adult patients with extensor hypertonus. Straps over the trunk, hips and feet secure the patient, and a table is attached for arm support (Fig. 6.11). The sup-

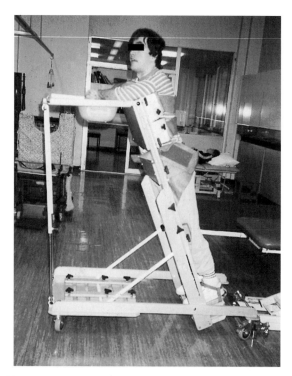

Figure 6.11 Prone standing table.

porting surface is on the flexor aspect, which prevents the patient pushing backwards and exacerbating his extensor tone. At the same time, this positioning may stimulate more normal extensor tone by providing secure and stable proximal support.

The stability afforded to the trunk, pelvis and lower limbs enables more specific intervention for facilitation of, for example, head control or increased range of movement of the upper limbs.

The main disadvantage of the prone standing table is the relative difficulty in positioning the patient in the frame and attaining the upright position. As with all moving and handling, careful assessment is necessary to determine the effectiveness of this standing aid. For adults, as opposed to children, with neurological disability the prone standing table is now rarely used.

Standing using two or more therapists

This is a more dynamic intervention, providing for instant response and adjustment on the part of the therapist to the patient's changing status. However, standing in this way is more demanding on staff and should only be attempted with patients who have some activity, are able to participate actively in the stand and with whom the therapist feels confident. Therapists new to working with neurological patients should not feel that this method of standing must be used at all costs. In most instances, therapists need time to develop their handling skills and confidence to attempt this more complex intervention.

Standing a patient with minimal activity requires greater input from the therapists and the benefit to the patient of this more dynamic stand must be weighed against the risk to the treating staff.

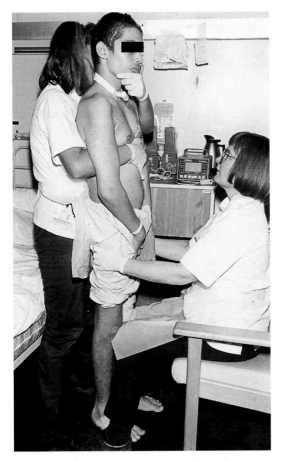

Figure 6.12 Standing, using two physiotherapists.

One therapist stands in front of the patient, supporting the knees and securing the position of the feet. Her hands are placed under the patient's ischeal tuberosities from where she guides him into standing. Once the patient is upright, the therapist in front of the patient can sit on a stool or chair, maintaining control of the hips, knees and feet (Fig. 6.12). The second therapist stands behind the patient supporting the patient's head and trunk as he is brought up into standing. Standing a patient with hypertonus may need adaptation, depending on the severity and distribution of tone, and more than two therapists may be required.

The advantage of standing the patient in this way is that it enables the therapists to feel and respond to any change in the patient's status. Movements may be facilitated from standing to sitting back on to the therapist behind, and up again into standing. Transfer of weight from one side of the body to the other, while maintaining the correct alignment, provides the sensation of movement between the two sides, which is of particular importance for patients with a hemiplegic presentation.

Summary. Standing patients in this more dynamic way is often of great benefit both to the patient and to the therapist. However, the therapist must be competent and confident to manage this technique. If there is any doubt in the mind of the therapist, or the patient shows concern, other means should be adopted, utilising equipment aids as indicated.

Many experienced neurological therapists continue to use either the tilt table or a standing frame, and with good reason. The persistent, insidious strain from heavy lifting and supporting patients with severe neurological deficit can have long-term consequences, particularly in relation to back injuries. Selection of the most appropriate treatment intervention must therefore always consider the therapist as well as the patient.

Use of back slabs

Back slabs, made from either plaster of Paris or fibreglass material, may be used to maintain the legs in an extended position to stand. Davies (1994) considers this the method of choice when

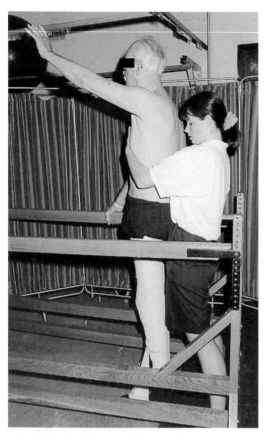

Figure 6.13 Standing with back slabs in parallel bars.

support is required to stand patients following head injury. They should be made specifically for the individual patient and be securely bandaged in place. (A detailed description is given in Ch. 10.)

The purpose of the back slabs is to enable the therapist to work for improved trunk and pelvic control while stabilising the lower limbs. The therapist may choose to stand in front of or behind the patient while stimulating head, trunk and upper limb control, or the patient may stand in the parallel bars to facilitate weight-bearing through the arms (Fig. 6.13). By maintaining a posterior tilt of the pelvis, shortening of the iliofemoral ligament and of the hip flexor muscles may be prevented.

Back slabs are mainly used in the treatment of patients with low tone and for those with flexor hypertonus.

For patients with severe flexor hypertonus of the legs, it may be impossible to secure the slabs without the use of excessive force. As previously discussed in relation to the tilt table, mobilising techniques must first be used to enable the patient to accept this support.

The use of a back slab has been advocated in the early management of stroke patients with lack of midline orientation (Davies 1985). These patients are often referred to as 'pushers' in that they overuse the sound side, pushing themselves off balance to the affected side. The back slab, applied to the affected leg, enables the patient to transfer weight through this limb and thereby regain more body awareness. This should be used with caution if flexor hypertonus becomes dominant in the lower limb.

The main disadvantage of using this method is that the patient cannot be taken up into standing through sitting. With the legs fixed in extension, the patient may need assistance to stand and the potential benefit to the patient must be weighed against the strain placed on treating staff. Once in standing, it is impossible to facilitate release of activity to allow the patient to move towards sitting by coordinating movement between the pelvis, hips, knees and feet. A further disadvantage is that there is little stimulation of the lower limb extensors.

Summary. The use of back slabs enables specific mobilisation of the trunk on pelvis and the pelvis on extended lower limbs. In this way, they are of benefit in preventing the onset of, or reducing, hip flexor contracture. The main disadvantage is that back slabs preclude normal movement from sitting to standing and, unless the patient has good arm function and is able to stand independently in parallel bars, standing the patient in this way places greater and possibly unacceptable demands on the treating staff.

MOVEMENTS

Orofacial movements

Patients with severe brain damage may demonstrate significant problems relating to impaired control and coordination of facial structures. The mouth is one of the most sensitive areas of the body and yet it is an area which is often neglected in rehabilitation (Davies 1994). There are many aspects which need to be considered in the maintenance of orofacial function. These include:

- The positioning of the head and trunk; if the head is held in extension, swallowing becomes difficult if not impossible.
- Many patients have increased tone of the tongue, which may be palpated as a tight ball behind the chin. As with other muscles dominated by hypertonus, restricted range of movement results unless passive movement of the tongue is undertaken by either the physiotherapist or speech and language therapist.
- Hypertonia of the facial muscles may produce grimacing and loss of range of movement of the jaw. In severe cases, the temporomandibular joint may sublux.
- A gag, swallowing or bite reflex may be in evidence. These will severely compromise the maintenance of oral hygiene and, where appropriate, feeding. Orofacial therapy is essential to prevent increasing sensitivity to touch of the area within and around the mouth (Davies 1994).

Therapists are often apprehensive about treating facial structures, particularly the mouth, tending to concentrate more on the trunk and limb movements. 'The patient who is unconscious or whose mouth is significantly paralysed, experiences an almost total sensory deprivation interrupted only by certain nursing or medical procedures, sometimes unpleasant ones' (Davies 1994). If something unpleasant is put into the mouth of a normal subject, the response is one of disgust registered by grimacing and possibly spitting the object out. The patient who is unable to respond in this manner may show signs of distress with a general increase in tone throughout the body.

Orofacial treatment is essential to desensitise these abnormal responses and to enable the patient to receive more appropriate feedback. Patients respond positively to mobilisation of facial structures, particularly within the mouth and the surrounding area. *Great care must be taken when working inside the mouth of a patient with a bite reflex and gloves should always be worn to minimise the risk of cross-infection.*

Examples of techniques which may be used to manage some of the problems listed above include:

- elongation of the cervical spine with extension of the trunk to prevent adaptive shortening of the cervical spine into extension; this is best achieved with the therapist behind the patient, supporting the trunk and holding the chin between the index and middle fingers with the thumb extending to the temporomandibular joint (Fig. 6.14).
- maintaining this grip and mobilising the tongue with the middle finger to facilitate swallowing
- taking hold of the tongue using a piece of cotton gauze and gently mobilising to maintain or regain its range of movement

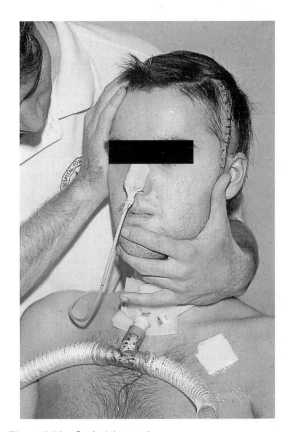

Figure 6.14 Orofacial control.

- massage/mobilisation of facial muscles to reduce hypertonus and maintain or restore symmetry
- massage of the gums and the interior aspect of the cheeks after immersing the finger in water, or using a wet piece of gauze.

These techniques and others are described in detail in Davies (1994).

Shoulder girdle and upper limb

The shoulder joint is particularly vulnerable to trauma, being the most mobile joint of the body in terms of its anatomical structure. It is dependent upon muscular activity for stability and therefore, when abnormal tone prevails, the mechanics of the joint are compromised (Lippitt & Matsen 1993).

Movements of the upper limb must be carried out with great care and with a detailed knowledge of the shoulder mechanism. The therapist must appreciate the holistic nature of functional activity. Movements of the upper limb cannot be viewed in isolation. Attention must be paid to the position in which the movements are performed, the stability afforded by the supporting surface, the patients' ability to maintain themselves or move against gravity and the ability of the trunk to respond effectively to the imposition of distal movement.

Potential problems affecting the shoulder girdle and upper limb function

The patient with low tone. In sitting or standing, the scapula rotates medially as there is little or no muscular activity to maintain its position of lateral rotation around the chest wall. The inferior angle of the scapula lies closer to the vertebral column than normal, as illustrated in Figure 6.15. This produces abnormal alignment of the glenoid fossa, leading to a degree of abduction at the shoulder joint.

In the adducted position, the capsule becomes taut, preventing downward displacement of the humerus (Cailliet 1980). The shoulder is vulnerable in a position of abduction, as the superior

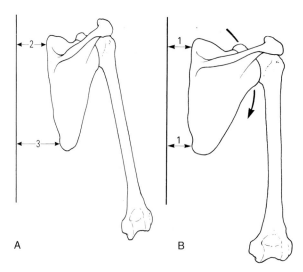

Figure 6.15 Relationship of the shoulder girdle and vertebral column: (A) normal; (B) abnormal (reproduced from Bromley 1998 with permission).

portion of the capsule is slack. In the patient with hypotonus the 'locking mechanism' is no longer effective, resulting in a subluxation of the glenohumeral joint, as shown in Figure 6.16. Preventive measures offering support to the

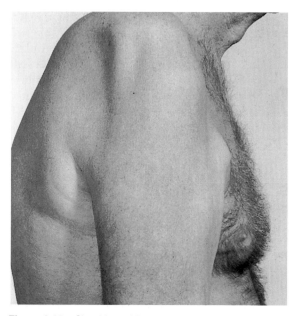

Figure 6.16 Shoulder subluxation.

upper limb should be employed before irreparable damage occurs.

The scapulohumeral rhythm is impaired and therefore movement performed by the therapist at the glenohumeral joint must include adequate excursion of the scapula.

Specific problems which may arise as a result of hypotonus include:

- hyperactivity of the upper fibres of trapezius in an attempt to support the flail arm
- loss of shoulder girdle stability due to weakness of the lower fibres of trapezius
- shortening of the pectorals leading to reduced range of horizontal abduction
- shortening of latissimus dorsi
- immobility of the scapula *or*
- hypermobility of the scapula should the medial rotators, namely latissimus dorsi, teres major and subscapularis, become shortened.

The patient with increased tone. In patients with hypertonia, the most commonly observed posturing of the upper limb is that of retraction of the scapula, adduction and medial rotation of the glenohumeral joint, flexion of the elbow, pronation of the forearm, flexion and ulnar deviation of the wrist, and flexion of the fingers with adduction of the thumb (Bobath 1990, Rothwell 1994).

Increased tone produces a degree of immobility; the dynamic co-contraction and stability afforded by the scapula as described in Chapter 3 is impaired. Reciprocal innervation is compromised; the grading of movement is lost with the static co-contraction of the dominant hyperactive muscle groups. Selective movement of the upper limb becomes difficult if not impossible due to impaired proximal stability. Shortening of the muscle groups, producing the stereotyped posturing, may result.

The scapula is pulled closer to the vertebral column by hypertonus of the rhomboids. This may be either in a vertical position or with a degree of medial rotation. The angle of the glenoid fossa becomes vertical or possibly even downward facing. This malalignment of the glenohumeral joint produces a degree of relative abduction at the shoulder joint, as seen in hypotonia. Increased tone of pectorals and medial rotators produces an anterior, rotational movement of the humerus, further distorting its position in relation to the glenoid fossa (Irwin-Carruthers & Runnalls 1980).

Movements undertaken by the physiotherapist to maintain range of movement must incorporate techniques of tone reduction. There is both malalignment of the joint surfaces and resistance from hypertonic muscle groups. Hypertonia invariably affects all muscle groups in spite of the predominance of flexion, adduction and medial rotation. Attention must be paid to the position in which the movements are performed. For example, movement of the arm into elevation will be more successful with adequate thoracic spine extension (Crawford & Jull 1993).

The scapulohumeral rhythm is altered, the extent to which this is disrupted being dependent upon the severity and distribution of hypertonia. For example:

- The excursion of the scapula may be limited by the increased tone of its extensive musculature. In this situation, attempted movement of the arm away from the body may traumatise the glenohumeral joint and the surrounding tissues.
- Hypertonia of the medial rotators may reduce the range of movement at the glenohumeral joint through shortening of latissimus dorsi, teres major and subscapularis in particular. In this instance, attempted movement of the arm away from the body produces hypermobility of the scapula to compensate for the immobility at the glenohumeral joint (Fig. 6.17).

Pain may be an additional complication which may develop as a result of the stereotyped posturing and/or forcing range without appropriate tone reduction, thereby traumatising the shoulder.

Prehension is dependent upon the proximal musculature of the shoulder for placing the hand in the correct spatial location to effect function. Neurological impairment affecting the shoulder mechanism will therefore affect the selective use of the hands for function.

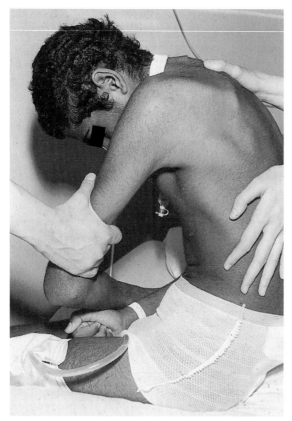

Figure 6.17 Reduced glenohumeral movement resulting in increased excursion of the scapula.

The elbow joint

Flexor hypertonus affecting the upper limb may result in shortening of the elbow flexors, most commonly in conjunction with pronation of the forearm. Where increased tone of biceps is dominant, this flexion may be seen in conjunction with supination.

Mobilisation/massage and stretching of the elbow flexors is beneficial for reducing flexor hypertonus and improving muscle flexibility, thereby facilitating movement into extension. However, it is important not to force range against the stereotyped resistance as this may be a causative factor of myositis ossificans. Passive movement of the arm into extension must ensure release and elongation of the elbow flexors to prevent excessive strain on the periosteum onto which the forearm muscles insert.

Prophylactic or corrective splinting by means of a drop-out cast (see Ch. 10) is the preferred option where there is excessive hypertonus and subsequent inability to maintain extension of the elbow.

The wrist and fingers

Flexor hypertonus of the wrist and finger flexors is most commonly seen with pronation of the forearm, ulnar deviation of the wrist and thumb adduction.

It is often difficult to prevent shortening of these structures unless splinting is used to maintain a functional position (see Ch. 10). However, the effects of this intervention must be carefully monitored. Inappropriate splinting may further reinforce the dominant hyperactivity if the patient is unable to accommodate the support. Ideally, the splint should be removable to allow mobilisation of the wrist and fingers to desensitise the grasp response. It is important to instruct family and friends in the most appropriate way of mobilising the wrist and hand, the hand being one of the most common points of contact between the patient and his relatives.

Movements of the wrist and fingers can only be effective with a reduction of flexor tone throughout the upper limb. Attempts to straighten the fingers, for example, or radially deviate the wrist, are singularly unsuccessful if the shoulder and elbow are still dominated by flexor hypertonus.

Movements of the wrist and hand for patients with cervical cord injuries must be performed with extreme care. For example, a patient with a lesion at the level of the sixth cervical vertebra loses control of the fingers and is dependent upon the wrist extensors to effect function by the use of a tenodesis grip. If the wrist and fingers are passively extended to the extreme of range, the finger flexors may become overstretched and the tenodesis grip ineffective. Contracture of the finger flexors is to be avoided, but overstretching can have catastrophic functional consequences.

Some stroke patients have a moderate amount of both proximal and distal selective movements. For these people, recent therapy approaches have included 'constraint induced movement therapy'. The patient is forced to use the affected upper limb for a significant proportion of waking hours by restraining the sound upper limb. This is believed to reverse the learned non-use of the affected upper limb and enables the patient to realise the full potential of recovering function (Wolf et al 1989, Taub et al 1993, Miltner et al 1999, Van der Lee et al 1999). In these studies, the key criteria is that patients have a minimum of 20 degrees of active wrist extension and 10 degrees of active finger extension.

However, in rats forced overuse of the affected forelimb in the early stages post-injury was found to cause severe motor deficits and enlargement of the lesion (Kozlowski et al 1996). Therefore, while forced use of the affected limb appears to have beneficial effects on motor recovery, extreme overuse during a critical period after injury can be detrimental, at least in rats. The optimal frequency, intensity and timing of forced use remains to be determined (Nudo 1999).

The lower limb

In a normal subject, in supine lying, there is a central stabilising effect if the leg is actively lifted on to the chest. Abdominal and erector spinae activity stabilise the lumbar spine and control the pelvis in a posterior tilt; this is essential to ensure effective action of the iliopsoas muscle as a hip flexor. As the leg is flexed, the pelvis should be posteriorly tilted and the sacrum remain in contact with the bed as the leg is then extended. In this way, normal range of psoas may be preserved. Patients with long-term immobility invariably lose range in the hip flexors so that in the supine position, with hips extended, the lumbar lordosis is exaggerated (Pope 1992) (Fig. 6.18).

Hip adduction may accompany either flexor or extensor hypertonus. Movements of the leg into abduction must ensure that the movement occurs at the hip joint and does not produce a lateral tilt of the pelvis. In severe cases, such as with the 'windswept hips' deformity (see Fig. 6.3), ipsilateral shortening of the hip adductors may result in displacement of the hip joint. Although this complication is more common in children with neurological impairment and with an immature musculoskeletal system, it has been known to occur in adults with severe hypertonia and contracture. In this situation, the patient may lose the ability to be positioned in a wheelchair or to stand in a standing frame. Genital hygiene and the management of continence may also be compromised.

The use of wedges and T-rolls as described above may prove beneficial in maintaining alignment and in preventing contractures. Appropriate seating systems (see Ch. 9) are also essential.

The foot and ankle

Movements to maintain muscle and joint range at the foot and ankle are often difficult, more so in patients with hypertonus of the triceps surae.

For patients with low tone, maintaining range of ankle movement is not as problematic as main-

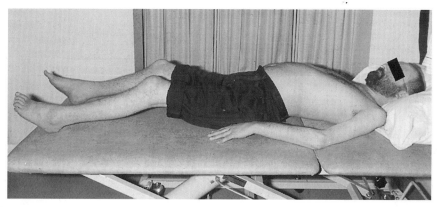

Figure 6.18   Flexion contraction of the hips.

taining mobility within the foot. The normal activity of the intrinsic foot musculature which occurs, particularly during standing and walking, is hard to replicate. Movements of the metatarsals and maintaining range at the metatarsalphalangeal joints, particularly of the great toe, is essential to enable effective stance and gait. Massage and mobilisation and stretching of the calf muscles may also be effective in improving range within these structures.

The effects of force imposed over the forefoot have been described on page 138. In patients with severe hypertonus, maintaining ankle range of movement is often best achieved with the use of prophylactic or corrective below-knee casting (see Ch. 10).

SUMMARY

Patients with neurological dysfunction resulting in abnormal posture and movement are at great risk of developing structural deformity (Yarkony & Sahgal 1987). Treatment to control body posture and movement must be initiated at the onset of neurological disease or damage and continued for as long as the danger of secondary complications exists.

Positioning and movement are interdependent on each other. Patients with restricted range of movement of the limbs also often have loss of range within the trunk and around the pelvis and shoulder girdles. Attempts to take the limbs through a full range of movement while there is impaired range proximally will almost certainly traumatise the joints and soft tissues. It is therefore essential that the person performing these movements is aware of established limitations in respect of obtainable range. Any forcing of range must be considered detrimental.

REFERENCES

Ada L, Canning C, Paratz J 1990 Care of the unconscious head-injured patient. In: Ada L, Canning C (eds) Key issues in neurological physiotherapy: physiotherapy foundations for practice. Butterworth-Heinemann, Oxford

Andrus D 1991 Intracranial pressure: dynamics and nursing management. Journal of Neuroscience Nursing 23(2): 85–91

Arbour R 1998 Aggressive management of intracranial dynamics. Critical Care Nurse 18: 30–40

Berré J, Moraine J, Mélot C 1998 Cerebral CO_2 vasoreactivity evaluation with and without changes in intrathoracic pressure in comatose patients. Journal of Neurosurgical Anesthesiology 10: 70–79

Bobath B 1990 Adult hemiplegia: evaluation and treatment, 3rd edn. Heinemann Medical Books, London

Brimioulle S, Moraine J, Norrenberg D, Kahn R 1997 Effects of positioning and exercise on intracranial pressure on a neurosurgical intensive care unit. Physical Therapy 77: 1682–1689

Bromley I 1998 Tetraplegia and paraplegia: a guide for physiotherapists, 5th edn. Churchill Livingstone, London

Brown P 1994 Pathophysiology of spasticity. Journal of Neurology, Neurosurgery and Psychiatry 57: 773–777

Brownlee S, Williams S J 1987 Physiotherapy in the respiratory care of patients with high spinal injury. Physiotherapy 33: 148–152

Brucia J, Rudy E 1996 The effect of suction catheter insertion and tracheal stimulation in adults with severe brain injury. Heart & Lung 25: 295–303

Butler D S 1991 Mobilisation of the nervous system. Churchill Livingstone, London

Cailliet R 1980 The shoulder in hemiplegia, 5th edn. F A Davis, Philadelphia

Carriere B 1999 The 'swiss ball': an effective physiotherapy tool for patients, family and physiotherapists. Physiotherapy 85: 552–561

Chitnavis B, Polkey C 1998 Intracranial pressure monitoring. Care of the Critically Ill 14: 80–84

Chollet F, DiPiero V, Wise R J, Brooks D J, Dolan R J, Frackowiak R S 1991 The functional anatomy of motor recovery after stroke in humans: a study with positron emission tomography. Annals of Neurology 29: 63–71

Chudley S 1994 The effects of nursing activities on intracranial pressure. British Journal of Nursing 3: 454–459

Ciesla N 1989 Chest physiotherapy for special patients. In: MacKenzie C F (ed) Chest physiotherapy in the intensive care, 2nd edn. Williams & Wilkins, London

Cordo P J, Nashner L M 1982 Properties of postural adjustments associated with rapid arm movements. Journal of Neurophysiology 47: 287–302

Crawford H J, Jull G A 1993 The influence of thoracic posture and movement on the range of arm elevation. Physiotherapy Theory and Practice 9(3): 143–148

Crosby L, Parsons L C 1992 Cerebrovascular response of closed head injured patients to suctioning. Journal of Neuroscience Nursing 24: 40–48

Cruz J 1998 The first decade of continuous monitoring of jugular bulb oxyhemoglobin saturation. Management strategies and clinical outcome. Critical Care Medicine 26: 344–351

Daud O, Sett P, Burr R G, Silver J R 1993 The relationship of heterotopic ossification to passive movement in paraplegic patients. Disab Rehab 15(3): 114–118

Davies P M 1985 Steps to follow: a guide to the treatment of adult hemiplegia. Springer-Verlag, Berlin

Davies P M 1990 Right in the middle. Springer-Verlag, Berlin

Davies P M 1994 Starting again. Springer-Verlag, Berlin

Dexter F 1997 Research synthesis of controlled studies evaluating the effect of hypocapnia and airway protection on cerebral outcome. Journal of Neurosurgical Anesthesiology 9: 217–222

Dickstein R, Heffes Y, Laufer Y, Ben-Maim Z 1999 Activation of selected trunk muscles during symmetric functional activities in poststroke hemiparetic and hemiplegic patients. Journal of Neurology, Neurosurgery and Psychiatry 66: 218–221

Dufosse M, Massion J 1992 Posturo-kinetic interactions: modeling and modes of control. In: Stelmach G E, Requin J (eds) Tutorials in motor behaviour II. Elsevier Science Publishers, London

Edwards S 1998 The incomplete spinal lesion. In: Bromley I (ed) Tetraplegia and paraplegia: a guide for physiotherapists, 5th edn. Churchill Livingstone, London

Ersson U, Carlson H, Mellstrom A, Ponten U, Hed-strand U, Jakobsson S 1990 Observation on intracranial dynamics during respiratory physiotherapy in unconscious neurosurgical patients. Acta Anaesthesiologia Scandinavica 34: 99–103

Feldman Z, Robertson L, Contant C, Gopinath S, Grossman R 1997 Positive end expiratory pressure reduces intracranial compliance in the rabbit. Journal of Neurosurgical Anesthesiology 9: 175–179

Ferner R, Barnett M, Hughes R A C 1987 Management of Guillain–Barré syndrome. British Journal of Hospital Medicine Dec: 526–530

Fisher D, Frewen T, Swedlow D 1982 Increase in intracranial pressure during suctioning: stimulation vs rise in $PaCO_2$. Anesthesiology 57: 416–417.

Frank C, Akeson W H, Woo S L-Y, Amiel D, Coutts R D 1984 Physiology and therapeutic value of passive joint motion. Clinical Orthopaedics and Related Research 185: 113–125

Friedli W G, Hallett M, Simon S R 1984 Postural adjustments associated with rapid voluntary arm movements 1. Electromyographic data. Journal of Neurology, Neurosurgery and Psychiatry 47: 611–622

Gardner B, Theocleous F, Watt J, Krishnan K 1985 Ventilation or dignified death for patients with high tetraplegia. British Medical Journal 291: 1620–1622

Garradd J, Bullock M 1986 The effect of respiratory therapy on intracranial pressure in ventilated neurosurgical patients. Australian Journal of Physiotherapy 32(2): 107–111

George R 1983 Duration of suctioning. An important variable. Respiratory Care 28: 457–459

German K 1988 Interpretation of ICP pulse waves to determine intracerebral compliance. Journal of Neurosurgical Nursing December 20: 344–349

Goldman J, Rose L, Williams S, Silver J, Denison D 1986 Effect of abdominal binders on breathing in tetraplegic patients. Thorax 41: 940–945

Goldspink G, Williams P 1990 Muscle fibre and connective tissue changes associated with use and disuse. In: Ada L, Canning C (eds) Key issues in neurological

physiotherapy: physiotherapy foundations for practice. Butterworth-Heinemann, Oxford

Hall T, Hepburn M, Elvey R L 1993 The effect of lumbosacral posture on a modification of the straight leg raise test. Physiotherapy 79(8): 566–570

Hasler D 1981 Developing a sense of symmetry. Therapy Aug 27: 3

Imle P, Mars M, Ciesla N, Anderson P, Delaney P 1997 The effect of chest physical therapy on intracranial pressure and cerebral perfusion pressure. Physiotherapy Canada Winter: 48–55

Irwin-Carruthers S, Runnalls M J 1980 Painful shoulder in hemiplegia: prevention and treatment. South African Journal of Physiotherapy 36: 18–23

Jackson J 1998 Specific treatment techniques. In: Stokes M (ed) Neurological physiotherapy. Mosby, London

Johnson S M, Omery A, Nikas D 1989 Neurological aspects of critical care, effects of conversation on intracranial pressure in comatosed patients. Heart and Lung 18(1): 56–63

Kelly B J, Luce J M 1991 The diagnosis and management of neuromuscular diseases causing respiratory failure. Chest 99: 1485–1493

Kerr M, Brucia J 1993 Hyperventilation in the head injured patient. An effective treatment modality. Heart & Lung Nov/Dec: 516–522

Kerr M E, Rudy E B, Brucia J, Stone K S 1993 Head injured adults: recommendations for endotracheal suctioning. Journal of Neuroscience Nursing 25(2): 86–91

Kerr M, Lovasik D, Dorby J 1995 Evaluating cerebral oxygenation using jugular venous oximetry in head injuries. AACN Clinical Issues 6: 11–20

Kerr M, Rudy E, Webber B et al 1997 Effect of short duration hyperventilation during endotracheal suctioning on intracranial pressure in severe head injured adults. Nursing Research 46: 195–201

Kerr M, Sereika S, Orndoff P et al 1998 Effect of neuromuscular blockers and opiates on the cerebrovascular response to endotracheal suctioning in adults with severe head injuries. American Journal of Critical Care. 7: 205–217

Klein-Vogelbach S 1990 Functional kinetics: observing, analysing and teaching human movement. Springer-Verlag, Berlin

Kozlowski D A, James D C, Schallert T 1996 Use-dependent exaggeration of neuronal injury after unilateral sensorimotor cortex lesions. Journal of Neuroscience 16: 4776–4786

Lee S 1989 Intracranial pressure changes during positioning of patients with severe head injury. Heart & Lung 18(4): 411–414

Leurssen T, Marshall F 1990 The medical management of head injury. In: Braakman R (ed) Handbook of clinical neurology: head injury. Elsevier, Amsterdam, pp 207–247

Lewis Y 1989 Use of the gymnastic ball in adult hemiplegia. Physiotherapy 75(7): 421–424

Lindsay K, Bone I 1997 Neurology and neurosurgery illustrated, 3rd edn. Churchill Livingstone, London

Lippitt S, Matsen F 1993 Mechanics of glenohumeral joint stability. Clinical Orthopaedics and Related Research 291: 20–28

Maitland G D 1986 Vertebral manipulation, 5th edn. Butterworth, London

Mansel J K, Norman J R 1990 Respiratory complications and management of spinal cord injuries. Chest 97: 1446–1451

March K, Mitchell P, Grady S, Winn R 1990 Effect of backrest position on intracranial and cerebral perfusion pressures. Journal of Neuroscience Nursing 22(6): 375–381

Marsden C D 1984 Motor disorders in basal ganglia disease. Human Neurobiology 2: 245–250

Miltner W H R, Bauder H, Sommer M, Dettmers C, Taub E 1999 Effect of constraint-induced movement therapy on patients with chronic motor deficits after stroke. A replication. Stroke 30: 586–592

Mitchell P H, Ozuna J, Lipe H P 1981 Moving the patient in bed: effects of turning on intracranial pressure. Nursing Research 30: 212–216

Nelles G, Spieckermann G, Jueptner M et al 1999 Reorganisation of sensory and motor systems in hemiplegic stroke patients. Stroke 30: 1510–1516

Nudo R J 1999 Recovery after damage to motor cortical areas. Current Opinion in Neurobiology 9: 740–747

Odell M 1996 Intracranial pressure monitoring: nursing in a district general ICU. Nursing in critical care 1: 245–247

Panturin E, Stokes M 1998 Musculoskeletal treatment concepts applied to neurology. In: Stokes M (ed) Neurological physiotherapy. Mosby, London

Paratz J, Burns Y 1993 The effect of respiratory physiotherapy on intracranial pressure, mean arterial pressure, cerebral perfusion pressure and end tidal carbon dioxide in ventilated neurosurgical patients. Physiotherapy Theory and Practice 9: 3–11

Parsons C, Shogan J 1984 The effects of the endotracheal tube suctioning/manual hyperventilation procedure on patients with severe closed head injuries. Heart & Lung 13: 372–380

Parton M, Lyall P, Leigh P 1999 Motor neurone disease and its management. Journal of the Royal College of Physicians of London 33: 212–218

Pope P M 1992 Management of the physical condition in patients with chronic and severe neurological pathologies. Physiotherapy 78(12): 896–903

Pope P M, Bowes C E, Tudor M 1991 Surgery combined with continuing post-operative stretching and management for knee flexion contractures in cases of multiple sclerosis – a report of six cases. Clinical Rehabilitation 5: 15–23

Prasad A, Tasker R 1990 Guidelines for the physiotherapy management of critically ill children with acutely raised intracranial pressure. Physiotherapy 76(4): 248–250

Pryor J, Webber B 1998 Physiotherapy for respiratory and cardiac problems. Churchill Livingstone, London

Reilly P, Lewis S 1997 Progress in head injury management. Journal of Clinical Neuroscience 4: 9–15

Rising C 1993 The relationship of selected nursing activities to ICP. Journal of Neuroscience Nursing 25(5): 302–307

Rosner M, Rosner S, Johnson A 1995 Cerebral perfusion pressure: management protocol and clinical results. Journal of Neurosurgery 83: 949–960

Roth E J, Lu A, Primacks S et al 1997 Ventilatory function in cervical and high thoracic spinal cord injury. American Journal of Physical Medicine & Rehabilitation 76: 262–266

Rothwell J C 1994 Control of human voluntary movement, 2nd edn. Chapman and Hall, London

Rudy E, Baun M, Stone K, Turner B 1986 The relationship between endotracheal suctioning and changes in intracranial pressure. A review of the literature. Heart & Lung 15: 488–494

Rudy E, Turner B, Baum M, Stone K, Brucia J 1991 Endotracheal suctioning in adults with head injury. Heart & Lung 20: 667–674

Shacklock M 1995 Neurodynamics. Physiotherapy 81(1): 9–16

Shalit M N, Umansky F 1977 Effects of routine bedside procedures on intracranial pressure. Israel Journal of Medical Science 13(9): 881–886

Shumway-Cook A, Woollacott M 1995 Motor control. Theory and applications. Williams & Wilkins, London

Silva A, Luginbuhl M 1981 Balancing act treatment. Therapy Aug 27: 3

Silver J R 1969 Heterotopic ossification: a clinical study of its possible relationship to trauma. Paraplegia 7: 220–230

Simmons B 1997 Management of intracranial hemodynamics in the adult: a research analysis of head positioning and recommendations for clinical practice and future research. Journal of Neuroscience Nursing 29: 44–49

Simonds A 1996 Non invasive ventilation in progressive neuromuscular disease and patients with multiple handicaps. In: Simonds A (ed) Non invasive respiratory support. Chapman and Hall, Oxford

Snyder M 1983 Relation of nursing activities to increases in intracranial pressure. Journal of Advanced Nursing 8: 273–279

Soryal I, Sinclair E, Hornby J, Pentland B 1992 Impaired joint mobility in Guillain–Barré syndrome: a primary or a secondary phenomenon? Journal of Neurology, Neurosurgery and Psychiatry 55: 1014–1017

Tardieu C, Lespargot A, Tabary C, Bret M D 1988 For how long must the soleus muscle be stretched each day to prevent contracture? Developmental Medicine and Child Neurology 30: 3–10

Taub E, Miller N E, Novack T A et al 1993 Technique to improve chronic motor deficit after stroke. Archives of Physical Medicine and Rehabilitation 74: 347–354

Thornton H, Kilbride C 1998 Physical management of abnormal tone and movement. In: Stokes M (ed) Neurological physiotherapy. Mosby, London

Tobin M J 1989 Essentials of critical care medicine. Churchill Livingstone, London

Van der Lee J H, Wagenaar R C, Lankhorst G J, Vogelaar T W, Deville W L, Bouter L M 1999 Forced use of the upper extremity in chronic stroke patients. Results from a single-blind randomised clinical trial. Stroke 30: 2369–2375

Wainwright S, Gould D 1996 Endotracheal suctioning in adults with severe head injury. Literature review. Intensive and Critical Care Nursing 12: 303–308

Ward T 1998 Spinal Injuries. In: Pryor J, Webber B A (eds) Physiotherapy for respiratory and cardiac problems. Churchill Livingstone, London

Warren J B 1983 Pulmonary complications associated with severe head injury. Journal of Neuroscience Nursing 15(4): 194–200

Weiller C, Ramsay S C, Wise R J, Friston K J, Frackowiak R S 1993 Individual patterns of functional reorganisation in the human cerebral cortex after capsular infarction. Annals of Neurology 33: 181–189

Williams A, Coyne S 1993 Effects of neck position on intracranial pressure. American Journal of Critical Care 2: 68–71

Williams P E 1990 Use of intermittent stretch in the prevention of serial sarcomere loss in immobilised muscle. Annals of Rheumatic Diseases 49: 316–317

Wolf S L, Lecraw D E, Barton L A, Jann B B 1989 Forced use of hemiplegic upper extremities to reverse the effect of learned nonuse among chronic stroke and head injured patients. Experimental Neurology 104: 125–132

Wong W P 1998 Use of body positioning in the mechanically ventilated patient with acute respiratory failure: application of Sackett's rules of evidence. Physiotherapy Theory and Practice 15: 25–41

Yarkony G M, Sahgal V 1987 Contractures: a major complication of craniocerebral trauma. Clinical Orthopaedics and Related Research 219: 93–96

Young C 1984 Recommended guidelines for suction. Physiotherapy 10(3): 106–108

7

Drug treatment of neurological disability

Alan J. Thompson

INTRODUCTION

The use of drugs in the treatment of neurological disorders falls broadly into two main groups. The first is the utilisation of drug treatment in order to influence the disease process itself. This may be:

- as replacement therapy, as is the case with dopamine-containing compounds in Parkinson's disease
- suppressing disease activity, as with the use of beta interferon in multiple sclerosis, or
- limiting damage, as in the acute treatment of stroke with fibrinolytic agents.

It is perhaps worth noting that in few, if any, of these conditions is drug therapy alone sufficient in the long-term management. There is almost invariably the need for input from therapists and other practitioners who make up the neurological multidisciplinary team.

The second indication for drug therapy is to manage symptoms common to many neurological disorders. While many of these symptoms, particularly those found in chronic and progressive conditions, are related to disorders of movement such as spasticity, rigidity, dystonia, myoclonus and ataxia with tremor, additional symptoms such as neuralgic pain, which can respond to carbamazepine (Tegretol), may also be major factors in influencing outcome. In some neurological conditions, two or more movement disorders may coexist. This has a cumulative effect on disability, making management even more complex: for example, spasticity and ataxia in multiple sclerosis (MS) and spasticity and chorea in cerebral palsy. When symptoms are very severe, it may be difficult to differentiate between them, for example spasticity and rigidity.

This chapter focuses on the drug treatment of this movement-related subset of symptoms, primarily spasticity, ataxia and extrapyramidal disorders, which have been discussed in Chapter 5. It will not discuss the treatment of Parkinson's disease in great detail, as this would warrant a chapter of its own. For a more detailed discussion of the comprehensive management of this condition the reader is referred to a recent review article by Colcher & Stern (1999). Discussion of any movement-related symptoms must be prefaced by the statement that the management of symptoms such as spasticity must be firmly based on therapy input, and incorporate patient education. Furthermore, the success or otherwise of drugs such as antispasticity agents is dependent on guidance by the therapist, who can evaluate their effect while also being aware of their potential disadvantages. An example of this is the potential of antispasticity agents to exacerbate an already weak hypotonic trunk.

SPASTICITY

Spasticity is a common, disabling symptom which is seen in a wide range of neurological disorders including spinal cord and head injury, stroke, multiple sclerosis (70% of patients) and the rarer hereditary spastic paraplegias (Reid 1999). It is a complex, poorly understood symptom which is a component of the upper motor neurone syndrome and is associated with structural changes in the muscles (thixotrophy) leading to further resistance to movement and shortening (see Ch. 5). Spasticity may be associated with pain and discomfort, which may be chronic or influenced/exacerbated by spasms.

In multiple sclerosis the lower limbs are more markedly affected by spasticity than the arms (Kesselring & Thompson 1997). Extensor hypertonus of the legs, particularly of the quadriceps, might be considered advantageous for standing, walking and transferring but this is at the expense of selective movement (Latash & Anson 1996,

---

Box 7.1 Impact of spasticity
Mobility 　Gait 　Transfers 　　bed to chair 　　toilet 　　car **Dexterity** 　Bed mobility 　Feeding 　Writing 　Personal care **Bladder management** **Bulbar function** 　Swallowing 　Respiration 　Communication

---

Dietz 1997). Sudden loss of tone may occur when the muscle reaches a certain crucial length as a result of increasing resistance and progressive stretching. Functionally, spasticity can reduce mobility and dexterity (Box 7.1), while spasms may prevent transfers and comfortable sitting and lying posture, and affect sleep.

Treatment of spasticity should not be aimed at its removal *per se* but rather at improving function, easing care or alleviating pain (Fig. 7.1). Key components in the management of spasticity include patient education and physiotherapy input. This should include awareness that noxious stimuli such as urinary tract infections, bowel impaction and ingrown toenails may worsen spasticity (Box 7.2) and should emphasise the importance of correct positioning in lying and sitting and the value of a standing programme.

Box 7.2 Spasticity: aggravating factors
Urinary tract infections Bowel impaction Skin irritation/ulceration Ingrowing toe nails Increased sensory stimuli from tight fitting clothes or orthoses Deep venous thrombosis

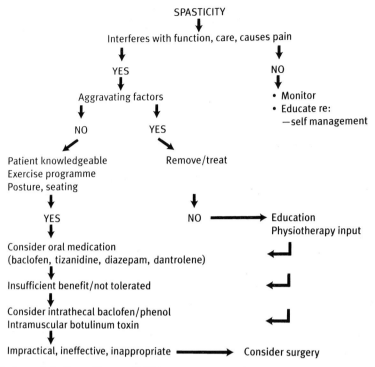

Figure 7.1   Treatment of spasticity (from Sheean 1998b).

Treatment may be divided into oral therapy, drugs given by other routes (intrathecal, intraneural and intramuscular) and surgery. The choice of agent will be influenced by the clinical setting. For example, intrathecal baclofen (ITB) may be more appropriate for severe spastic paraparesis, as occurs in multiple sclerosis, while intramuscular botulinum toxin may be used in more focal spasticity. It must be remembered that whatever treatment is chosen it should be associated with therapy input. Furthermore, in chronic progressive conditions such as MS, spasticity tends to change over time and it is important to re-evaluate treatment at regular intervals.

There are relatively few trials of antispasticity agents and those that exist are usually of small numbers where the pattern of spasticity is inadequately described, the objectives of treatment are not specified and only short- to medium-term outcomes are assessed. In clinical practice, it is suggested that only one substance at a time be used, although there may be rationale for combining drugs if a single agent is ineffective or

only partially effective. Of the agents available, baclofen has undergone most evaluation, both of the oral and intrathecal routes, and tizanidine has been the most recently licensed drug in the UK and the USA. Most of the studies have been carried out 20–30 years ago and many have focused on spinal cord injury. Recent studies have provided data for the use of botulinum toxin and intrathecal baclofen. The management of severe spasticity may be best provided by a multidisciplinary clinic which incorporates neurological, physiological and physiotherapy expertise and can provide a wide range of treatment options (Thompson 1998).

Oral therapy

Baclofen

This γ-aminobutyric acid (GABA) B receptor agonist acts mainly on the presynaptic and postsynaptic terminals of primary fibres of the spinal cord both to reduce the release of amino acids and to antagonise their actions. It is particularly useful in the treatment of painful spasms and increased tone of spinal origin, though functional benefits have been more difficult to demonstrate. In a large study of 759 patients with MS, 70% of patients showed marked improvements in spasticity (defined as a two-step reduction on the Ashworth Scale) and flexor spasms (Sachais et al 1997). A beneficial effect on spasms and hypertonicity was also seen in a small double-blind placebo-controlled cross-over study which involved 22 patients (Duncan et al 1976). The efficacy of baclofen has been shown to be equal to, if not greater than, that of diazepam (Jones et al 1970, Roussan et al 1985). Baclofen is given three times a day in doses starting at 5–10 mg in stepwise increases until the desired effect is achieved and/or side-effects such as drowsiness, fatigue and muscle weakness become unacceptable, usually reaching a dose of between 40 and 80 mg a day. Side-effects are reported in up to 45% of patients (Hattab 1980). Abrupt discontinuation may result in withdrawal symptoms, which include hallucinations and seizures.

Tizanidine

This imidazoline derivative, which is closely related to clonidine, acts by stimulating α_2-adrenergic receptors in the spinal cord (Wagstaff & Bryson 1997). A number of studies have suggested that its efficacy is similar to baclofen (Stien et al 1987) and more recently it was evaluated in two double-blind, placebo-controlled trials in the UK and USA involving 187 and 220 patients, respectively (Smith et al 1994, UK Tizanidine Trial Group 1994). In the American trial, tizanidine reduced spasms and clonus significantly but had no effect on spasticity as measured on the Ashworth Scale and, although the patients rated the drug significantly better on efficacy, the assessing physician did not. In the UK trial, a 20% reduction in spasticity was reported and 75% of patients on tizanidine reported a subjective benefit without an increase in muscle weakness. However, no improvement in mobility-related activities of daily living was found. The sug-

gestion that it may not cause weakness is of therapeutic value (Emre 1990). It is suggested that it be started at a low dose, 2 mg three times a day, and increased gradually up to a maximum of between 18 and 36 mg. The most frequent side-effects are tiredness, drowsiness and dry mouth. Liver function tests need to be checked before and after treatment, as transient hepatotoxicity may occur.

Dantrolene and benzodiazepines

Few studies have evaluated the role of these drugs or compared their efficacy in the management of spasticity. Dantrolene has a peripheral target of action and exerts its effect within the muscle itself by inhibiting the release of calcium ions from the sacroplasmic reticulum, and thereby preventing muscle contraction. Therefore it is, theoretically, a useful additional agent if centrally acting drugs are not effective. It is thought to be more useful in treating spasms and clonus than hypertonicity (Joynt 1976) and long-term benefit has been documented (Ketel & Kolb 1984). However, it is poorly tolerated, with side-effects including drowsiness, weakness and fatigue, and occasionally hepatotoxicity, which may be irreversible.

Benzodiazepines have three potential anti-spasticity actions: suppression of sensory impulses from muscle and skin receptors, potentiation of GABA action postsynaptically and inhibition of excitatory descending pathways (Cook & Nathan 1967, Bakheit 1996). Benzodiazepine efficacy has been evaluated in a small, double-blind, cross-over trial of 21 patients with spastic paraparesis (Wilson & McKechnie 1966). It may be used as additional therapy in resistant cases of spasticity; its role is limited by side-effects, including drowsiness and dependence.

Other oral agents

A range of drugs have been tried in spasticity, and reports involving small numbers have appeared in the literature. These include clonazepam, memantine, glycine, L-threonine, vigabatrin and, more recently, gabapentin (Dietz &

Young 1996). There is an increasing pressure to evaluate the role of cannabinoids in spasticity in MS, and a major study is about to commence in the UK.

Other routes

Intrathecal baclofen and phenol

In very severe spasticity, high doses of oral agents are likely to be either ineffective or not tolerated and drugs may be best given intrathecally, via a subcutaneously placed infusion pump. Although this may be considered an invasive treatment, it is very efficient and less than one-hundredth of the oral dose is required to achieve the required effect. This route was originally described by Kelly & Gautier-Smith (1959) for the use of phenol and has more recently been evaluated by Penn et al (1989) for baclofen. Dramatic effects on both tone, as measured by the Ashworth Scale, and spasm frequency were seen in MS and spinal cord injury. Some effect on function, particularly relating to transfers and self-care, has also been reported but few investigators have evaluated a potential effect on quality of life (Campbell et al 1995). The effect is initially tested by bolus injection of 25–100 mg given via a lumbar puncture before continuous drug application through an electronically programmed drug delivery system. Long-term treatment using ITB has been evaluated and found to be beneficial (Ochs et al 1989). The main complications are technical and include pump malfunction, catheter-related problems (kinking, breaking, displacement), local inflammation and, rarely, spinal meningitis. Although the original studies were restricted to patients who were wheelchair bound, ITB is now being used with encouraging results in more ambulant patients. It should be used as part of a goal-orientated rehabilitation programme and careful assessment and selection is essential (Leary et al 2000).

There has been a recent resurgence in interest in intrathecal phenol (4 mg or 2.5 mg in glycerine) which may be useful in improving care and posture in severely disabled patients who no longer have bowel and bladder functio.. .... whom sensation in the lower limbs is absent. In a recent retrospective study of 21 patients, 16 of whom had MS, benefit was seen in all patients, which translated into functional gains in 18 (Pinder & Bhakta 1999).

Intramuscular botulinum toxin (BTX)

Although initially introduced for focal dystonia (see page 109), it was not long before the potential of BTX to reduce focal spasticity was recognised. The current situation has been summarised in a number of recent reviews (O'Brien 1997, Sheean 1998b, Richardson & Thompson 1999). Its use has been evaluated to a greater or lesser extent in stroke, MS (Hyman et al 2000), spinal cord injury (Burbaud et al 1996) and in a range of conditions resulting in upper limb spasticity (Richardson et al 1997, Simpson et al 1999) and in both upper and lower limb spasticity (Richardson et al 2000). Intramuscular botulinum toxin weakens muscles by producing neuromuscular junction blockade. It is taken up by the presynaptic nerve terminal where it prevents binding of acetylcholine vesicles to the presynaptic membrane, inhibiting their release and causing the muscle to become functionally 'denervated'. Thus it is possible to produce focal, selective, graded muscular weakness, which is temporary. The transient effect may be seen as a potential disadvantage in some clinical scenarios but there is a fundamental difference in the treatment philosophy of spasticity from that of focal dystonia. In spasticity it is anticipated that the reduced tone will facilitate the therapy input such that there will be a functional change which will in itself prevent the tone increasing when the effect of the toxin wears off. The advantages and disadvantages of botulinum toxin treatment are listed in Table 7.1.

Studies to date tend to have small patient numbers and limited statistical evaluation. They vary in dosing regimes, electromyographic (EMG) guidance, follow-up regimes and clinical outcomes. Some utilise a cross-over regime (without always having a washout period), which may not be appropriate in this clinical context where patients often do not return to

Table 7.1 Advantages and disadvantages of botulinum toxin treatment

Advantages	Disadvantages
Effects are focal, selective, graded	Biological effects last only 3–4 months – repeated injections required
No CNS side-effects (e.g. sedation)	Effects are non-reversible during period of action
Works independently of pathophysiological mechanism of motor overactivity	Injection (painful) Limited maximal dose
No sensory disturbance[a]	May require EMG guidance
Non-destructive[a] Closed procedure[a] Weakness resolves spontaneously Safe and well tolerated	

[a] Compared with phenol injection

baseline. The largest study carried out to date, that of Richardson et al (2000), looked at 57 patients with distal spasticity of either the upper or lower limb resulting from a single incident affecting the brain or the spinal cord. Benefits were seen in the Ashworth Scale, Rivermead Mobility Assessment (lower limb) and a subjective problem rating scale. No effect was detected in upper limb function or goal achievement.

This paper raised a number of clinical issues which are essential for the optimum use of this therapy (some of which have already been mentioned in the context of other interventions but warrant repetition):

1. *Identification of the clinical problem.* This may include (a) pain; (b) restriction of movement, for example, at the elbow or wrist; (c) excessive/inappropriate movement, such as a positive support response or an associated reaction. This may limit function, prevent physiotherapy input including the use of an orthosis, or prevent personal/nursing care.
2. *Evaluation of the clinical problem.* The treatment of focal spasticity must consider the clinical context which is invariably complex and is best evaluated by a multidisciplinary team, which includes a neurophysiotherapist, neurologist/neurorehabilitation physician and

neurophysiologist. Experienced neurophysiotherapists have invaluable knowledge of the functional anatomy and dynamics of movement and can, perhaps, best predict the consequences of weakening muscles. They also play an essential role in ensuring appropriate therapy to maximise the effect of the toxin. Electromyographic assessment can be helpful by (1) establishing the relative contribution of neural and biomechanical components to the hypertonia – hypertonia predominantly due to soft tissue changes is unsuitable for BTX injections; (2) identifying the overactive muscles, as not all agonists may behave the same way – this helps to select the muscles and dose; (3) providing some indication of the muscle activity, particularly the antagonists. The neurologist/neurorehabilitationist guides therapy and integrates BTX injections with other medical treatments.

3. *Setting treatment goals.* A double-blind, placebo-controlled, dose-ranging study of botulinum toxin in 74 patients with multiple sclerosis and severe adductor spasticity demonstrated benefit over placebo in muscle tone, distance between knees and hygiene scores (Hymen et al 2000). Generally, however, botulinum toxin is considered to be more useful in the treatment of distal muscles in the arms and legs and most practitioners are discouraged by the frequent large doses required for adductor spasticity in MS.

ATAXIA

Ataxia may be defined as a lack of or reduction in coordination and is invariably associated with tremor, i.e. an involuntary, rhythmic, oscillatory movement of a body part. These symptoms occur in patients with multiple sclerosis (up to 75%), the hereditary ataxias and any pathology affecting the cerebellum, including vascular disease and tumours. They are severely disabling and embarrassing, affecting upper limb function, gait and, in severe cases, standing and sitting balance. In MS, tremor is frequently just one component of a complex movement disorder which includes dysmetria and other ataxic features, and the

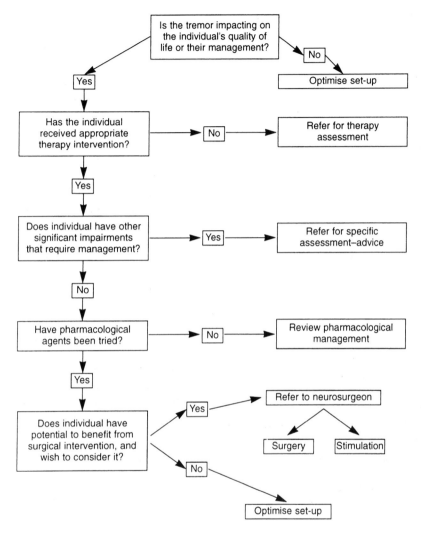

Figure 7.2   Management of ataxia.

underlying mechanisms are poorly understood (Alusi et al 1999). Although inflammatory demyelination in different parts of the cerebellum and related areas may produce a distinct tremor, nonetheless it is extremely difficult to classify individual tremors in patients. It remains one of the most difficult symptoms to manage and is associated with a poor outcome in rehabilitation (Langdon & Thompson 1999).

As with spasticity, there are practical components to the management of ataxia, which must be considered prior to other interventions (Fig. 7.2).

These include patient education, improving posture and proximal stability during activities and the provision of equipment (see Ch. 5). Weights have not proved to be very successful, although they may be more beneficial if a computer damping device is incorporated (Aisen et al 1993), and a small exploratory study of therapy input suggested modest benefit (Jones et al 1996). Other treatments may be divided into drug therapy, which is limited and often not well tolerated, and more invasive surgical intervention which includes thalamotomy and thalamic stimulation.

Medical treatment

Few drugs have been evaluated and none adequately. Isoniazid (with pyridoxine) has been shown to be of limited benefit in a number of small studies (Duquette et al 1985), producing some effect in 10 of 13 patients, although this did not translate into improved function, while four of six patients showed sufficient benefit that they wished to continue the drug (Hallett et al 1985). It is thought to be more useful in postural tremor with an intention component rather than pure intention tremor. Up to 1200 mg a day in divided doses has been used, increasing gradually from 200 mg twice a day. This drug is not well tolerated and causes gastrointestinal disturbance.

There has been even less evaluation of other drugs, including carbamazepine, clonazapam and buspirone. Ethyl alcohol and propranalol have not been found to be useful (Koller 1984). A single-blind cross-sectional study evaluated the role of carbamazepine in cerebellar tremor in 10 patients and suggested some benefit (Sechi et al 1989). More recently, the 5-HT3 antagonist ondansetron has been evaluated, given both by intravenous (Rice et al 1997) and oral routes (Rice et al 1999). Although the intravenous studies looked promising, the more recent placebo-controlled, double-blind parallel group study was negative. Fifty-two patients, the majority of whom had MS, were randomised and the treatment arm received 8 mg per day for 1 week. While some benefit in the nine-hole peg test was seen in the treated arm, there was no difference between the groups on the global ataxia rating scale. However, some benefit was seen in patients with hereditary ataxia.

Surgical intervention

Thalamotomy of the ventral intermediate nucleus (VIM) has been shown to be beneficial in controlling tremor in Parkinson's disease. There has been limited evaluation of its role in tremor relating to MS but it does not appear to be as effective in this condition. In selected patients with MS, thalamotomy has been reported to alleviate contralateral limb tremor, initially in about 65–96% of cases, although in about 20% tremor returns within 12 months (Obeso et al 1997). Functional improvement is estimated to occur in only 25–75% of patients. However, these results are not based on controlled studies, and no prospective study has evaluated the influence of this procedure on overall disability, handicap and quality of life, nor have side-effects been quantified, though they may occur in up to 45% of cases. Serious side-effects, including hemiparesis, dysphasia and dysphagia, occur in up to 10% of patients. Experience suggests that in MS optimum results are obtained in patients with relatively stable disease, good mobility and minimal overall disability status – an extremely small group.

Three recent papers have suggested that thalamic stimulation can also alleviate tremor in up to 69% of patients in studies involving 13, 5 and 15 patients, respectively (Geny et al 1996, Whittle et al 1998, Montgomery et al 1999). These were carefully selected patients; for example, the 5 patients reported by Whittle et al (1998) were from an initial group of 17 patients and no control study has as yet been carried out. Serious side-effects were seen in 2 of 15 patients in the study by Montgomery et al (1999). No trial has compared thalamic stimulation versus lesioning, though it is suggested that stimulation is associated with fewer side-effects (Nguyen et al 1996, Haddow et al 1997, Schuurman et al 2000). Other approaches, including extracranial application of brief AC pulsed electromagnetic fields, dynamic systems with multidegrees of freedom, orthoses and robotic arms based on virtual reality, have not been adequately evaluated.

EXTRAPYRAMIDAL DISORDERS

Parkinsonism, which consists of tremor, rigidity and bradykinesia, is the most common disorder involving this area. The most common cause is Parkinson's disease (70% of cases), which usually results in major disability across all areas of function including mobility, self-care and communication. Treatment of the clinical manifestations of the condition is essentially by dopamine replacement therapy although input from a wide range of therapies may also be appropriate at specific stages of the condition (Colcher & Stern 1999).

There are other extrapyramidal disorders which produce a variety of movement disorders. They include multisystem atrophy and corticobasal degeneration and do not have a specific treatment (Quinn 1995). Features which should alert the clinician that the diagnosis may not be Parkinson's disease include:

- presence of early instability or falls
- pyramidal or cerebellar signs
- downgaze palsy
- early autonomic failure
- dementia.

Extrapyramidal movement disorders may also occur in isolation. These include the dystonias, which may be generalised but are more often focal, myoclonus, hemiballismus, chorea and athetosis.

Parkinson's disease

Levodopa treatment remains the mainstay of the therapeutic management of Parkinson's disease and is the most effective drug for the alleviation of symptoms and signs of the condition (Marsden 1994, Bhatia et al 1998, Olanow & Kollar 1998). It is usually prescribed in association with a dopa-decarboxylase inhibitor which reduces conversion of levodopa to dopamine outside the brain, so limiting peripheral unwanted side-effects and increasing the delivery of levodopa to the brain. The most common early side-effect is nausea, which usually responds to ingestion with meals. Long-term treatment is associated with fluctuations in level of mobility, a variety of dyskinesias and psychiatric manifestations including hallucinations and confusion.

After using levodopa for 3–8 years, patients often develop motor fluctuations and peak-dose dyskinesias and these can prove extremely difficult to manage (Stocchi et al 1997). It has been suggested, though not proven, that these may be delayed by using slow-release formulations. The monoamine oxidase type B inhibitor selegiline reduces the breakdown of endogenous dopamine and has a modest beneficial effect on symptoms. Its use in early Parkinson's disease may delay the need for levodopa therapy. However, it has been suggested that its use, together with levodopa, may be associated with increased mortality (Lees 1995, Parkinson Study Group 1996). Dopamine receptor agonists may also be used. These include existing agents such as apomorphine, bromocriptine, lysuride and pergolide and three newer agents: cabergoline, pramipexole (Clarke 2000) and ropinirole. Bromocriptine and lysuride have been used in early disease but with limited effect, while apomorphine tends to be used in the management of refractory motor fluctuations (Chaudhuri & Clough 1998, O'Sullivan & Lees 1999). This potent dopamine agonist is useful in advanced Parkinson's and reliably reverses levodopa induced off-period motor disability. It needs to be given parenterally (subcutaneously) because of its frequent adverse reactions and has a rapid onset and short duration of action. It can be given in an intermittent or continuous fashion, which is usually preceded by a challenge dose. The threshold dose determined during the apomorphine challenge is usually doubled to determine the therapeutic dose, which is typically between 1 and 5 mg. Injections using insulin-type syringes are usually given into the lower abdominal wall. However, continuous subcutaneous infusions are sometimes used in patients who require very frequent intermittent injections. A number of groups have demonstrated a reduction of at least 50% of the time spent 'off' per day after commencing intermittent or continuous subcutaneous apomorphine with efficacy maintained for up to 5 years (Frankel et al 1990). Anticholinergic agents, including biperiden, procyclidine, orphenadrine, benzhexol and benztropine, mildly improve parkinsonian symptoms and are used to treat tremor and rigidity rather than bradykinesia.

In the last decade there has been a resurgence of interest in the neurosurgical treatment of Parkinson's disease. Current targets for lesion operations include the motor thalamus (thalamotomy), the internal segment of the globus pallidus (pallidotomy) and the subthalamic nucleus (Obeso et al 1997). Thalamotomy is useful in drug-resistant tremor, but not for bradykinesia and rigidity, while it has been suggested that pallidotomy may be helpful in levodopa-induced dyskinesias. Deep brain stimulation of these areas may be as effective and cause less tissue destruction.

Dystonia

The dystonias are a group of neurological conditions characterised by sustained involuntary muscle contractions which lead to abnormal postures and movements (Fahn et al 1987). The spectrum of severity ranges from focal dystonia (affecting one part of the body) to generalised dystonia. Focal dystonia makes up 70% of cases and includes blepharospasm, torticollis or cervical dystonia (50% of all cases), spasmodic dysphonia and writers' cramp (Warner 1999). Cervical dystonia is characterised by involuntary activity of the neck muscles that results in abnormal head movements and pain. The mainstay of treatment for cervical dystonia and the other focal dystonias is botulinum toxin (Blackie & Lees 1990) which provides relief for up to 80% of patients for 3–4 months. In contrast to the use of this agent in spasticity, the toxin has to be given on a regular basis. This raises a number of issues, including the development of antibodies which may shorten the duration of the effect.

Other forms of treatment for cervical dystonia, which are usually considered when individuals do not respond to botulinum toxin, include selective peripheral denervation (Bertrand & Moligna-Negro 1988) and even deep brain stimulation (Krauss et al 1999).

Other agents are also available, including the anticholinergics mentioned above. Generalised dystonia, otherwise known as primary generalised idiopathic dystonia, usually begins in childhood and is an extremely difficult condition to treat. The best results have been obtained with high-dose anticholinergic therapy, but a minority of patients show some response to baclofen, carbamazepine, benzodiazepines or, paradoxically, both dopamine agonists and antagonists. There is a small group of patients with juvenile-onset dystonia which is exquisitely sensitive to levodopa. Botulinum toxin may be useful for focal problems, and both surgery and electrostimulation have been used.

Myoclonus

Among the other motor disorders, myoclonus is the most common and can present under a number of different guises including essential myoclonus, which presents in the first two decades and rarely progresses; nocturnal myoclonus, which covers a variety of different types of movement, not least of which is hypnic or hypnagogic jerks; post anoxic action myoclonus; and segmental myoclonus (Quinn 1996). There are some distinguishing clinical features among these, and readers are referred to the recent edition of *Neurology in Clinical Practice* for a review of these (Riley & Lang 2000). The most effective treatment for essential myoclonus is clonazepam, and sometimes anticholinergics may be beneficial. One of the forms of nocturnal myoclonus, termed periodic movements of sleep (PMS), may cause distress particularly if associated with restless legs syndrome; PMS may respond to levodopa, although agonists such as pergolide or ropinirole may provide a more sustained response. Other effective agents include clonazepam, gabapentin or opiates such as codeine.

Post anoxic action myoclonus emerges following coma and is often associated with epilepsy. It may severely curtail mobility and interfere with rehabilitation. It is thought to relate to serotonin deficiency and dramatic relief may be achieved by giving the serotonin precursor L-5-HTP together with carbidopa to prevent peripheral decarboxylation. Valproic acid and clonazepam are equally effective and piracetam may also be useful (Werhahn et al 1997). Segmental myoclonus, which includes palatal and spinal myoclonus, may respond to clonazepam, although it is often resistant to treatment. Tetrabenazine, 5-HTP, trihexyphenidyl, and carbamazepine may also be helpful.

COMBINATION OF PYRAMIDAL AND EXTRAPYRAMIDAL DYSFUNCTION

This combination poses particular problems and is seen following head injury and in cerebral palsy. The latter is a particularly challenging condition which is often poorly managed in adulthood. There is a suggestion that some people with this condition show functional deterioration over time, although it is unclear if this relates to neurological change or simply poor management of its motor symptoms (Green et al 1997). Careful assessment is essential in this patient population before deciding which, if any, of the current treatment options is appropriate. For example, both ITB and botulinum toxin are now licensed for the treatment of this condition.

SUMMARY

Drug therapy has a useful place in the overall management of neurological disability. Just as with any other intervention, to be effective, the selection or drug therapy needs to be based on a clear understanding of the presenting problem, and with an awareness of the potential advantages and disadvantages it may have for the patient's functioning and quality of life. Of crucial importance, communication between the neurologist, therapists and nursing staff must occur to ensure optimal drug treatment throughout the course of the disease.

REFERENCES

Aisen M L, Arnold A, Baiges I, Maxwell S, Rosen M 1993 The effect of mechanical damping loads on disabling action tremor. Neurology 43(7): 1346–1350

Alusi S H, Glickman S, Aziz T Z, Bain P G 1999 Tremor in multiple sclerosis (editorial). Journal of Neurology, Neurosurgery and Psychiatry 66: 131–134

Bakheit A M O 1996 Management of muscle spasticity. Critical Reviews in Physical Medicine and Rehabilitation 8(3): 235–252

Bertrand C B, Moligna-Negro P 1988 Selective peripheral denervation in 111 cases of spasmodic torticollis by selective denervation. Advances in Neurology 50: 637–643

Bhatia K, Brooks D J, Burn D J et al; The Parkinson's Disease Consensus Working Group 1998 Guidelines for the management of Parkinson's disease. Hospital Medicine 59: 469–476

Blackie J D, Lees A J 1990 Botulinum toxin treatment in spasmodic torticollis. Journal of Neurology, Neurosurgery and Psychiatry 53: 640–643

Burbaud P, Wiart L, Dubos J L et al 1996 A randomised, double blind, placebo controlled trial of botulinum toxin in the treatment of spastic foot in hemiparetic patients. Journal of Neurology, Neurosurgery and Psychiatry 61(3): 265–269

Campbell S K, Almeida S, Penn R D, Corcos D M 1995 The effects of intrathecally administered baclofen on function in patients with spasticity. Physical Therapy 75: 352–362

Chaudhuri K R, Clough C 1998 Subcutaneous apomorphine in Parkinson's disease. British Medical Journal 316(7132): 641 (editorial)

Clarke C E 2000 Management of early Parkinson's disease. Hospital Update supplement June

Colcher A, Stern M B 1999 Therapeutics in the neurorehabilitation of Parkinson's Disease. Neurorehabilitation and Neural Repair 13: 205–218

Cook J B, Nathan P W 1967 On the site of action of diazepam in spasticity in man. Journal of Neurological Science 5: 33–37

Dietz V 1997 Neurophysiology of gait disorders: present and future applications. Electroencephalography and Clinical Neurophysiology 103: 333–355

Dietz V, Young R R 1996 The syndrome of spastic paresis. In: Brandt T, Dichgans J (eds) Neurological disorders: course and treatment. Academic Press, New York

Duncan G W, Shahani B T, Young R R 1976 An evaluation of baclofen treatment for certain symptoms in patients with spinal cord lesions. Neurology 26: 441–446

Duquette P, Pleines J, du Souich P 1985 Isoniazid for tremor in multiple sclerosis: a controlled trial. Neurology 35(12): 1772–1775

Emre M 1990 Review of clinical trials with Tizanidine (Sirdalud) in spasticity. In: Emre M, Benecke R (eds) Spasticity. The current status of research and treatment. Cairnforth United Kingdom and Park Ridge USA, pp 153–184

Fahn S, Marsden C D, Calne D B 1987 Classification and investigation of dystonia. In: Fahn S, Marsden C D (eds) Neurology 7: Movement disorders 2. Butterworths, London

Frankel J P, Lees A J, Kempster P A, Stern G M 1990 Subcutaneous apomorphine in the treatment of Parkinson's disease. Journal of Neurology, Neurosurgery and Psychiatry 53: 96–101

Geny C, Nguyen J P, Pollin B et al 1996 Improvement of severe postural cerebellar tremor in multiple sclerosis by chronic thalamic stimulation. Movement Disorders 11(5): 489–494

Green C, Proch C, Gara S E 1997 The changing face of cerebral palsy: a review of the disorder and its treatment. Journal of Neurological Rehabilitation 11(4): 245–253

Haddow L J, Mumford C, Whittle I R 1997 Stereotactic treatment of tremor due to multiple sclerosis. Neurosurgery Quarterly 7: 23–34

Hallett M, Lindsey J W, Adelstein B D, Riley P O 1985 Controlled trial of isoniazid therapy for severe postural cerebellar tremor in multiple sclerosis. Neurology 35(9): 1374–1377

Hattab J R 1980 Review of European Clinical Trials with baclofen. In: Feldman R G, Young R R, Koella W P (eds) Spasticity: disordered motor control. Year Book, Chicago, pp 71–85

Hyman N, Barnes M, Bhakta B et al 2000 Botulinum toxin (Dysport®) treatment of hip adductor spasticity in multiple sclerosis; a prospective, randomised, double-blind, placebo-controlled, close-ranging study. Journal of Neurology, Neurosurgery and Psychiatry 68: 707–712

Jones L, Lewis Y, Harrison J, Wiles C M 1996 The effectiveness of occupational therapy and physiotherapy in multiple sclerosis patients with ataxia of the upper limb and trunk. Clinical Rehabilitation 10: 277–282

Jones R F, Burke D, Marosszeky J E, Gillies J D 1970 A new agent for the control of spasticity. Journal of Neurology, Neurosurgery and Psychiatry 33: 464–468

Joynt R 1976 Dantrolene sodium: long-term effects in patients with muscle spasticity. Archives of Physical Medicine and Rehabilitation 57: 212–217

Kelly R E, Gautier-Smith P C 1959 Intrathecal phenol in the treatment of reflex spasms and spasticity. Lancet ii: 1102–1105

Kesselring J, Thompson A J 1997 Spasticity, ataxia and fatigue in multiple sclerosis. In: Miller D H (ed) Baillière's clinical neurology: multiple sclerosis. Baillière Tindall, London, pp 429–445

Ketel W B, Kolb M E 1984 Long-term treatment with dantrolene sodium of stroke patients with spasticity limiting the return of function. Current Medical Research and Opinion 9: 161–169

Koller W C 1984 Pharmacologic trials in the treatment of cerebellar tremor. Archives of Neurology 41: 280–281

Krauss J K, Pohle T, Weber S, Ozdoba C, Burgunder J M 1999 Bilateral stimulation of globus pallidus internus for treatment of cervical dystonia. Lancet 354: 837–838

Langdon D W, Thompson A J 1999 Multiple sclerosis: a preliminary study of selected variables affecting rehabilitation outcome. Multiple Sclerosis 5: 94–100

Latash M L, Anson J G 1996 What are 'normal movements' in atypical populations? Behavioral and Brain Sciences 19: 55–106

Leary S M, Jarrett L, Porter B, Richardson D, Rosso T, Thompson A J (2000) A multi-disciplinary, goal-orientated approach to intrathecal baclofen therapy in progressive neurological disease. Journal of Neurology, Neurosurgery and Psychiatry 69: 412–413

Lees A J on behalf of the Parkinson's Disease Research Group of the United Kingdom 1995 Comparison of therapeutic effects and mortality data of levodopa and levodopa combined with selegiline in patients with early, mild Parkinson's disease. British Medical Journal 311: 1602–1607

Marsden C D 1994 Parkinson's disease. Journal of Neurology, Neurosurgery and Psychiatry 57: 672–681

Montgomery E B, Baker K B, Kinkel R P, Barnett G 1999 Chronic thalamic stimulation for the tremor of multiple sclerosis. Neurology 53: 625–628

Nguyen J, Feve A, Keravel Y 1996 Is electrostimulation preferable to surgery for upper limb ataxia? Current Opinion in Neurology 9(6): 445–450

Obeso J A, Guridi J, DeLong M 1997 Surgery for Parkinson's disease. Journal of Neurology, Neurosurgery and Psychiatry 62: 2–8

O'Brien C F 1997 Overview of clinical trials and published reports of botulinum toxin for spasticity. European Journal of Neurology (suppl 2) S11–13

Ochs G, Struppler A, Meyerson B A et al 1989 Intrathecal baclofen for long-term treatment of spasticity: a multi-centre study. Journal of Neurology, Neurosurgery and Psychiatry 52: 933–939

Olanow C W, Koller W C 1998 An algorithm for the management of Parkinson's disease: treatment guidelines. Neurology 50(suppl 3): 551–557

O'Sullivan J D, Lees A J 1999 Use of apomorphine in Parkinson's disease. Hospital Medicine 60: 816–820

Parkinson Study Group 1996 Impact of deprenyl and tocopherol treatment on Parkinson's disease in DATATOP subjects not requiring levodopa. Annals of Neurology 39: 29–36

Penn R D, Savoy S M, Corcos D et al 1989 Intrathecal baclofen for severe spinal spasticity. New England Journal of Medicine 320: 1517–1521

Pinder C, Bhakta B B 1999 Intrathecal phenol for severe lower limb spasticity – is there still a role? Joint meeting of BSRM and VRA

Quinn N 1995 Parkinsonism – recognition and differential diagnosis. British Medical Journal 310: 447–452

Quinn N 1996 Essential myoclonus and myoclonic dystonia. Movement Disorders 11: 119–124

Reid E 1999 The hereditary spastic paraplegias. Journal of Neurology 246: 995–1003

Rice G P A, Lesaux J, Vandervoort P, Macewan L, Ebers G C 1997 Ondansetron, a 5-HT3 antagonist, improves cerebellar tremor. Journal of Neurology, Neurosurgery and Psychiatry 62: 282–284

Rice G P A, Lescaux J, Ebers G 1999 Ondansetron versus placebo for disabling cerebellar tremor: final report of a randomized clinical trial. Abstract. Annals of Neurology 46: 493

Richardson D, Thompson A J 1999 Botulinum toxin: its use in the treatment of acquired spasticity in adults. Physiotherapy 85: 541–551

Richardson D, Edwards S, Sheean G L, Greenwood R J, Thomson A J 1997 The effect of botulinum toxin on hand function after incomplete spinal cord injury at the level of C5/6: a case report. Clinical Rehabilitation 11: 288–292

Richardson D, Werring D J, Sheean G et al (2000) A double blind, placebo controlled trial to evaluate the role of electromyography guided botulinum toxin type A in adults with focal limb spasticity. Journal of Neurology, Neurosurgery and Psychiatry 69: 499–506

Riley D E, Lang A E 2000 Movement disorders. In: Bradley W G, Daroff R B, Fenichel G M, Marsden C D (eds) Neurology in clinical practice. Vol 2, 3rd edn. Butterworth-Heinemann, Boston

Roussan M, Terrence C, Fromm G 1985. Baclofen versus diazepam for the treatment of spasticity and long-term follow-up of baclofen therapy. Pharmatherapeutica 4(5): 278–284

Sachais B A, Logue N, Carey M 1997 Baclofen: a new antispastic drug. Archives of Neurology 34: 422–428

Schuurman P R, Bosch D A, Bossuyt P M M et al 2000 A comparison of continuous thalamic stimulation and thalamotomy for suppression of severe tremor. New England Journal of Medicine 342(7): 461–468

Sechi G P, Zuddas M, Piredda M et al 1989 Treatment of cerebellar tremors with carbamazepine: a controlled trial with long-term follow-up. Neurology 39(8): 1113–1115

Sheean G 1998a Pathophysiology of spasticity. In: Sheean G (ed) Spasticity rehabilitation. Churchill Communications, Europe Ltd, London

Sheean G 1998b The treatment of spasticity with botulinum toxin. In: Sheean G (ed) Spasticity rehabilitation. Churchill Communications, Europe Ltd, London

Simpson D M, Alexander D N, O'Brien C F et al 1999 Botulinum toxin type A in the treatment of upper extremity spasticity: a randomized, double-blind, placebo-controlled trial. Neurology 46: 1306–1310

8

Case histories

Susan Edwards

INTRODUCTION

Rehabilitation is a problem-solving and educational process aimed at reducing the disability and handicap experienced by someone as a result of a disease, always within the limitations imposed by available resources and by the underlying disease (Wade 1992).

The definition of rehabilitation from the Oxford Dictionary is 'to restore to a good condition or for a new purpose'. This is most apt in describing the process of neurological rehabilitation where the aim is to maximise and maintain the residual capability. For this reason rehabilitation must be viewed along a continuum, from the preventive, early-stage management to the ongoing, continuing care of patients with chronic, residual disability.

Patients with different and varied pathologies require neurological rehabilitation. The patient, in most instances, is medically stable and able to participate in a rigorous programme of treatment. This is undertaken by all members of the multidisciplinary team and includes physiotherapists, occupational therapists, speech and language therapists, the nursing and medical staff and, in many cases, a social worker and clinical psychologist. It is therefore impossible to view neurological rehabilitation in professional isolation. Physiotherapy is but a part of the whole and unless the different members of the team complement one another's interventions, patients are unlikely to achieve their optimal level of recovery.

Most importantly, the patient must be involved in the planning of treatment, and in the setting of goals and objectives. This has been shown to increase the motivation and compliance of patients facing what is often an extensive course of rehabilitation (Kaye 1991). The long-term goal may be that the patient will walk independently, but it is important to provide stepping stones along the way, in the form of short-term goals, to enable the patient to realise that perhaps only small, but substantial progress is being made. Family and friends must also be involved in the treatment programme. This is especially important in the rehabilitation of patients with cognitive deficit. These patients may not be able to comply actively with treatment and it is often through the more constant input of the carers that positive changes can be implemented.

Many rehabilitation centres have been established to cater for the needs of people with neurological disability. Inevitably these units are more able to provide the full gamut of multi-disciplinary intervention and in so doing cater more effectively for the needs of the patients. However, it must be appreciated that not all patients who would benefit from neurological rehabilitation are successful in obtaining a place in such a unit. Many people with neurological disability continue to be treated in general hospitals where the emphasis is more on illness than on the promotion of independence. In this environment it is even more important to co-ordinate the professional/patient/carer intervention and, where appropriate, to enable the person with the disability to have responsibility for their management.

A problem-solving approach is of value in:

- the analysis of the prevailing symptoms
- the prevention of unwanted and unnecessary compensations
- the promotion of useful, necessary compensatory strategies to attain the optimal level of function.

The majority of patients with neurological disability demonstrate a complex and varied picture which is potentially changeable depending on the existing pathology and the environment in which they function. For example, a patient with an incomplete lesion of the spinal cord, in many instances, demonstrates an imbalance of muscle activity. If the less-affected muscle groups are allowed to dominate in the attainment of function, these muscles will become even stronger at the expense of potential recovery of the weaker muscle groups (Edwards 1998). Even if the muscle strength were to remain unaltered throughout the course of rehabilitation, the patient must be made aware of the danger of contracture and given advice as to the maintenance of range of movement. Recovery of weakened muscle groups is even more difficult if joint and muscle range is compromised.

The following case histories describe the rehabilitative process which may be instigated for patients with neurological disability.

PATIENT WITH A RIGHT HEMIPLEGIA FOLLOWING SURGERY FOR LEFT MIDDLE AND POSTERIOR FOSSA EXPLORATION AND REMOVAL OF CLIVUS MENINGIOMA

This patient presented with a dense right hemiplegia following his surgery. Physiotherapy commenced immediately post-surgery, his problems being identified as including:

1. inability to communicate
2. dysphagia
3. impairment of respiratory function
4. dense right hemiplegia
5. severe sensory impairment of the right side
6. lack of midline orientation, with neglect of the right side
7. overactivity of the left side, constantly pushing him over to his right
8. difficulty in sustaining an appropriate sitting posture due to the overactivity of his left side
9. inability to accept weight on his right side, making positioning in bed extremely difficult
10. lack of bladder and bowel control.

This patient illustrates the need for multi-disciplinary treatment, each member of the team being made aware of the others' roles and supporting recommended intervention. During the early stages of rehabilitation, while receiving treatment in the acute environment, the patient was totally dependent upon others for all his functional needs. All problems were immediately addressed.

1. A personalised communication booklet with pictures was issued by the speech and language therapist to provide a means of communication. The patient was unable to speak but was able to recognise pictures.

2 and 3. The speech and language therapist and physiotherapist worked together to facilitate swallowing and maintain and restore his respiratory function.

4–9. Treatment intervention for the paralysis of his right side; the sensory impairment and the overactivity of his left side were managed primarily by the physiotherapist, the nursing staff and the occupational therapist. The main problem for the patient was his fear of accepting weight on the right side, which no longer provided appropriate sensory input. Basic management such as turning the patient from side to side in bed, transfers from bed to chair and positioning in a wheelchair was particularly difficult for patient and staff alike. All movements had to be carried out with great care to allow the patient time to accommodate to and accept the change of position.

10. The lack of bladder and bowel control was primarily due to his movement impairment and communication difficulties and was initially managed by means of an indwelling catheter and regular toileting. This problem was of relatively short duration. Once the patient was able to communicate and was able to be moved more readily, the situation was largely resolved. While the catheter was in situ, a leg bag attached to the lower leg, under his trousers, was used whenever the patient was out of bed.

The patient was transferred to a rehabilitation unit 4 weeks after the surgery.

Following a joint assessment involving the patient and all relevant staff, which included the nurse, physiotherapist, occupational therapist and speech and language therapist, the short- and long-term goals were agreed. The problems listed as numbers 4–9 on the original list were considered to be a true reflection of the patient's condition, although improvements could be identified.

Problem 1. His inability to communicate had resolved although his speech remained dysarthric.

Problem 2. Dysphagia remained a problem but had improved in that he was now able to take a soft diet with supervision.

Problem 3. Respiratory dysfunction had resolved.

Problem 10. The lack of bladder and bowel control had resolved.

Physiotherapy intervention was largely directed towards improving the coordination of activity between the two sides of the body. The sensory impairment continued to give rise to severe difficulties in terms of movement, in particular the patient's ability to respond to being moved and handled.

The long-term goal was that the patient would return home independent of a wheelchair in all activities of daily living, he would be able to take a few steps within his own home, with close supervision, and he would have intelligible speech to his family. The timescale for this achievement was 4 months.

The short-term goals were identified as enabling the patient:

1. to accept the left side-lying position and to be positioned in bed on alternate sides with the assistance of one person
2. to be moved from lying to sitting and from sitting to lying over both sides with the assistance of one person
3. to be transferred between the bed and wheelchair to either side using a sliding board
4. to maintain a symmetrical position in the wheelchair.

The timescale for the attainment of these goals was 3 weeks.

These goals were specifically aimed at improving the patient's sensory awareness and restoring his midline orientation. All members of the multidisciplinary team were involved in these activities, each one being aware of the necessity to constantly reinforce the agreed means of achieving these goals.

1. Turning from side to side was reinforced in the physiotherapy treatment area by slowly facilitating the patient on to his right side. Movements of the left side were encouraged while the patient maintained the right side-lying position (Fig. 8.1). This activity stimulated an active response of the right side through his dependency on the weight-bearing side for balance.
2. Movements from lying into sitting and from sitting into lying over the right and left sides were performed with support and facilitation at the right shoulder. This enabled the patient to move his body away from the right upper limb, thereby preventing potential problems of shortening of the pectorals and medial rotators. These movements were performed slowly to allow the patient time to respond appropriately. This was of particular relevance in ensuring weight transfer over the right buttock while stimulating activity of the right trunk side flexors. The patient's tendency was to stabilise himself by overuse of the left trunk side flexors, which in turn inhibited recovery of the right side of his trunk. At each stage of the movement, integrated activity between the two sides of the body was facilitated. The patient was also assisted to lie down and sit up over his left side, thereby actively using this side rather than merely pushing.
3. Transfer from the bed to chair and from chair to bed was carried out using a sliding board. This was agreed to be the preferred option in that attempts by the patient to transfer himself without this support required excessive effort. This transmitted itself into overactivity of the left side, pushing him across and beyond the right side. Use of the sliding board in the early stages enabled staff to move the patient fairly passively, thereby preventing the excessive use of the left side. In this way the patient accommodated to being moved prior to actively

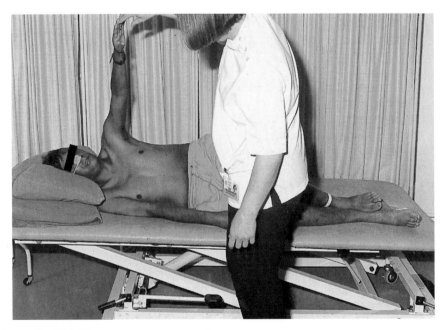

Figure 8.1 Lying on the right side.

participating in the transfer. Transfers were carried out to both left and right sides.

4. Positioning in the wheelchair ensured that the patient was symmetrical and had appropriate support within the chair. The arms rested forwards on a fitted tray attached to the wheelchair. A Jay cushion was provided, which gave a basis of stability while ensuring adequate pressure control. A foam wedge was placed at the back of the chair to provide appropriate support and to counteract sagging. The tray was felt to be essential to support the arms and thereby control subluxation of the right glenohumeral joint, and to improve the patient's awareness of the right upper limb. The tray further encouraged the patient to lean for-

wards in the chair, thus inhibiting the tendency to push backwards. An electric wheelchair was provided after 2 weeks in the unit to allow increased independence (Fig. 8.2).

All members of the multidisciplinary team ensured each of these goals; all functional requirements at this time were carried out in the way described. Activities such as eating, dressing and toileting complemented this approach.

In physiotherapy, the patient was facilitated into standing and supported in this position by means of a vari-table. This gave the patient a feeling of security and allowed the therapist to work independently with the patient upright against gravity. Without the vari-table, another

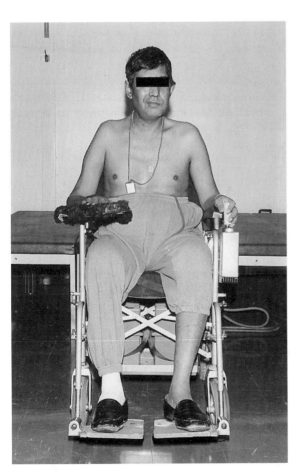

Figure 8.2 Sitting in an electric chair.

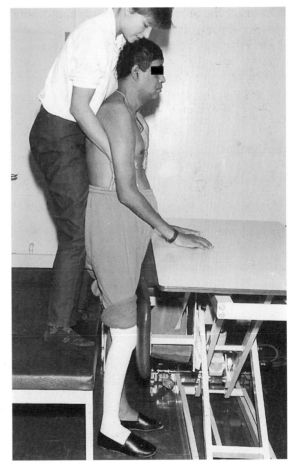

Figure 8.3 Using a vari-table

person was required to stabilise the right knee. The patient was taken up into standing with the therapist standing immediately behind, providing direction and full support (Fig. 8.3). The knee pad maintained the knees in extension, enabling the therapist to work for activity in the trunk with improved midline orientation.

This activity was not used purely for the patient to attain standing but also to facilitate movement to and from standing and sitting. Static positioning in standing tended to make the patient fix, overusing the left side in an attempt to attain stability. Slow, repetitive movements such as letting go into sitting back on to the therapist from the standing position were used as a means of preventing the development of unnecessary fixation.

This additional intervention further helped to restore the patient's midline orientation and sensory awareness, thereby assisting in the achievement of the agreed short-term goals.

Within the 3-week timescale, the patient was able to be:

- turned and could lie securely on alternate sides
- moved from lying into sitting and from sitting into lying over both sides with the assistance of one person
- transferred to and from bed to chair over both sides using a sliding board with the assistance of one person
- positioned appropriately in a wheelchair and able to manoeuvre independently by means of electric controls.

Throughout the rehabilitation process new short-term goals were set in conjunction with the patient, to indicate progress. These goals were in many cases specific to one profession, such as a physiotherapy goal of being able to stand symmetrically using the vari-table. Each new short-term goal was discussed with the team on a weekly basis to ensure continuity and consistency of care.

Summary

This patient returned home after a 4-month period of rehabilitation. He was able to walk with a stick within the home but required a wheelchair for outdoor use. There was no significant recovery in the right upper limb. In spite of this, the limb was involved in many functional activities: for example, when eating, the arm was positioned forwards on the table and, when dressing, the arm was brought forwards when putting on or taking off clothing. In standing, the patient had sufficient awareness to recognise changes in tonus which depended primarily on the degree of effort used and his ability to transfer weight confidently over the right side. He was generally able to release unwanted activity by ensuring he had adequate weight over his right side. This control enabled him to have a free arm as opposed to one which, with uncontrolled hypertonus, may have adversely affected his walking by impairing balance.

A major factor in the outcome was that the patient regained his awareness of the right side in spite of there being little objective change on testing of sensory modalities. Sensory impairment is recognised as a limiting factor in neurological recovery. The treatment of this patient is an example of what may be achieved with consistency of approach by all members of the team, including his wife and family, and constant reinforcement of the involvement of the right side in all functional activities (Fig. 8.4).

PATIENT WITH AN INCOMPLETE SPINAL LESION AT THE T12-L2 LEVEL

This patient was admitted to hospital for embolisation of a spinal arteriovenous malformation (AVM) at the T12-L2 level. The impairment was one of marked sensory loss, bladder dysfunction and severe muscle weakness affecting all muscle groups innervated from below L2. Following the embolisation, muscle charting using the Oxford Scale was documented weekly for a period of 2 months. After this time, measurement of muscle strength was reduced to fortnightly and, within a further 2 months, to monthly. The initial reading and a further one taken 6 months post-embolisation show little change in terms of the strength of individual muscles.

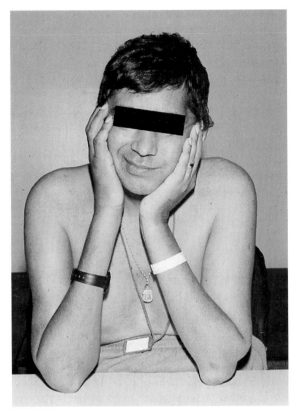

Figure 8.4 Hands on face to increase sensory awareness of the right side.

Specific problems identified

1. Severe weakness of the gluteal muscles. Active extension of the hips was not possible.
2. Attempts to stand without full leg support resulted in flexion of the hips, hyperextension of the knees, lateral rotation of the legs and inversion of the feet. Correct alignment in standing could only be controlled by the physiotherapist ensuring that extension of the hips was maintained.
3. Danger of contracture of the iliopsoas muscle and the foot invertors and plantar flexors.
4. Overactivity of the upper body as a result of wheelchair dependency.
5. Lack of bladder control necessitating self-catheterisation three times daily.
6. Sensory impairment below the knees.

Goal setting

Realistic goals were agreed with the patient, which were a compromise between his determination to achieve an independent gait and the therapist's perspective that this may only be realised, if at all, following a period of gait re-education using long leg calipers. The key to this compromise was the detailed anatomical description of the affected muscle groups and the potential complications, specifically in terms of loss of joint and muscle range, which may have resulted from overuse of the less severely affected muscle groups, particularly the hip flexors.

Treatment plan

1. Active assisted exercises to facilitate recovery of the affected muscle groups, most notably gluteus medius and maximus and the hamstrings. This incorporated exercises in prone (Fig. 8.5), supine and side-lying to stimulate hip extension and knee flexion.

   The gymnastic ball was also used to facilitate general activity, particularly at the trunk and pelvis and of the quadriceps and hamstrings.
2. Sitting to standing and the maintenance of standing with assistance as required from the physiotherapist (Fig. 8.6). With correct alignment of the hips, the lateral rotation of the legs, hyperextension of the knees and inversion of the feet could be controlled.

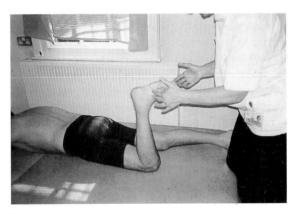

Figure 8.5 Hamstring strengthening in prone lying.

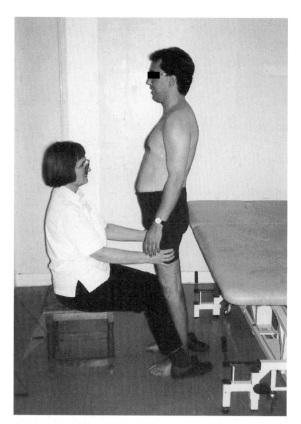

Figure 8.6 Standing with support from physiotherapist.

3. Bilateral back slabs were made of fibreglass material extending from the line of the hip joint to 1 inch above the malleoli. Hinged, ankle–foot orthoses (AFOs) were supplied to allow dorsiflexion but otherwise control the feet in the plantigrade position. (These were designed in such a way that they could be incorporated into a long leg caliper if this was felt to be appropriate at a later stage.)

Walking using back slabs ensured full extension of the hips during the stance phase of walking. This maintained the extensibility of the iliopsoas muscle and of the iliofemoral ligament. The patient utilised a four-point gait which, with the hinged AFOs, allowed for dorsiflexion but prevented loss of range into plantar flexion. Correct alignment of the legs and feet within the back slabs and AFOs maintained the feet in a neutral position, preventing inversion.

4. Overactivity of the upper body was not discouraged in that this was essential for independence in the wheelchair and for caliper walking. However, while facilitating active standing and sitting to standing, the emphasis was to ensure maximal activity of the legs. Progress was monitored by the reduction in upper limb activity in the maintenance and attainment of standing.
5. Bladder control was monitored by the urology department.
6. No specific intervention was carried out to facilitate sensory recovery. Increased activity and function improved the patient's lower limb awareness although he continued to be dependent on his vision to compensate for his sensory loss.

Treatment progression

Within 6 weeks the patient had achieved an independent gait using back slabs, hinged AFOs and a rollator walking frame. Throughout this period of gait re-education, an intensive exercise programme was continued to facilitate maximal activity of all muscle groups, most notably through sitting to standing and the maintenance of standing with support from the therapist. At this stage of his rehabilitation, he was discharged home and continued his treatment as an outpatient.

Having mastered an independent gait, the patient progressed to alternately removing first the left back slab, the left leg being the stronger, and later the right. The potential danger of this progression was shortening of the iliopsoas muscle due to the patient's inability to extend his hip during the stance phase of gait. Having grade 3 quadriceps, the patient was able to maintain his leg in an extended position but only with the hip in a flexed position. This was discussed between the patient and therapist, the result being that walking with only one back slab in situ was always followed by a period of standing with both legs fully supported to ensure a full range of hip extension. In most instances this was carried out by the patient on his return home. Kneel standing (Fig. 8.7) was recommended as an additional means of maintaining the length and extensibility of the psoas muscle.

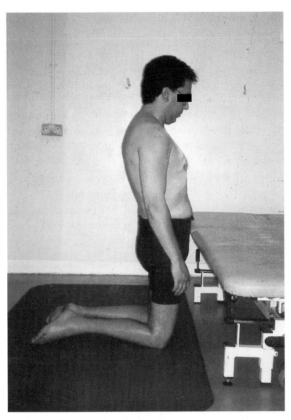

Figure 8.7 Kneel standing to facilitate hamstring activity and to maintain range of movement at the hip to extension.

Three months after the embolisation, in consultation with the patient, his wife, orthotist and consultant neurologist, it was decided to issue bilateral long leg calipers. There had been little recovery of the affected muscle groups and it was felt that wearing calipers would enable the patient to walk more consistently and functionally in his home environment. The patient's concern that this may reduce the potential recovery of the more impaired muscles was dispelled with assurance that his treatment sessions while in physiotherapy would be almost exclusively directed towards strengthening these muscle groups.

Summary

As with many patients following neurological damage, the prognosis for this patient in terms of functional recovery is uncertain. At worst, he is independent in his wheelchair and has the ability to 'walk' using long leg calipers and a four-point gait. The ethical dilemmas which play an increasing part in health care provision may well ultimately determine the outcome. For how long does, or can, therapy intervention continue? At what stage does further neurological or functional recovery become an impossible goal?

With continued physiotherapy intervention, combined with a home programme of exercises, this patient may achieve an independent gait with only AFOs as opposed to long leg calipers. Whatever the outcome, cessation of treatment must be agreed with the patient. In this instance, if there is insufficient recovery of the hip extensors to enable the patient to walk without long leg calipers, the patient must appreciate the need to continue with the calipers or standing in a frame. Were he to attempt to walk without this support following his discharge from treatment, contracture of the iliopsoas muscles would be the likely outcome. It is the therapist's responsibility to ensure that the patient fully understands the implications of his decision. The functional consequence of contracture of the hip flexors is the inability to stand in alignment. Additional stress is then imposed on the lumbar spine and lower limbs with increasing dependency on the arms to maintain an upright posture. However, it remains the prerogative of patients to decide whether or not they wish to accept this advice.

PATIENT FOLLOWING HEAD INJURY

This patient was admitted for rehabilitation 3 months after sustaining a head injury while living and working in America. Due to the severe nature of his injuries, he had not yet been out of bed. He was in considerable pain and very aggressive towards all personnel including his family.

Following discussion between the patient, his wife and family, medical and nursing staff and therapists, the problems were identified as including:

1. reduced range of movement throughout the body with severe contractures of:

a. both feet in plantar flexion and inversion
b. the knees in extension
c. the right hand, wrist and elbow in flexion
d. the left hip fixed in 30 degrees flexion through heterotopic ossification

2. pain
3. inappropriate and aggressive behaviour
4. inability to sit unsupported due, primarily, to the immobility of his left hip
5. inability to stand or be placed in standing due to the deformity of his feet
6. dysarthria
7. total dependency on others for all activities of daily living
8. loss of short-term memory.

Treatment plan

1. Reduced range of movement. Splints were made for the feet and the right hand in an attempt to regain movement and prevent further deterioration in muscle and joint range. Below-knee casts made from fibreglass material were applied to the feet, maintaining the available 10-degree range of movement and controlling against inversion of the feet. The intention was to serially cast, changing the splint on a weekly basis, to support any increase in range. A cone-shaped splint made of thermoplastic materials was applied to the right hand with a view to constant adjustment as the contracted tissues were lengthened. Splinting was not used for the knees or right elbow as it was agreed that his increased level of activity should, in itself, result in an improved range of movement.

2 and 3. Pain and behavioural problems. Pain management was instigated. This was felt to be an integral part of the behavioural problems. He associated therapy with pain and was therefore somewhat reluctant to participate in treatment, his initial reaction being one of aggression. Detailed discussion and explanation of the proposed procedures, analgesia prior to physiotherapy and a guarantee from the therapist that there would be no forcing of joint range resulted in almost immediate compliance. Because he felt that he was now in control of his treatment, the aggressive behaviour ceased, with the

exception of the occasional outburst which was rarely associated with difficulties arising in treatment.

The analgesia prior to treatment was required for only 1 week, after which time he himself suggested that it was no longer necessary.

The clinical psychologist provided support and advice in the most appropriate way to manage the patient's mood and behaviour, to all personnel involved in his care. This was of particular relevance for his wife and family who would often take the brunt of his outbursts of temper.

On admission, the patient had been described as being depressed. This was felt to be related more to his pain and general inactivity in being confined to bed than to clinical depression. From

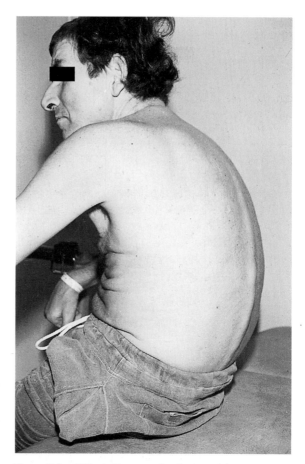

Figure 8.8 Sitting with excessive flexor activity to maintain balance.

the moment that what he considered to be appropriate and purposeful intervention was instigated, depression was no longer a problem.

4. Seating difficulties. Radiography of his left hip revealed extensive heterotopic ossification, fixing the joint in a position of 30 degrees of flexion. The patient had not been out of bed since his accident and his body reflected the position which earlier hypertonus had dictated and enforced. This, according to his medical notes, was one of extension with flexion of the upper limbs. The extension of his left leg had been compounded by a debulking injury to the left quadriceps necessitating a skin graft.

Attempts to sit the patient, initially over the side of the bed, presented tremendous problems in that it was impossible to bring the trunk and pelvis forwards over the hips. In addition, the legs had to be supported, as the knees had a restricted range of movement from full extension to 20 degrees of flexion. This enforced posture at the hips with the pelvis in a position of posterior tilt resulted in the patient having to overcompensate with flexion of the trunk to prevent falling backwards (Fig. 8.8).

For these reasons, active sitting without support was discouraged and a wheelchair provided which accommodated the deformities. The back of the chair was angled backwards with a wedged seat further reducing the hip angle. The legs were supported on elevating leg rests positioned at the maximum range of flexion which the patient could tolerate.

While the limitations imposed by the immobility of his left hip were recognised, other restrictions in range of movement throughout the body, most notably of the trunk, were not of a permanent nature. An intensive programme of treatment was instigated to regain available range by means of mobilisation of the trunk in sitting and on the gymnastic ball (Fig. 8.9) and by positioning on alternate sides when in bed. Prone lying over a wedge was used to stimulate extensor activity within the trunk which would provide proximal stability to free the arms for function.

Although the patient was in a position of predominant extension, this was not enforced by excessive extensor hypertonus. The patient had control of virtually all muscle groups but these were weak through disuse. In effect, the patient had become trapped within his own body as a result of the loss of range of movement which had arisen from his immobility and the earlier hypertonus, now virtually resolved. As his aware-

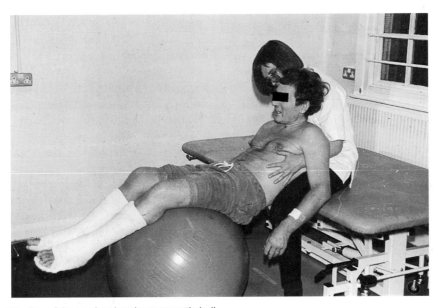

Figure 8.9 Mobilisation of the trunk using the gymnastic ball.

ness improved, attempts to move were dominated by flexion in his efforts to counteract his enforced extended position. It was therefore important to regain range into flexion but at the same time to stimulate extensor activity and reciprocal innervation.

5. Difficulty with standing. Standing was considered to be an optimal means of stimulating normal extensor activity throughout the body. The below-knee splints provided stability at the ankles, albeit in a position of extreme plantar flexion. A heel wedge was positioned to accommodate the deformity. The Oswestry standing frame was used to provide additional stability, with two therapists assisting him up into standing from a high plinth. This procedure was

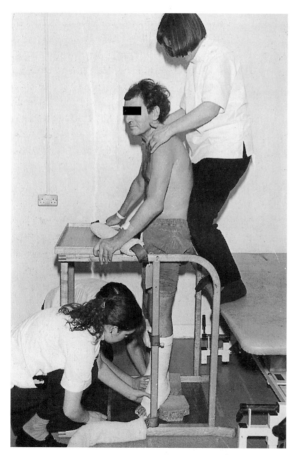

Figure 8.10 Standing in the Oswestry standing frame, wearing below-knee casts.

undertaken with great care, the patient feeling naturally apprehensive. This feeling of apprehension was compounded by the fact that, due to the lack of flexion at the knees, the patient was unable to transfer his weight forwards over his feet to stand, or be brought up into standing, in the normal way.

This position was found to be most effective in facilitating trunk control and improved body awareness (Fig. 8.10). Within 3 days the patient was able to lift his hands alternately off the table, demonstrating his improved proximal control and the inherent capability of his upper limbs. This demonstrated quite clearly that the movement impairment, although initially one of hypertonus, was now one of disuse and subsequent weakness. The underlying tone was relatively normal, there being only minimal hypertonia affecting the right side. Even in these early stages of rehabilitation it was felt that, with increased mobility and resolution of his contractures, the patient had the potential to achieve an independent gait and functional use of his hands.

6. Dysarthria. The patient was severely dysarthric on admission and was assessed and subsequently treated by the speech and language therapist. However, his speech problems were compounded by both his behavioural state and his impaired respiratory control caused by his general immobility. As with all aspects of his care, although in this instance the speech and language therapist played a major role, all staff and his family contributed to the improvement in both his psychological state and mobility. The underlying speech impairment was significantly less than that initially thought.

7. Dependency for activities of daily living. The patient's total dependency on others for all activities of daily living resulted in tremendous frustration which was a causative factor of his inappropriate and aggressive behaviour. This provides a perfect illustration of how the environment can influence disability. For example, it was impossible for him to feed himself when lying in bed and yet, when sitting in a wheelchair, he was independent in this activity. He was unable to dress himself sitting unsupported but, when supported in the wheelchair, he was able to put on and take off a T-shirt. These achievements, accomplished with no intervention other than providing the appropriate support, had a dramatic effect in terms of the patient's attitude to his disability and to treatment. Much of his behaviour resulted from his lack of self-esteem and subsequent negativity with regard to possible improvement in his condition. Realisation that there were many things he could do for himself given the right environment created a more positive approach towards his treatment and management.

The attainment of function was dependent on restoration of range of movement. With improved mobility came an increase in functional achievement. The nursing staff and family were closely involved in utilising the gains made through the improved mobility. Transfers from the wheelchair to the bed, toilet and the car became much easier for the patient, staff and carers with improved trunk mobility and as he became able to place his feet closer in towards his body. Within 4 weeks, the patient was able to transfer virtually independently with the use of a sliding board.

8. Memory. The loss of short-term memory was addressed by all staff and his family following advice from the clinical psychologist. The setting of short-term goals, agreed with the patient, which were written down, provided a constant reminder to the patient as to what were the main objectives in terms of restoration of function. By breaking down the functional goal to the component parts, the patient was able to concentrate on specific aspects of everyday life, making continual reference to his written objectives. For example, when eating, his right arm was to be positioned forwards on the table while he fed himself with the left hand. All staff and his family were aware of this agreed objective and would ask him if he had forgotten something if the right arm was not on the table. In the early stages, the patient would often need to refer to his written instructions to find out what it was he had forgotten. With this constant reinforcement, a simple reminder became sufficient for him to ensure the correct positioning of the right arm.

The patient was very aware of this problem, which added to his frustration. All staff, and his family in particular, were encouraged to give him time and appropriate prompts to help him find his own answers, rather than responding for him immediately or telling him what to do.

The agreed long-term goal was that, in 3 months, the patient would return home independent in all activities of daily living and that he would achieve an independent gait using a rollator subject to the management of his foot contractures. (The ossification of his left hip would inevitably restrict activities such as putting on and taking off socks and shoes.)

Plan of action

1. To provide effective pain relief.
2. To influence his predominantly extended posture by providing appropriate seating.
3. To restore range of movement of the right hand and the feet by means of serial splinting.
4. To improve trunk and lower limb mobility to enable transfer as opposed to the patient having to be lifted into and out of the chair.
5. To maintain standing in the Oswestry standing frame for 10 minutes while lifting alternate hands off the support.

Three attempts were made to improve range of movement at the feet and ankles by means of serial splinting over a period of 3 weeks. No objective change was noted and it was apparent that this intervention alone would not be adequate to influence the established contractures. The patient was assessed by an orthopaedic surgeon who agreed to lengthen the Achilles tendons. This surgery was carried out 4 weeks after admission. The initial casts applied following surgery held the patient in 30 degrees of plantar flexion. Instructions were given by the surgeon that the casts should be changed on a weekly basis until plantigrade position was achieved.

Within 4 weeks this position was attained and the casts were then bivalved. The patient had continued to stand while in the casts within 1 week of the surgery. Following bivalving of the casts, progressive short-term goals were set for

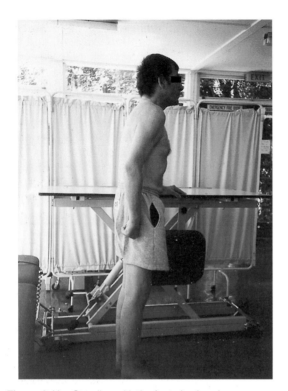

Figure 8.11   Standing with the feet plantigrade.

him to gradually increase the length of time he was able to stand without the support of the casts. This was carefully monitored, particularly in respect of pain and swelling. Analgesia was given as needed and support stockings used to control the swelling. The casts were discarded within 1 week.

This surgical intervention was the most significant factor in his rehabilitation in terms of his ability to walk. Being able to place the feet in the plantigrade position (Fig. 8.11) enabled him to transfer independently, bring himself from sitting to standing with minimal assistance from one person and initiate walking in the parallel bars, again with the assistance of one person.

Within physiotherapy, continued mobilisation was specifically directed at improving his gait pattern. Although the range of movement in his knees had improved significantly – he now had 100 degrees of flexion – he was not yet able to utilise this increase of range in the release of the leg prior to stepping through. The patient had to

be constantly reminded to bend the knee, which at this stage he was only able to do with active flexion as opposed to releasing the limb into flexion.

Summary

The patient was discharged home following 3 months of intensive rehabilitation. His status on discharge was full independence from his wheelchair and walking with a rollator with the supervision of one person. He still had the occasional outbursts of temper, most notably when he was challenged to do something with which he was not confident. His speech remained dysarthric but was intelligible to all if he spoke slowly. The problems with short-term memory persisted but, with written and verbal feedback, the patient felt that this had improved.

Following discharge, the patient attended for outpatient physiotherapy with the aim of further improving his gait. By this stage he was able to release his leg prior to stepping through, but this still required conscious effort. The potential to achieve a more fluent gait increased as the mobility of his feet and ankles improved. At this time there was a passive range of 5 degrees of dorsiflexion at his ankles.

No surgical intervention was contemplated for the heterotopic ossification of his left hip at this stage of his rehabilitation. At a later stage, surgical management may be contemplated with a view to removing the bony mass and potentially increasing the available range of movement. However, as surgery is also associated with the development of heterotopic ossification, there is understandably some reservation amongst surgeons to operate (Andrews & Greenwood 1993).

Unless this problem is addressed, it is inevitable that the patient compensates for the lack of range at the left hip, particularly when sitting. For this reason it is important that standing and walking become functional and are used on a frequent and spontaneous basis. Sitting with the pelvis in a fixed posterior tilt will result in increased flexor activity within the trunk and upper limbs for all functional goals. Constant reinforcement of flexion over a period of time will be reflected in the patient's posture and a potential reduction in functional capability.

PATIENT WITH MULTIPLE SCLEROSIS

This 38-year-old patient had a 10-year history of multiple sclerosis (MS). She presented with spastic paraparesis with progressive weakness affecting both legs and increasing difficulty with walking. There had been a marked reduction in function particularly over the last year. Her level of mobility had deteriorated to such an extent that, having been able to walk up to 100 metres using a frame, at the time of admission she had been bed-bound at home for 5 months. She also complained of back pain, which contributed to her increased disability.

The patient lived with her parents, who were her main carers, in a council-owned, semi-detached house. Her bedroom was on the ground floor with an en-suite bathroom with a wheelchair accessible shower. There was a stair lift in situ to the first floor and, up until 6 months prior to admission to the rehabilitation unit, the patient was working full time, doing administrative duties for a car company, and was able to drive. In her leisure time she enjoyed shopping, watching television and reading.

She was admitted to hospital to investigate her back pain and was immediately started on a low dose of oral baclofen. An MRI (magnetic resonance image) of the spine concluded that the appearance was compatible with spinal MS, without any compressive lesions. Following these initial investigations, it was decided that this lady would benefit from a period of inpatient rehabilitation to improve her level of function. Her main problems were identified as being:

Impairments

1. quadraparesis, with the lower limbs being more affected than the upper limbs and the left side being more affected than the right
2. weakness and stiffness of the trunk and pelvis
3. alternating flexor and extensor lower limb spasms with shortening of hip flexors, adductors, hamstrings and plantar flexors

4. compensatory overuse of the head and shoulder girdles
5. back pain
6. bladder and bowel dysfunction
7. right sixth nerve palsy, mild visual impairment
8. low mood.

Disabilities

1. dependent on maximal assistance of two people or a hoist for all bed mobility and transfers
2. unable to be seated for longer than 10 minutes: this was limited by back pain
3. unable to stand or walk
4. dependent for all domestic tasks
5. unable to leave the home
6. limited leisure activities
7. prone to incontinence and dependent on pads
8. irregular bowel regime.

A treatment plan was formulated in conjunction with the patient and all relevant personnel. This included the medical staff, nursing staff, the physiotherapist and the occupational therapist. Full consultation was held with the local community services managing the patient at home.

The aims and objectives of physiotherapy with regard to her impairments and disabilities were to:

- improve mobility and control of the trunk and pelvis
- reduce the hypertonus in the lower limbs
- reduce the pain in her back
- improve bed mobility and transfers
- provide an appropriate seating system
- enable standing and possibly walking.

The instability and stiffness of the trunk and pelvis were considered to be major contributors to the lower limb hypertonus and back pain. Treatment initially concentrated on realigning and mobilising the trunk and pelvis in a variety of postures. Her lumbar spine was flexed, with restricted range of movement into extension and a posterior tilt of the pelvis. The instability and stiffness of the trunk made it difficult for her to maintain an upright posture or to lie comfortably (Fig 8.12 and Fig. 8.13). The patient found sitting particularly uncomfortable as this exacerbated her back pain.

Trunk mobilisations were used to improve symmetry and to enable more equal weight-bearing through the ischeal tuberosities. This intervention had to be performed slowly, allow-

ing time for the patient to adjust to being moved and to participate in the activity.

Following this preparatory work in sitting and lying, there was improved alignment and there-fore a better basis from which to recruit more appropriate muscle activity in the trunk. This resulted in a reduction in the lower limb hyper-tonus and an improvement in her back pain.

In spite of marked asymmetry, standing was used early on in treatment to stimulate activity in the trunk and to counter her flexed lower limb posture (Fig 8.14). This flexed posture appeared to be due to a combination of predominant flexor hypertonus and underlying weakness. The pro-longed stretch to shortened structures, most notably the hip flexors, hamstrings and plantar flexors, reduced the intensity and severity of the flexor spasms but initially revealed severe under-lying weakness to the extent that the patient was dependent on the straps of the standing frame to maintain an upright posture. However, within 3 weeks of standing, she had developed suf-ficient strength to control her legs in extension.

There was also a definite psychological benefit to standing for this patient who had been bed-bound for 5 months and was understandably very low in mood.

In conjunction with the occupational therapist, a detailed posture and seating assessment was carried out and a variety of wheelchairs and cushions were used to determine the most effect-ive means of support. A timetable was initiated to gradually increase the length of time the pa-tient was able to tolerate being positioned in the wheelchair. Following 2 weeks of therapy the patient was able to sit in the wheelchair for periods of up to 2 hours without experiencing any back pain (Fig. 8.15).

With improved trunk control and reduced back pain the patient was able to transfer using a sliding board, taking gradually more weight through her feet. She was also able to dress independently. Following a bladder assessment which was carried out by the nursing staff, the patient used intermittent self-catheterisation once during the day, voiding on the commode at other times. However, she had persistent dif-ficulties with getting her clothes down and up

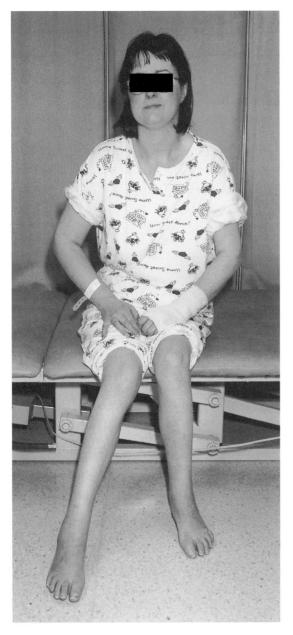

Figure 8.12 Difficulty in maintaining upright posture.

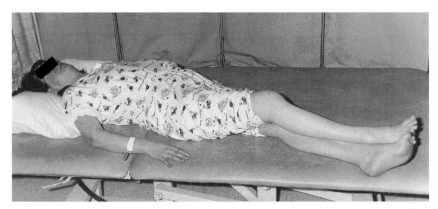

Figure 8.13   Difficulty in lying comfortably.

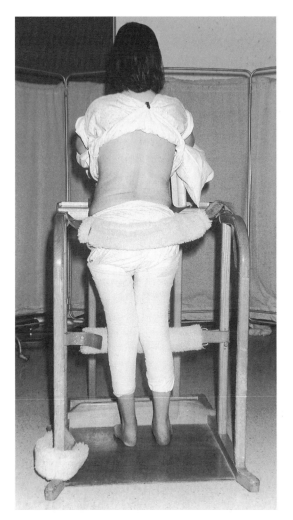

Figure 8.14   Standing was used to stimulate trunk activity and to counter the patient's flexed lower limb posture.

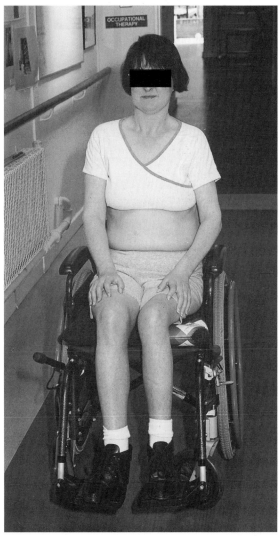

Figure 8.15   Sitting in a wheelchair following 2 weeks of therapy.

As the patient gained more independent control in standing it was possible to facilitate some selective movement in the lower limbs. At the end of a treatment session she was able to take automatic steps with the support of two people. The patient was also able to transfer through standing using a rollator frame and to take steps for up to 10 metres using the frame and a dorsiflexion bandage (see Ch. 10) on her left foot (Fig 8.16).

In addition to standing, she also had improved bed mobility, increased independence in some aspects of her personal care and experienced a significant reduction in her pain and spasms. A range of outcomes was measured: hypertonicity (Modified Ashworth Scale); disability (Barthel Index); and handicap (Handicap Assessment Scale). Each measure demonstrated a positive improvement.

Summary

As reported by Freeman et al (1997), inpatient rehabilitation can be effective in improving the level of disability and handicap in patients with multiple sclerosis, in spite of unchanging impairment. This lady was discharged home into the care of her parents after 8 weeks of rehabilitation. She was referred to the community neuro-rehabilitation team in her area, so the functional gains made while she was an inpatient could be applied in the home environment.

DISCUSSION

Rehabilitation following an acute episode resulting in neurological impairment and subsequent disability is an accepted part of patient management in the Western world. However, where this rehabilitation takes place and for how long varies, depending on the facilities available and, increasingly, on financial constraints.

In many instances, the neurological damage gives rise to permanent disability, such as quadraplegia following spinal cord injury or residual hemiplegia following stroke. The restoration of normal movement is neither a realistic nor an attainable goal in these circumstances. The ulti-

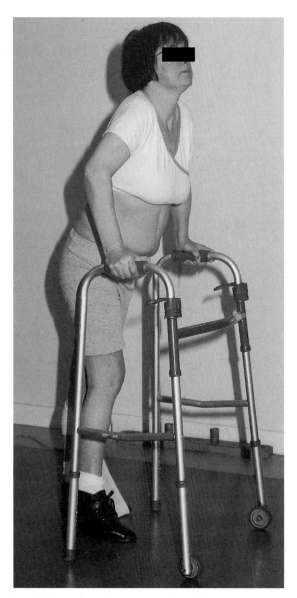

Figure 8.16   Standing, using a rollator frame.

again following voiding and the possibility of a suprapubic catheter was discussed with the patient and, with her agreement, referral was made to the relevant medical personnel. The combination of this more appropriate bladder regime, the improved trunk alignment and the significant reduction in the lower limb spasms resulted in a gradual reduction and, after 5 weeks, cessation of baclofen.

mate goal for all personnel involved in the rehabilitative process is to maximise the patient's level of function and, perhaps more import- antly, to ensure that this optimal outcome is maintained.

REFERENCES

Andrews K, Greenwood R 1993 Physical consequences of neurological disablement. In: Greenwood R, Barnes M P, McMillan T M, Ward C D (eds) Neurological rehabilitation. Churchill Livingstone, London

Edwards S 1998 The incomplete spinal lesion. In: Bromley I (ed) Tetraplegia and paraplegia: a guide for physiotherapists, 5th edn. Churchill Livingstone, London

Freeman J A, Langdon D W, Hobart J C, Thompson A J 1997 The impact of inpatient rehabilitation on progressive multiple sclerosis. Annals of Neurology 42: 236–244

Kaye S 1991 The value of audit in clinical practice. Physiotherapy 77(10): 705–707

Wade D 1992 Measurement in neurological rehabilitation. Oxford University Press, Oxford

9

Posture management and special seating

Pauline M. Pope

INTRODUCTION

Posture as a subject is of particular interest to the physiotherapist and is a prominent feature of textbooks on neurology. Special seating, on the other hand, is a relative newcomer in the field of neurological physiotherapy. The linking of posture and special seating in the same chapter serves to emphasise the relationship between them.

The population under consideration incorporates the relatively small number of people with motor and posture impairment who require a degree of external support to stabilise body posture and position relative to the supporting surface in lying, sitting and, where appropriate, standing. The problems presented by this group challenge the expertise of many experienced therapists.

Posture in the able-bodied person has occupied the minds of medical practitioners over the centuries. Faulty posture was thought to be responsible for a variety of maladies. Great emphasis was placed on correct posture habits, particularly in Victorian times. There are many who would agree with Zacharkow (1988) who stated in his comprehensive review that much of the literature of that period is equally valid and pertinent today.

Studies of posture in the able-bodied population intensified in the last century, culminating in more appropriate support for the body in a wide range of activities from sleeping to motor car racing. The disabled person, unfortunately, has not benefited in any comparable way.

Changes in the epidemiology of disease and injury have triggered the need to redress the balance. Advances in medical science and technology are responsible for the increase in numbers of people surviving severe trauma and disease. Further, the increased longevity in those with progressive diseases is accompanied by an increase in the severity of conditions. This situation has not stabilised. The numbers surviving with profound and complex disability in urgent need of posture support are increasing.

The physiotherapeutic approach is evolving from a position of treating the impairment to one of managing the physical condition (Condie 1991, Pope 1992, 1997a). This concept incorporates control of body posture within the context of the whole environment and recognises the fundamental necessity of posture stability for effective functional performance.

Special seating, in cases of neurological impairment, supplements or substitutes for impaired mechanisms of posture control, with the aim of reducing secondary complications associated with the impairment while at the same time facilitating remaining functional ability.

It is important to emphasise that although this chapter is largely concerned with the analysis of problems associated with posture in sitting and the principles underlying their resolution, isolation of the subject in this way should never be considered in practice. To be effective it is imperative that posture management extends to all aspects of lifestyle throughout 24 hours. More damage to the body system is likely to arise from uncontrolled lying than from uncontrolled sitting.

POSTURE

The word and the subject have suffered from imprecise definition and over-generalised application. Lack of precision is aggravated by association with adjectives such as 'good' and 'bad' without defining the terms of reference.

Whitman (1924), described man's erect posture as a constant struggle against the force of gravity. While acknowledging this, a more precise defin-

ition of posture competence is offered here in terms of the ability to:

- conform to the supporting surface symmetrically and with weight distributed equally through the load-bearing surfaces
- select and adopt the alignment of body segments appropriate to the efficient performance of a specific activity
- balance and stabilise the selected body attitude relative to the supporting surface
- adjust to changes within the body or support while maintaining balance and stability
- free the parts of the body required for movement from their load-bearing role
- secure a fixed point about which the muscles can act.

'Good' posture is that body attitude which facilitates maximum efficiency of a specific activity in terms of effectiveness and energy cost without causing damage to the body system. Thus a 'bad' posture can be demonstrated in different ways: for example, the unskilled lifting of a load which results in a lesion of the inter vertebral disc, or the increased difficulty in writing when the arm is inadequately supported.

The achievement of the objective for the minimum expenditure of energy is the prime concern, not the manner of the performance.

Energy-conserving strategies

It is generally accepted that the so-called 'correct' postures in sitting and standing (Fig. 9.1A & B) cannot be sustained other than for short periods of time. They are energy consuming and are rarely employed in everyday life. Postures such as those illustrated in Figure 9.2A & B are more usually adopted, conserving energy and maintaining a balanced stable posture by astute use of the skeleton and soft tissues. These postures are intrinsically 'bad', as they are potentially damaging to the body system. However, damage is avoided as discomfort eventually signals overload and stress within the tissues, forcing a change of posture. Alternative tissues are then loaded until they too signal distress.

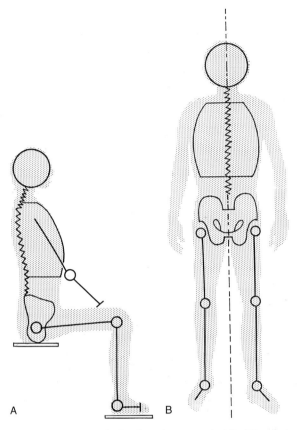

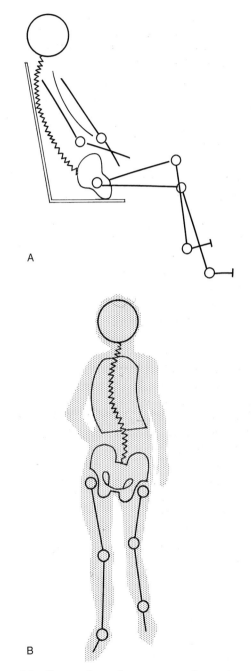

Figure 9.1 Anatomically aligned postures in (A) sitting and (B) standing.

Posture as a prerequisite to movement

The number and amplitude of discrete movements of body segments is a function of the degree of control of the centre of mass over the supporting base area (Massion & Gahery 1978). The gymnast and ballet dancer illustrate the ultimate in this control.

The anticipatory and preparatory nature of posture adjustments which enhance the efficiency of motor function is now well recognised. Posture is concerned with balance and stability. It is a primary function taking precedence over other activities. When balance is threatened, all body segments are recruited to maintain equilibrium. This is a familiar phenomenon: for example, when walking on a slippery surface, discrete

Figure 9.2 Commonly used energy-conserving postures in (A) sitting and (B) standing.

movement of specific body segments is difficult if not impossible.

Figure 9.3 illustrates a comparable situation in the individual with impaired posture striving to

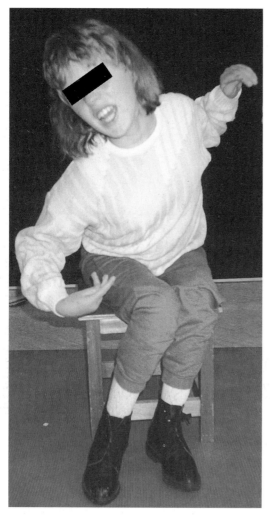

Figure 9.3 A typical posture demonstrating use of the limbs as an aid to balance in a girl with cerebral palsy.

Organisation of body segments develops sequentially, starting with the ability to control the trunk, which acts as a stable base about which movement can occur (Pountney et al 1990). Associated development of purposeful movement is, according to Edelman (1993), the result of initial trial and error. 'Successful' random movements are reinforced, gradually achieving a level of efficiency consistent with the maturity, needs and wishes of the individual. Efficiency develops gradually as the individual learns to move within the external and internal constraints imposed by the environment and the body structure itself (Massion 1992). The precise moulding of the intrinsic structures and mechanisms of posture and movement control is governed by these constraints (Kidd 1980) in a manner analogous to that by which the magnitude and direction of the stresses and strains determines final bone structure.

This knowledge is of profound significance when attempting to analyse so-called abnormal movement such as is observed in the child with cerebral palsy. In these cases, initial impairment limits the ability to achieve a sufficiently stable base from which to move. As a result, the child develops strategies of movement designed to maximise efficiency from an inadequate base, a view endorsed by Latash & Anson (1996) and Latash & Nicholas (1996). Thus, learning can be considered in essentially the same way as in the healthy child, but the movement/function which results differs and corresponds to the prevailing, less advantageous, mechanical conditions.

The important point to recognise is that these movements are appropriate to the particular circumstances of the child. The imposition of so-called normal posture may well reduce performance, at least in the short term. This is not to imply that intervention directed to improve posture is inappropriate; functional progress is dependent upon such intervention, but a lengthy period of relearning a new strategy may be necessary. A golfer, for example, may be advised to alter his technique when a plateau is reached. Initially, performance deteriorates but, with practice, remoulding of internal neural pathways occurs and progress is facilitated beyond a previous best.

maintain balance over a reduced area of support, in this case one side of the buttocks. An adequate base must first be established if functional progress utilising the limbs is to be realised.

Learning control of posture

The basic components of the sensorimotor mechanism are present at birth in the healthy child. The integrity of these components, central activator and control mechanisms together with an intact effector and feedback apparatus, is essential to the learning of posture control.

Rapidly increasing knowledge of plasticity within the human system, the extent of this and the means by which it can be enhanced, support the view that appropriate intervention can be expected to improve performance in many cases. Form and function are closely related but practice is required to bring about physiological change. Theories of learning and clinical experience suggest that time and motivation in addition to practice are fundamental to a successful outcome (Shadmehr & Holcomb 1997, Karni et al 1998).

Radical change imposed on highly developed actions in the older child or adult, however inefficient, should be undertaken with caution. Some activities may have developed in a far from normal way but, as such, are relatively successful strategies which have adapted to the disadvantageous conditions operating at the time of learning. A notable example is swallowing in some cases of cerebral palsy.

Posture deficit in sitting

A deficit of posture control is recognised in the inability to organise the attitude of the body. It is manifest as follows:

- The body slumps or arches.
- The trunk rolls to one side; lateral flexion is accompanied by rotation within the spine.
- The head falls forwards, sideways or backwards depending upon the direction of forces acting upon it.
- The trunk leans against the back support increasing the tendency to slide, predisposing to frictional damage to the skin. Where friction prevents sliding, shear and tensile stresses are high, deformation and mechanical damage occur within the tissues and between tissue layers.
- The tissues are subjected to unequal loading with resultant localised high-pressure areas.
- Body segments buckle and bend, finding their own level of support (Fig. 9.4).

The precise attitude of the limbs and head may vary and is dependent upon the severity and location of the impairment, released neural

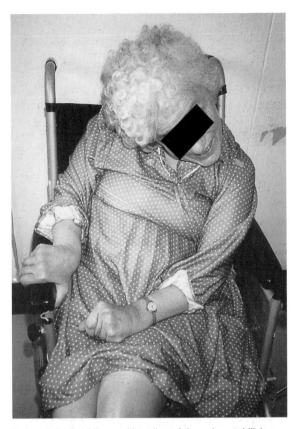

Figure 9.4 Buckling and bending of the spine stabilising one body segment against another.

activity, and the magnitude and direction of forces acting on the body. When these conditions are sustained, the tissues adapt, leading to 'preferred' postures and positional deformity (Fulford & Brown 1976, Pope et al 1991). The basic characteristics noted above are not exclusive to any particular neurological pathology, suggesting a strong environmental influence on their development. If such is the case, it follows that the deleterious effects of the uncontrolled environmental forces on the paralysed patient can be avoided or at least reduced.

Strategies adopted by the disabled person to maximise performance

The ways in which performance may be enhanced are many and varied. The following exam-

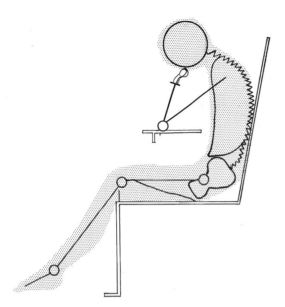

Figure 9.5　Strategy used to facilitate feeding, gaining segmental stability, lowering the centre of gravity and reducing the distance travelled.

ples illustrate two different but quite common strategies.

1. When paralysis or weakness increases the difficulty in feeding independently, the patient will achieve the requisite stability of posture by slumping and using the body structure and table for support. The overall height is reduced and the centre of mass is lowered, facilitating balance; the distance from plate to mouth is decreased (Fig. 9.5). In this way the aim is achieved for minimum energy cost.

2. The use of so-called 'extensor thrust' as a basis for action is shown in Figure 9.6. In this, the shoulders and feet are used as the fixed (loaded) points about which movement/ function develops, instead of the more appropriate base for sitting, i.e. the pelvis and thighs. Extension of the spine is the only possible option for any movement from such a starting point, with the result that attempts to sit back in the seat are ineffective.

It is essential that the therapist recognises that these attempts are voluntary and not 'spasms'.

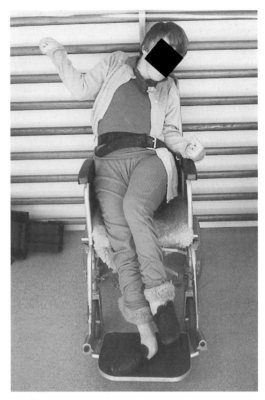

Figure 9.6　Young woman with cerebral palsy attempting to sit back in the wheelchair.

Given the inability to flex the trunk any movement or function can only be executed in extension.

It is not the postures per se which are 'bad'. In the first example paralysis or fatigue prevents a change of posture, thus predisposing to structural damage. In the second case, the inability to organise the body posture more appropriately for the task reduces the effectiveness of performance and limits the potential repertoire of functional activity.

The significant feature common to both these examples is the fundamental need to establish stability of position and a fixed point about which to move.

The solution lies in the design of equipment which controls alignment, provides an appropriate and stable base, and relieves stress on loaded structures while at the same time maintaining a posture or position which will maximise remaining functional activity. A somewhat daunting task!

Complications associated with 'bad' posture

- Tissue adaptation, leading to contracture and deformity.
- Tissue breakdown due to necrosis or mechanical damage.
- Reduced efficiency of performance.
- Respiratory distress.
- Respiratory/urinary tract infections.
- Discomfort.

In addition, increased neural activity and some forms of movement disorders, such as in spastic and athetoid cerebral palsy, multiple sclerosis and brain injury, appear to be functions of imbalance and instability of posture.

The sequence of development of complications may be represented as in Figure 9.7.

The situation is self-reinforcing and, if left, the disabled person will eventually become bedfast (Fig. 9.8) It must be remembered that these complications arise from lack of posture control in both sitting *and* lying.

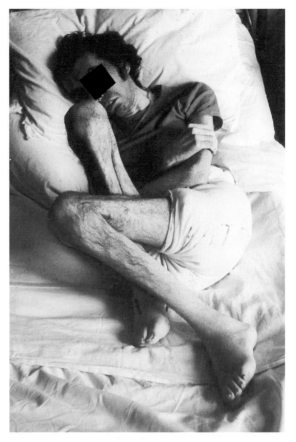

Figure 9.8   The bedfast state.

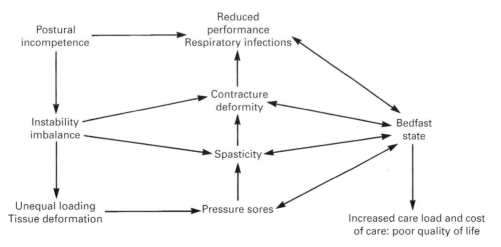

Figure 9.7   Development of complications associated with deficit of posture control.

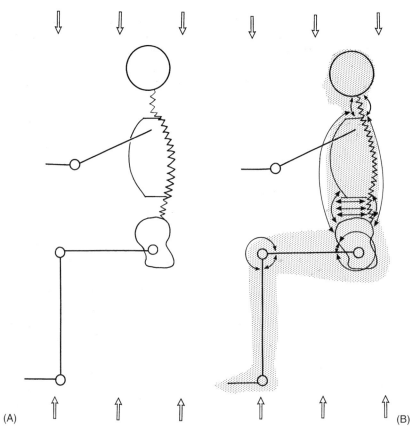

Figure 9.9 Diagrammatic representation of the structure of the body: (A) as a system of segments and linkages; (B) with the muscles, soft tissues and body cavity pressures involved in support and stability.

BIOMECHANICS OF THE SEATED POSTURE

Some understanding of the complexity of the body structure is essential prior to discussion of posture problems. A review of the main points is considered here but further detail is given in Pope et al (1988) and Norris (1995).

Structure

The body is multisegmental and highly flexible. It is inherently unstable in the erect posture. The degree of flexibility is readily appreciated when attempting to lift or support the unconscious or paralysed person and may be likened to that of lifting a fluid-filled balloon.

The body structure may be described as a series of segments of variable stiffness with linkages of varying mobility (Fig. 9.9A). The segments identified are the head, thorax, pelvis, thighs, lower limbs and feet. The upper limbs here are considered as one segment as they do not normally transmit load. The linkages are the spinal joints, hip, knee, ankle and shoulder joints.

Of the segments, the pelvis and head, together with the long bones, are relatively rigid components. The head is heavy in proportion to the other segments and is balanced on the highly flexible cervical spine. The cage-like structure of the thorax and the multiple components of the feet render these segments more vulnerable to deviation, yielding readily to prolonged stress.

The upper limb segment is additional weight carried by the trunk. The loading on the spine will vary according to the position of the arms at any given time.

Structure and movement of the linkages vary. The isolated spine is highly unstable and will buckle and bend under loads exceeding 2 kg (Morris et al 1961) and when subjected to eccentric loading (Koreska et al 1977). The result of sustained stress is irreversible damage within the disc and spinal ligaments.

The spine is a highly sophisticated compromise between stability and flexibility. The movements between the vertebrae are complex, combining flexion, rotation and gliding. The movement combination depends upon the particular spinal segment (Shirazi-Adl et al 1986, Putz & Muller-Gerbl 1996).

Shearing is resisted by facet joints and intervertebral discs. The structure is likened to a complex helical spring, the plane and degree of movement varying with the spinal segment. Although movement between adjacent vertebrae is small, even in the more mobile cervical and thoracolumbar sections, the composite movement of the whole significantly extends the range.

The pivot joints at hip and shoulder allow extensive multiplanar movement controlled by muscle action. The shoulder joint linkage relies on soft tissues for stability and, in cases of diminished or absent muscle control, connecting tissues are particularly vulnerable to damage in handling procedures. Knee and ankle joints are more limited in movement range and are predominantly uniplanar.

All linkages, with the exception of the shoulder joint, normally transmit load.

The base in sitting is formed by the pelvis and thighs. The superstructure above the pelvis is balanced on the rockers formed by the ischial and pelvic rami, the whole rotating about the highly mobile pivot joint of the hip. Sagittal movement of the pelvis is limited only by contact of the trunk on the thigh in flexion and the tension of soft tissues in extension. In the absence of muscle control, the pelvis is free to rotate forwards or backwards about the hip joint according to the forces acting upon it. Kelly (1949) likened the erect posture above the pelvis to balancing a one-legged stool. Even worse, the one leg, the spine, is itself highly flexible and unstable.

Factors influencing stability

The skeleton, connective tissue and the co-ordinated action of the muscles combine to give most of the support to the erect body posture (Fig. 9.9B).

The bones themselves, together with the locking mechanisms of some joints, notably the facet joints of the spine, afford a degree of stability (Oda et al 1996, Putz & Muller-Gerbl 1996, Onan et al 1998). The stability provided by these joints is reduced on certain movements, particularly during flexion and rotation.

The connective tissues of the body, particularly the ligaments and tendons, assist in limiting joint movement. They are most effective at joints that are subject to minimal movement: for example, those of the pelvic basin. Their effectiveness is limited at joints which have a wide range of movement, being vulnerable to damage when subjected to rapid or strong forces and to lengthening under prolonged stress.

Muscle action is crucial to the intrinsic stability of the body structure. It provides most of the stability at linkages. The cervical spine relies heavily on coordinated muscle action in balancing the head on the shoulders. As muscles require a fixed point about which to act at any time, head control can best be maximised if the trunk and shoulder girdle are stable.

Much of the trunk stability is gained through the coordinated action of the abdominal and erector spinae muscles (Zacharkow 1988). The intersegmental trunk muscles are found to be important stabilisers of the lumbar spine (Quint et al 1998). It is of interest to note that the isolated cadaveric spine held in the normal orientation at the base requires a loading of half body weight to maintain the upright position. Without this loading, the lumbar spine tends to spring back into full lordosis (Deane 1982, personal communication), an observation made during investigation into idiopathic scoliosis. This feature is considered to conserve energy in maintaining an erect posture but emphasises the crucial role of the abdominal muscles in achieving balance, stability and forward flexion of the spine.

Body cavity pressures provide a major contribution to the stability of the trunk. Abdominal cavity pressure, in conjunction with surrounding musculature, is responsible for the support of and prevention of damage to the spine (Morris et al 1961). Bartelink (1957) likened the abdomen to a fluid ball in which the pressure within, and therefore the support, is enhanced by muscular activity as effort increases.

Distribution of body weight appears to be a significant factor influencing stability of posture. Abdominal 'bulk' has been observed to support the spine and stabilise the trunk in sitting in some disabled individuals. In addition, in such cases, the centre of mass is lowered and base stability is increased. Conversely, amputation of a lower limb or reduction of muscle bulk in paralysed lower limbs raises the centre of mass with the suggestion of a corresponding increase in difficulty of balancing the trunk over the base.

The lower limbs and feet are said to contribute to stability in sitting (Son et al 1988). However, their effectiveness as stabilisers will be reduced when load transmission through the joints is not controlled by muscle action.

The achievement of a dynamic yet stable erect posture is a magnificent feat of structural design in combination with a perfectly synchronised control system responding to the changing demands of the body and the environment at all stages in life.

Primary areas of deviation

Where control of posture is inadequate, the body will bend and buckle between the opposing forces of gravity and the reaction of the supporting surface, aptly described by Hare (1990) in *The Human Sandwich*.

The areas where initial deficit of posture is observed are:

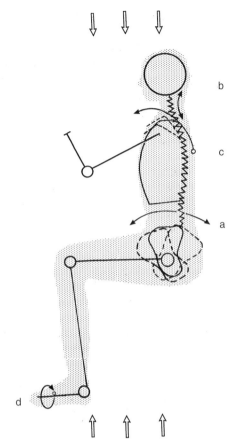

Figure 9.10 Primary areas of deviation: (a) pelvis about the hip joint; (b) cervical spine; (c) mid-thoracic spine; and (d) feet.

- the pelvis about the hip joint
- the mid-thoracic region of the spine
- the cervical spine
- the feet.

Due to its instability in sitting, the pelvis rocks forwards or backwards about the hip joint producing an anterior or posterior tilt (Fig. 9.10a), with a corresponding flexed or extended spine. In this way the hip joint linkage is stabilised. Tilting is not necessarily symmetrical, as when restriction of flexion in one hip introduces a torsion element within the pelvis and spine, predisposing to scoliosis and eventual structural deformity.

The mid-thoracic region of the spine between T6 and T9 has been found to be a point of high stress in the slumped posture (Pope 1985). Forward flexion of the head, shoulders and upper limbs exerts large bending moments about this region of the spine; the ligaments stretch, producing an exaggerated kyphosis and structural change (Fig. 9.10c).

Overstretched spinal tissues in the cervical region will reflect muscle weakness, fatigue and the weight of the head. When some head control remains but the trunk posture is slumped, the result is a compensatory cervical lordosis with tilting of the head (Fig. 9.10b). Keeping the head erect under these conditions requires increased effort and is difficult to maintain. Swallowing and speech mechanisms are also compromised. The child with cerebral palsy, unable to maintain the head erect position or when tired, may rest his head backwards on his shoulders, effectively stabilising the cervical spine linkage.

The delicate balance of weight-bearing through the feet is not easily achieved passively and without muscular control of limb position. Any deviation from the line of weight-bearing will be compounded by the reaction of the supporting surface, resulting in strained ligaments and deformity (Pope 1992).

ASSESSMENT

Purpose

Information is required in order accurately to identify the problems within the context of the particular clinical condition and lifestyle of the disabled person. With this information, realistic goals are set and recommendations made.

With particular reference to posture and special seating it is important that the client is accompanied by a person closely involved with his care. Ideally, as the posture being examined is a reflection of the support or lack of it, the client should be assessed first in the seat or support most used. It is not satisfactory, but sometimes unavoidable, to see the client in, say, a transit wheelchair when he spends most of the day in an armchair. Information required and the assessment process are illustrated in Figure 9.11. Social and environmental information is critical to the information required in assessment of people who are dependent and/or wheelchair users.

Sequence of assessment

It is very important to check personal details and note the date of assessment together with the name of the assessor. Written permission for photographs is necessary. It is important to ask the client and/or carer what they feel are

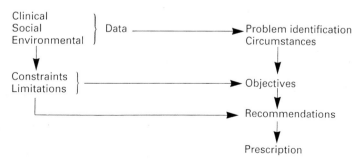

Figure 9.11 The assessment process.

their problems and how they would like them resolved. This information is extremely useful in establishing at the outset the perceived problems and whether the expectations are realistic.

- Gather relevant medical, social and environmental data.
- Establish what equipment and solutions have been tried in the past and the reasons for failure, as well as what measures are currently used to relieve a problem.

- While questioning, observe the client in his seat or wheelchair, noting the posture, any sign of discomfort, the degree of support, freedom and use of the upper limbs, areas of apparent loading, communication, comprehension, and, not least, the relationship with the person accompanying the client.
- Observe independent mobility: self-propulsion or powered.
- Photograph the presenting posture, without adjustment, removing items only if they obscure the picture.

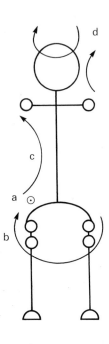

(A)

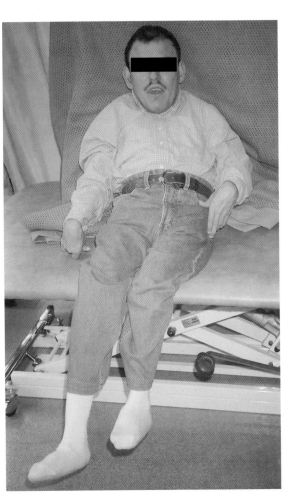

(B)

Figure 9.12 (A) Diagrammatic representation of anterior posture presenting in a photograph (B) of a young man with cerebral palsy showing (a) pelvis rotated forwards and elevated on right side; (b) windsweeping of the lower limbs; (c) lateral flexion of the trunk towards the right side; (d) position of the head.

- Examine in detail the quality of the presenting posture, in terms of alignment, overall attitude, contact surfaces and areas of support.

    It is helpful to superimpose this information on a diagram, as in Figure 9.12.
- Transfer to plinth.
- Immediately observe the seat for signs of localised high loading.
- Observe and note body posture in lying, again without correction. The overall attitude tends to reflect that in sitting when the condition is long standing.
- Establish whether the presenting posture is correctable. It is helpful to examine the trunk with hips and knees flexed as this gives the assessor greater control.
- Measure trunk symmetry. A useful clinical means is to measure vertical and diagonal lines between the coracoid process and the anterior superior iliac spine (ASIS).
- Measure range of movement, paying particular attention to hip, knee, ankle, foot and shoulder.
- Hip flexion is tested with the pelvis in mid-position. If knee flexion contractures interfere with examination of hip extension, the lower limbs are placed over the edge of the plinth, being careful to give support if needed as, if unsupported, severe back pain can be experienced.
- Knee extension is tested with the hip in 90 degrees of flexion.

    (Hip flexion and knee extension are critical measures for seating. The former determines the alignment of trunk to base and the latter the position of footrest to seat.)
- Examine the skin for signs of pressure.
- Assess posture ability in lying and then in sitting over the edge of the plinth (Fig. 9.12B) or sitting on a stool with feet supported. Note if arms or external support are required to maintain position.
- Determine the degree of head control.
- The client is then placed and if necessary supported in the optimum corrected sitting position. Photographs taken at this stage are a useful reference when carrying out recommendations.

- The amount of effort needed by the assessor(s) to hold and maintain the client in this posture is a guide to determining where and how much support is required and in what overall configuration. As an example, a hand required to hold the leg in abduction or foot alignment indicates that additional control is required.
- Transfer back to own seat/chair.

When all data are gathered, the problems are identified and set within the context of the lifestyle and circumstances of the client. Realistic objectives are made and the limitations and constraints are identified and recorded. The options are discussed and recommendations made.

Final prescription will depend upon consideration of the physical condition, lifestyle constraints and limitations together with the resources available. It will also depend upon what the client/carer will accept. Invariably, compromise of some sort is necessary.

It is strongly advised that where recommendations and prescription differ the reason should be documented together with any problems anticipated from, in the assessor's opinion, a less satisfactory prescription.

A review of the client should be automatic.

Measurement of posture ability

Quantification of ability is essential for effective evaluation of input. The Chailey Levels of Ability (Mulcahy et al 1988), developed from the original Physical Ability Scale devised by Hare (Hallett et al 1987), are useful.

However, the quality of the posture is likely to be as important as the quantity in the identification of problems, prescription and evaluation of outcome. The scale has been modified to address this deficit (Pope 1993, 1997b; Fig. 9.13).

BUILDING A STABLE POSTURE

Given the inherent instability and complexity of the body system, the difficulty of substituting for even the smallest deficit in posture ability will be appreciated. The aim of intervention is to use the anatomical structure and intrinsic support where

Quantity (circle appropriate level)		Quality (tick correspondingly)	
Level 1	Unplaceable in sitting	Trunk symmetrical	
Level 2	Placeable with support	Head midline	
Level 3	Can balance, not move	Arms resting by side	
Level 4	Can move forwards within base, cannot reach sideways	Knees mid-position	
Level 5	Can sit independently, move arms freely and reach sideways	Feet flat on floor	
Level 6	Can transfer across surface, cannot regain sitting position	Weight evenly distributed	
Level 7	Can move into and out of sitting position	Score number of ticks	

Figure 9.13 Physical ability scale – measurement of quality and quantity of sitting ability.

possible, applying external aid where it is likely to be most effective and least restrictive. Gravity is used to assist stability rather than using measures to counter it. It is important that the result is aesthetically acceptable.

Specific objectives of posture control

- Support and stabilise body segments and linkages in a symmetrical and appropriate posture for sitting.
- Minimise the load through the sections most vulnerable to deviation.
- Minimise tensile and shear stresses within the tissues.
- Equalise pressures over loaded tissues.
- Facilitate function.
- Provide comfort.
- Provide for an easy change of position.
- Ease the care load.

There are times when it is not possible to satisfy all the criteria. Objectives may conflict: for example, when external support is necessary to maintain alignment but this compromises functional ability.

It has already been noted that uncontrolled mobility of the pelvis and hip joint, weight and position of the head, drag of the upper limbs and shoulder girdle and alignment of the foot give rise to problems when inherent control of posture is impaired. Efforts are directed to control these regions.

A step-by-step approach to a stable posture

For purposes of description and clarity it is assumed that the client can be placed in anatomical alignment of the seated posture, with no significant tissue adaptation interfering with positioning.

Each body segment and linkage is controlled in turn. The extent of the support given will depend upon the degree of impairment.

It is logical to begin with the pelvis, as the orientation and location of the pelvis is 'a major controlling factor in attitude and motion due to its relationship to the centre of mass' (Reynolds 1978). The pelvis may be considered the keystone of the structure, the control of which is fundamental to balance, stability and alignment.

Step 1. Position a level symmetrical pelvis (Fig. 9.14a). Correct alignment is achieved after the client is seated by flexing the trunk about the hip joint in order to ensure an anterior tilt. The buttocks are then tucked as far back in the seat as possible. Check the position.

Step 2. The thighs are placed parallel and horizontal. The seat surface must accommodate the tapering shape of the thigh from buttock to knee thus preventing 'drag' on the seat position (Mulcahy et al 1988) (Fig. 9.14b).

Step 3. Feet are positioned in plantigrade and supported along the entire length of the foot (Fig. 9.14c). External control may be required to secure the position.

(The current tendency to design many wheelchairs with forward-positioned footrests is unsatisfactory for all but a small percentage of the more athletic wheelchair users. Any tightness in the hamstrings causes the feet to fall backwards off the footrest, or, if strapped, to pull the hips forwards on the seat, predisposing to a slumped posture.)

Step 4. Knees are separated and flexed to 90 degrees, the lower leg hanging as near vertical as possible. The position is controlled, if necessary by restraint exerting a pull backwards, downwards and outwards (Fig. 9.14d).

Knee and foot restraint can be considered complementary forms of control. It is rare that the foot alone requires fixation as any tightness in the foot inverters will cause the knees to adduct. It is not unusual to secure knee position alone.

Step 5. Hip and pelvic stability are secured by a strap with Y-shaped attachments exerting a force downwards and backwards, more effectively preventing posterior tilt of the pelvis (Letts 1992) (Fig. 9.14e).

Step 6. Support is applied to the pelvis in the upper sacral region, to prevent posterior tilt, to direct the line of the lumbar curve and to act as a pivot on raising the trunk (Fig. 9.14f). A posteriorly tilted pelvis and flattened lumbar curve prevent extension of the upper trunk and alignment of the head and shoulders.

Step 7. The trunk is raised and supported against the backrest. The dimension of the thorax differs from that of the pelvis; therefore support for the upper trunk should be angled to correspond with this difference (Fig. 9.14g). Contouring of the surface increases comfort and stability. A vertical backrest offers minimal support as there is little loading of the surface; the best that this can achieve is to prevent falling backwards. It is interesting to note that the vertical backrest is a

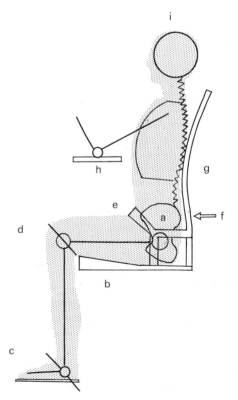

Figure 9.14 (a) Position of the pelvis; (b) accommodating the shape of the thigh; (c) feet in plantigrade, with control if necessary; (d) knees flexed and separated; (e) Y-shaped pelvic strap to assist in securing seat position; (f) posterior support for the pelvis directing lumbar curve; (g) profiling of upper and lower trunk segments; (h) support for the upper limbs; (i) head position – slightly posterior to midline.

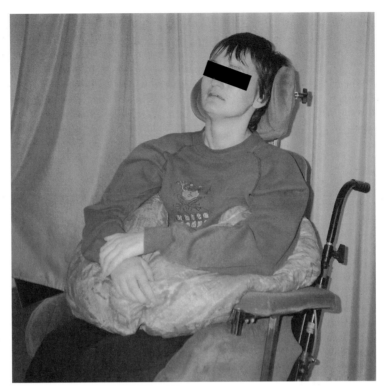

Figure 9.15 Arms supported using a bead bolster when a tray is unacceptable or inappropriate.

common feature of seating for the disabled person but rarely for the able-bodied!

Step 8. Weight of the arms is taken by support anteriorly, thus preventing drag on the shoulders and preventing a rolling forwards of the trunk. The upper limbs are supported at a height which facilitates contact of the extended upper trunk with the back support (Fig. 9.14h).

In less severe cases, adjustment of the height and widening the armrests may be sufficient, but it is quite inadequate for those with little posture control. A 'wrap-around' tray gives more effective support but must be level. A 'wrap-around' bolster filled with polystyrene beads serves as a useful alternative to a tray when the latter is not accepted, or for socialising. It can be made to suit individual tastes and is less conspicuous (Fig. 9.15). It is important to stress that the arms are not recruited to prop the trunk as this can cause pressure on the elbows and/or painful shoulders.

Step 9. Control of the head position usually provides the most challenging task. Considering the weight of the head and flexibility of the cervical spine this is not surprising. Effective control of the head is dependent upon satisfactory control of all parts of the body first. It is important to recognise the limitations of a headrest when used in the upright position. Little or no support is given to the head but it does prevent the head from falling backwards.

The optimum position for supporting the head is slightly posterior to the vertical midline while maintaining horizontal vision (Fig. 9.14i). Additional support may be necessary in the form of a collar or a head band. The latter is a last resort and, if used, should incorporate an elastic insert to prevent jarring the neck in instances of, for example, coughing. Both of these measures are aids to holding the position and are not the support itself.

Step 10. Finally, the difficult question of the overall orientation of the whole support system must be addressed, that is, the position(s) most likely to meet the specification, taking into account the level of posture ability and circumstances of the client. The erect anatomically aligned seated posture is difficult to secure over extended periods of time in spite of the means already outlined and the addition of a variety of straps and harnesses. Bending and buckling of the body occurs over time in most cases. Thus, criteria such as posture stability, alignment, comfort, tissue viability and function are met by use of differing configurations and orientations. It is essential that the support required is appropriate to each configuration, as has been described elsewhere (Pope et al 1988, 1994).

Alternative configurations to the upright posture are as follows:

- Forward lean (Fig. 9.16A) – base stabilised as in steps 1–5. The trunk leans forwards, pivoting about the hip joint, the knees are allowed to flex correspondingly (as hamstring muscles tighten), the trunk is supported anteriorly with the arms resting on a wedge placed on a tray. A pyramidal shape to the body structure is created, thus increasing inherent stability.

- Tilted (Fig. 9.16B) – fully supported as in the complete step-by-step approach described above with the whole system tilted backwards. The head is supported in a flexed position for horizontal vision. (Reclining the backrest without a corresponding adjustment to the seat is contraindicated as it leads to instability and a tendency to slide forwards.)
- Straddle/forward lean (Fig. 9.16C) – resembles the posture adopted by the conventional motorcyclist and incorporated into the design of the SAM system (Pope et al 1994). The support given follows the segment-by-segment control of position, but the means of support corresponds to the differing requirements of the configuration: i.e. straddle seat to fix the pelvis and anterior support for the trunk. The pelvic position is secured by a strap through the lower border of the anterior support which fastens to the back of the seat. The arms are supported on a tray, feet rest on the base (Fig. 9.17) The posture created is a modified pyramidal shape and is stable with support.

The ideal recommended, particularly in the severest cases, is a combination of forward lean,

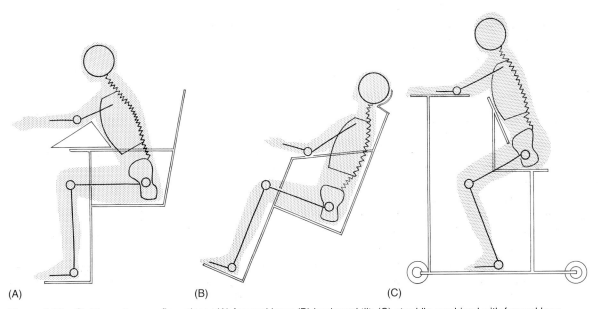

Figure 9.16 Stable posture configurations: (A) forward lean; (B) backward tilt; (C) straddle combined with forward lean.

(A)　　　　　　　　　　(B)　　　　　　　　　　(C)

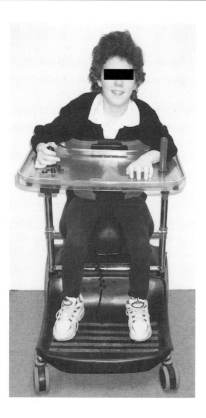

Figure 9.17 SAM seat incorporating a saddle seat and anterior support in a forward lean posture.

backward tilt and, where appropriate, upright. The latter is used only when some posture ability remains and for brief periods of time. There are many more wheelchairs available with a built-in tilt-in-space facility which accommodates posture function and rest needs without having to transfer out of the system.

Matching the level of ability to the support required

Hard and fast rules dictating the amount of support required in a specific case cannot be given. Much will depend on the circumstances of the individual and, not least, what he/she or the carer will accept.

The categories below relate the amount of posture support required to the Chailey Levels of Sitting Ability (see Fig. 9.13). As such, they are not necessarily appropriate to the lifestyle of the individual (see 'The art of compromise' p 212).

Level 1. Unplaceable; established contracture and deformity prevent alignment of body segments as in, for example, scoliosis.

Custom seating is the preferred option, usually moulded with optimum correction. The upright position is not recommended as support and control are much reduced in this position and progression of deformity continues. A tilting mechanism incorporated into the seating system offers the best compromise, allowing gravity-assisted positioning to maximise stability and segmental control together with brief periods in a more, but rarely full, upright position.

While the consensus opinion in the literature suggests that external supports do little to reduce the eventual magnitude of scoliosis, it is the view of this author, based on clinical experience, that containment and even some correction of deformity is possible, given the appropriate and consistent posture management in both lying and sitting.

Level 2. Placeable with support. This level of posture ability requires complete step-by-step build-up of support, described above (pages 203–204). It is unlikely that the erect position can be used other than for brief periods. Gravity-assisted positions (Fig. 9.16) are required to maintain alignment and stability of posture, preferably alternating between the forward lean and tilt, for function and rest, respectively.

Level 3. Can maintain position when placed but the quality of the posture may differ from the normal configuration (Fig. 9.3).

A good stable base is fundamental for maximum holding of thighs and pelvis. Additional support will be required for trunk and arms. Upright sitting will be possible for short periods only. An alternative supported position, either tilted or leaning forwards, will be required to counter the effects of weakness and fatigue.

Level 4. Can maintain position and move within the base. The support given is similar to that for level 3 but the trunk support may be reduced and the upright posture may be tolerated for longer.

Level 5. Can sit independently, use either hand freely and can recover balance.

A firm shallow contoured base, incorporating pelvis and thighs and feet stabilised, is the essential requisite, facilitating a wider range of postural adjustments and peripheral movement. A contoured backrest and support for the arms will be required for prolonged periods of sitting.

Level 6–7. Sitting ability is sufficiently developed to allow movement out of position and to regain position.

Well-designed seating for the able-bodied person is suitable, incorporating a firm contoured base and back support. Similarly, the arms will require support: a table or desk to lean on, armrests, tray or bolster on a wheelchair. If this support is not available, fatigue and drag on the shoulders results in a slumped C-shaped spine with poking head, a posture not exclusive to the disabled person!

The higher levels of sitting ability may still require periods of rest in controlled configurations as a means of countering or preventing selective tissue adaptation. The necessity for 'therapeutic positioning' is judged by the ability of the individual to change his posture regularly.

The decision to use the upright position and the time for which it can be used, particularly with the lower levels of ability, depend largely on the quality of the posture. Independent sitting achieved by deviation of alignment, asymmetrical loading and a lowering of the centre of mass predisposes to established contracture and deformity and perpetuates use of the limbs as an aid to balance. The indication in these cases is for more rather than less support. Further, it has been observed that the appropriate support does not prevent the development of independent control where the potential for this exists (Fulford et al 1982, Pope et al 1994) and may facilitate it.

The shape of the supporting components is important. The body itself is contoured in all planes. Much of the seating for able-bodied people reflects this, with the result that comfort and stability of posture are improved. Conversely, much of the seating for the disabled population incorporates flat surfaces or inappropriate contouring such as the 'hammock' seats of many folding wheelchairs. Comfort and support are minimal. Even the shallowest contouring will assist in channelling or guiding body segments to the correct position, provided that the overall shape corresponds/conforms to that of the occupant. Contouring also demands correct positioning of the client in the system. Incorrect positioning will do more harm than good and is likely to cause localised high pressure.

To summarise, a secure base is essential for prolonged sitting in every case. Additional support is dependent upon the quality and quantity of sitting ability. The appropriate support will not necessarily interfere with development of intrinsic posture control. Access to alternative resting positions is necessary and reasonable, recognising that few of us can sit in one position for any length of time.

CUSTOMISED SEATING

Customised seating can take many forms, from simple modifications to standard systems to intimately moulded systems. In the context of this section it refers to those systems moulded to the individual – for example, thermoplastic and foam carved moulding – together with linkage systems such as Matrix and Lynx.

It is not possible in this chapter to deal with the subject of custom-moulded seating in depth. However, there are certain points related to this form of seating which need to be mentioned.

When to use it

Strict prescriptive rules are not possible but, in general, custom-moulded seating is used in the following situations:

- in cases of structural deformity – for example, significant scoliosis and/or windsweeping of the limbs
- where predominant unilateral movement destabilises trunk position in those people with little ability to recover a midline position – for example, in hemiplegia, following brain injury.

Purpose of customised seating

- To arrest the progression of deformity. Custom moulding is used to give maximum support for the control of segmental alignment. If made correctly and used consistently it is this author's experience that arrest of deformity is possible and on occasion some correction is achieved.

- To stabilise the trunk and thereby free the limbs for movement.
- To distribute pressure over the maximum area.

The therapist must be aware that it is not the particular material used nor even the technical expertise with which the support is made which ensures a satisfactory result. The critical factor is that the shape corresponds to the particular individual. This is dependent upon correct analysis of the problems in the presenting body posture and identification of the overall body shape to be achieved together with the exact areas which can be used for support and control of the required posture. For example, if hip flexion is sig-

nificantly limited, the leg is not useful in stabilising position and other areas of support must be identified and used. Contouring the shape to correspond with the shape of the individual, correcting what is realistically possible and accommodating what is not is critical to the success of this form of support (Fig. 9.18A, B).

For a successful outcome, a tilted orientation is almost always necessary. This ensures the loading of the different areas of the mould which contribute to support and control of posture alignment.

Custom-moulded support systems require a depth of knowledge and skill not always available, with the result that many are unsatisfactory. The material from which they are made is usually blamed rather than the shape and orientation of the mould which is, in general, the real cause of failure.

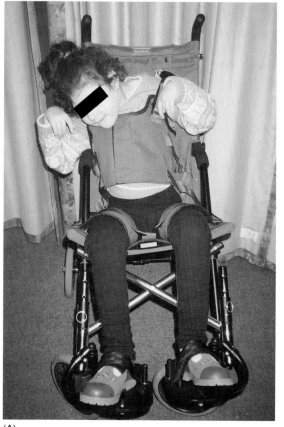

(A)

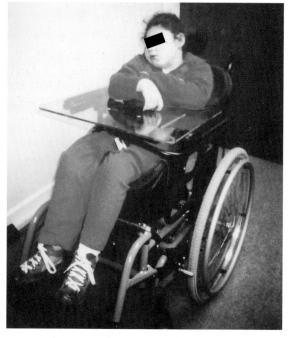

(B)

Figure 9.18 (A) Child without appropriate support – note position of arms and head; (B) with customised contoured support – head raised and arms relaxed.

SIT-TO-STAND WHEELCHAIRS

Wheelchair technology has developed extensively in recent years with an increase in the variety of wheelchairs available. Among these developments are a variety of systems which raise the user from sitting to standing. There are advantages to this facility which combines mobility with the therapeutic value of standing. Most of the systems currently available incorporate a powered elevating mechanism that encourages regular use of the standing posture by those unable to use it of their own accord.

A significant advantage of these wheelchairs lies in their ability to accommodate varying degrees of the erect posture in those with knee flexion contractures. They may even be used to stretch these tissues, but great care is necessary to prevent overstretch, pain and discomfort.

A further use of sit-to-stand wheelchairs is in those rare but difficult to manage cases where there is little or no hip flexion and a sitting posture is not possible. In such situations the supported standing position facilitates functional and social activity together with an, albeit limited, mobility.

In clinical practice a further advantage of standing with the aid of a sit-to-stand wheelchair has been observed: rising through the vertical plane produces less vertigo, less anxiety and less 'fainting'.

However, there are a number of disadvantages to these systems:

- The elevating mechanism adds to the weight and complexity of the machine.
- If the posture when standing is not aligned symmetrically, standing will compound the deviation.
- Perhaps the most significant caution relates to the forces acting on the ligaments of the knee joint in the process of rising from sitting to standing. In most of the existing systems the lower limb is fixed just below the knee joint such that excessive shearing occurs across the knee joint, which is particularly high in the mid range. While transient forces exerted during sitting to standing may not be deleterious, the sustained force exerted during partial standing may be excessive and lead to tissue

overstretch and damage. Research is required to clarify the mechanical conditions prevailing during sit to stand when using these wheelchairs.

SPECIFIC PROBLEM SOLVING

Pelvic obliquity. The level of the seat should only be altered to accommodate structural deficit such as amputation with disarticulation at the hip joint or when established deformity such as scoliosis makes compromise unavoidable. In all other cases the aim should be to achieve a level pelvis by correct alignment relative to the supporting surface. The technique when positioning the pelvis in cases of non-structural obliquity is to combine forward flexion of the trunk about the hip joint with bending into the concavity of the scoliosis. This position is held while the lower limbs are positioned and the pelvis secured. The

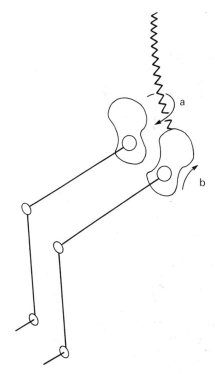

Figure 9.19 A seat-to-backrest angle greater than the available hip flexion angle induces (a) forward rotation on the side of the limited movement with (b) posterior tilting of the pelvis.

trunk is then raised, maintaining alignment while the rest of the support is secured.

Reduced hip flexion. Limitation in range of flexion at the hip joint is probably the greatest constraint on achieving balance of the upper trunk over the pelvis and thighs. If hip flexion is less than 90 degrees bilaterally and the seat-to-backrest angle is more acute, the pelvis will tilt posteriorly and slumping and sliding will occur. If hip flexion is limited on one side only, ipsilateral posterior tilting and rotation forwards of the pelvis occurs (Fig. 9.19). Frequently, the pelvis is forced upwards on the same side, predisposing to scoliosis concave to the side of limited hip flexion which, if not remedied, progresses to impingement of the thorax on the pelvis (Pope 1997b).

The existing hip angle determines the seat-to-backrest angle. If the backrest alone is reclined to accommodate a more open hip angle, sliding forwards will occur. The position is stabilised by ramping the seat without compromising the reduced hip flexion and/or by tilting the whole system to the point where stability of position is achieved. Where appropriate, the ramp can be adjusted to accommodate any differential in flexion between hip joints.

'Windswept' lower limbs. These can lead to pelvic rotation predisposing to spinal deformity. In lying, the lower limbs rotate the pelvis, in the same direction as the windsweeping. In sitting, if the deviated lower limbs are confined within the conventional seat the pelvis will appear to be rotated forwards in the opposite direction to the windsweeping (Fig. 9.20). In general, maintaining pelvic symmetry is the priority and deviation of the lower limbs must be accommodated.

Supporting the feet. Any bias of tissues towards plantar flexion and inversion will prevent the foot from maintaining alignment when placed on the footrests and will require additional control. The transmission of load when the foot is malaligned will compound the problem (Fig. 9.21A). Control should be applied as in Figure 9.21B: i.e. proximal to the talocalcaneal joint.

Complete removal of support is recommended in some situations when the feet are used as the fixed point for movement and activity, the so-called extensor thrust. Under these conditions, harnesses and straps do little to secure the posi-

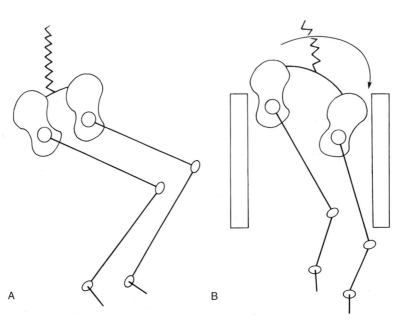

Figure 9.20 (A) 'Windswept' deformity of the lower limbs in lying. (B) When confined within the armrests of a conventional seat, the constraint imposed on the lower limbs rotates the pelvis.

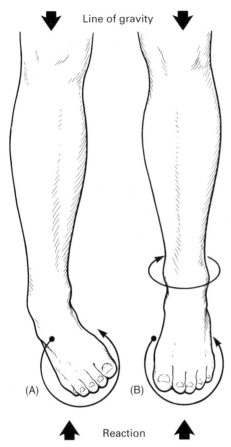

Figure 9.21 In (A) line of gravity falling medial to the normal compounds in the deformity; (B) location and direction of control required to correct deviation.

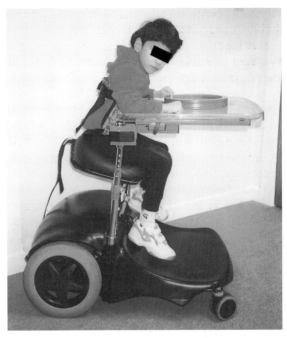

Figure 9.22 Feet unsupported to encourage learning to move about a sitting base rather than using the feet as the point about which movement occurs.

tion. Removing the point of fixation may encourage learning to sit, provided it is combined with an appropriately supported configuration as in the SAM system (Fig. 9.22, Pope et al 1994).

When not using the feet for support, particular attention must be given to the maintenance of a plantigrade foot by use of orthoses, supportive footwear and frequent stretching of tissues. The standing posture is the most effective means of stretching the tissues and thus helping to maintain a plantigrade foot, provided the foot is correctly aligned.

In conjunction with raising the seat in children whose repertoire of movement is limited to extension, lowering the tray or removing it altogether for limited periods has been found to facilitate activity in forward flexion (Fig. 9.22). An extending footrest which dissipates the force of the thrust can be a useful alternative to not supporting the feet in cases where extensor activity is a problem.

Knee flexion contractures. When very severe, knee flexion contractures can lead to the disabled person becoming unseatable. Even mild reduction in range of extension is a major constraint to achieving a stable sitting posture. The configuration of the conventional wheelchair seat, framework and footrests prevents accommodation of contracted lower limbs and feet. Feet will continually fall backwards off the footrests and if prevented from doing so by straps or restraint, the hips are pulled forwards, the pelvis tilts posteriorly, the spine flexes and a slumped unstable sitting posture results with all its concomitant problems (Pope 1985, Pope et al 1991).

Kyphosis. A long-standing, passively correctable, round-shouldered posture with overstretch of spinal ligaments may not be adequately controlled by the step-by-step approach described earlier. A continuing tendency of the upper trunk and/or head to roll forwards may be rectified by increasing the anterior tilt of the pelvis. The resultant increase in lumbar lordosis facilitates extension of the upper trunk. In addition, it may be necessary to raise the support for the arms. These measures will only be effective in combination with some degree of gravity-assisted positioning, i.e. tilting.

An effective yet simple and comfortable means of countering a mobile kyphosis is the use of the forward lean position, arms resting on a table or tray as in Fig. 9.16A. An adequate range of shoulder elevation is, however, required.

An established kyphosis will require accommodation of the curvature posteriorly in order to bring the head to vertical midline, thus ensuring horizontal vision. If the backrest is reclined in order to achieve this, sliding will occur. Tilting the system and/or increasing the rake of the seat will be necessary. In general, customised contouring of the backrest to the kyphotic trunk, combined with a degree of tilt, provides the most satisfactory solution.

Asymmetrical movement. Development of asymmetrical movement or recovery of movement on one side only, as in cases of cerebral palsy or following brain damage, can give rise to considerable posture problems in sitting. Each active movement tends to disturb balance and the body falls to the side of the movement. As the individual is unable to recover alignment, the posture is maintained. Further activity compounds the malalignment, increasing the curvature with eventual tissue and structural changes (Fig. 9.23). The problem is addressed by giving maximum trunk support, with particular attention directed to control at shoulder level on the side of the movement. Custom moulding is recommended in order to achieve the desired control.

Heightened neural activity and some movement disorders. These are symptoms which can be modified by treating them as a disorder of posture, directing effort to restore equilibrium, stability and alignment of body segments relative to the supporting surface outlined earlier (Pope 1992, 1994, Pope et al 1994). Conversely, dysto-

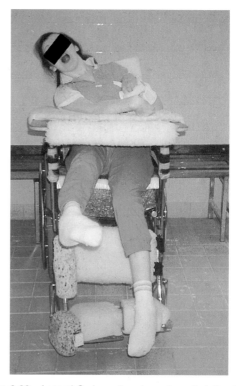

Figure 9.23   Lateral C-shaped posture characteristic of asymmetrical recovery of movement in the brain-damaged patient.

nias, chorea and rigid syndromes such as those found in Huntington and Parkinson's disease are less amenable, if not impossible, to control by these measures.

THE ART OF COMPROMISE

There is rarely, if ever, any intervention related to the imposition of external posture control which does not have some disadvantage. Compromise is almost always inevitable.

It is, on the whole, relatively easy to analyse the condition, identify the problem and even to recognise the solution. The difficulty arises when the solution has to be applied within the context of needs, wishes, lifestyle and environment of the disabled person and those caring for him. These are the factors setting the limits on intervention and preventing a rigid prescriptive practice. The particular answer to a problem remains specific to the individual and his circumstances. It is never more challenging than in the circumstances of the home, as opposed to the institutional environment (Pope 1997a). Clearly, this is the area which requires the greatest knowledge, skill, experience and tact.

The art of compromise lies, first of all, in the recognition that compromise is necessary and is accepted. The skill lies in determining the priorities. Setting these and discussing them is an exercise in cooperation with the client and those most involved with his care. This can be very demanding as each individual views the problem from a different perspective.

The data gathered at assessment are fundamental to the processes of setting priorities and of compromise. Perhaps the most useful clue to the needs and wishes of the client and carers is the response to the initial question at assessment: 'What is your problem and what would you like done about it'. It becomes apparent during assessment if the real problem has been recognised and if the expectations are realistic and/or feasible. Where choices have to be made, the options are discussed, clearly explaining the advantages and disadvantages of each. The final decision rests, as a rule, with the client and his carer.

There are cases in which it is advisable to accommodate the wishes of the client or carer against the better judgement of the professional, provided that safety is not compromised. As an illustration, consider the athletic young man confined to a wheelchair following traumatic brain injury. He has little or no independent sitting ability. The understandable desire of parents/relatives is for a system which fits the premorbid image, i.e. 'sporty'; thus a lightweight wheelchair is requested. Relatives may not be convinced of its unsuitability unless it is tried.

Any external support will, by definition, be restrictive to a greater or lesser degree. Best efforts in this respect are a poor substitute for inherent dynamic and highly sophisticated normal posture control mechanisms. Such support tends to attract attention and highlights the disability.

It is not within the scope of this chapter to cover the whole area of compromise, nor would it be possible to do so. There are, however, situations which are frequent and difficult to resolve, none more so than when the solution calls for a 'trade-off' between posture and function. The following are a few examples of such cases.

Support versus freedom of movement

As a general rule, function takes precedence over symmetry of posture. There is little point in achieving a symmetrical and stable posture if the disabled person is functionally less able than before the intervention. The most difficult decision in relation to this situation is when function is dependent on the adoption of balance strategies which predispose to the development of secondary complications. This situation is frequently encountered in progressive conditions where such strategies gradually develop to overcome the increasing weakness and instability, most notably in multiple sclerosis, muscular dystrophy and the spinal atrophies. Any interference with these strategies compromises function.

However, much can be done to satisfy both support and freedom of movement needs by judicious use of appropriate support together with alterations and adjustments to the environment, including angles and height of working surfaces. When little can be done to give the support necessary to control alignment, other procedures must be incorporated into the daily routine to counter the deleterious consequences of the particular posture adopted. There are occasions when some sacrifice of movement by restraint and control is both desirable and permissible.

High amplitude tremors. These are encountered in some conditions such as multiple sclerosis. Movements are spontaneous, and attempted functional activity is frustrating and futile. These wild fluctuations of movement, particularly of the head and limbs, result in damage to the person concerned and to those caring for him. Such symptoms are acutely distressing. The symptoms are alleviated by giving full support and containing the posture in the tilted position. It is a measure of satisfactory control of central body segments when distal segments require minimal support.

Severe ataxia. This is found in cerebellar disease, for example. The dysmetria, on attempted activity, may be so severe that voluntary movement becomes functionally ineffective. The degree of dysmetria is a function of the number of intervening joints, the length of the limb and the distance to be travelled in execution of the task. Support and restraint applied to proximal segments and intervening joints, together with a decrease in the distance to be travelled, may enhance functional performance. For example, independent feeding may be possible if the disabled person leans forward on to a raised table with the arms and shoulders well supported.

Spastic diplegia. This is characterised by the inability to secure a satisfactory stable base (i.e. pelvis and thighs) above which to balance and control the trunk. These clients frequently require knee and foot restraint in addition to securing a stable base, which inevitably compromises movement of the lower limbs. Benefit is seen, however, in the facilitation of balance and functional activity in trunk, head and upper limbs. In addition, learning to sit is probably helped rather than hindered, especially in the child.

Self-inflicted damage and mutilation. This is seen in cases of Lesch–Nyhan syndrome, and may require a system of total restraint. These conditions, together with the dystonias, are some of the least responsive to control through management of posture and are exceedingly distressing and frustrating for everyone concerned.

Support versus mobility

The addition of a ramp, wedge or contouring may impede transfer into and out of a seat, affecting the client or the carer. Adjustment is made in an attempt to satisfy mutually exclusive criteria: i.e. a secure postural base and easy transfer. In most cases the latter takes priority.

Support for the arms to relieve drag on the shoulders and upper trunk is frequently necessary. The client, however, may still wish or need to self-propel, in which case stability of the upper trunk is lost when the arms are not supported. The best compromise will depend on the individual case. Lever-type self-propulsion offers a solution to trunk instability and is ergonomically efficient (Glazer et al 1980), but involves compromise of a technical nature.

Client versus carer needs

Solutions which significantly increase the time and effort of care are unlikely to be adhered to in the long term. Consultation between all parties will enable the prescriber to arrive at the most appropriate solution in the particular circumstances. Therapists must always bear in mind the difficulties encountered and the stresses involved in the everyday care of a disabled person, particularly for a relative. While many relatives are keen to provide optimal care, they are frequently under intense stress when the addition of even a simple task is too much (Pope 1997a, Murphy 1999).

Aesthetics versus efficacy

Posture support or control is achieved in a number of ways, ranging from the simple and unobtrusive to the complex and obvious. There are few disabled people who wish to draw attention to their disability. This may account for much of the non-compliance with recommendations when posture control is the issue. The following examples illustrate the point.

- The mother with a disabled child is content with a 'buggy' as it is commonplace for all small children. She is less able to accept a more conspicuous system, even while recognising the necessity for both the control of posture and promotion of function.
- The teenager, perhaps suffering from muscular dystrophy, with a collapsing spine, who wishes to be as functional and inconspicuous as possible in a wheelchair will reject additional, albeit effective, but necessarily restrictive, support.

Such cases require extreme care, sensitivity, and delicacy in handling discussions. It is frequently necessary to proceed gradually, perhaps over a long time, in order to reach the best compromise.

Check list to aid prescriptive practice

The following questions have been found useful in helping to avoid inappropriate prescription of supportive equipment:

- Is it needed?
- Is it wanted?
- Do(es) he/she/they know how to use it?
- Can he/she/they manage it?
- Does it fit in with the home environment?
- Is it socially acceptable?
- Does it look good?
- What are the 'trade-offs' and are they acceptable?

Counter-strategies

There are times when, for one reason or another, intervention is not appropriate, possible, or acceptable. In these cases, strategies are used to counter or minimise the deleterious effects of sustained 'bad' posture in sitting.

The stresses and strains on the spine may be relieved by the following:

- A period of time in prone lying with the arms elevated to mid-position and a pillow under the chest.

- Leaning forwards over a firm foam wedge or pillow placed on a tray or table, provided that the forward inclination is achieved by flexion about the hip joint and not by flexion of the spine.
- Early signs of asymmetry within the trunk may be relieved by side-lying over a pillow or small roll. Care is essential to ensure the correction is being applied to the appropriate tissues. Surface marking of the spinous processes will help to clarify this.

A programme of daily standing ensures a change of position, relieving pressure and maintaining length in those tissues vulnerable to shortening with prolonged sitting. The hip and knee flexors and plantar flexors of the feet are particularly at risk.

Perhaps the most effective countermeasure of all is control of posture in lying. The majority of the more severely disabled people spend considerably more time in lying than in sitting. It is here that many of the initial problems arise and tissue adaptation occurs, as in the case of 'windswept' lower limbs.

Control of posture in lying is essential, even when the sitting posture is supported adequately. It is a vital part of the overall physical manage-

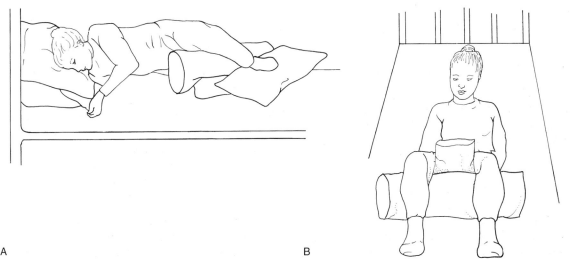

A   B

Figure 9.24 Control of posture in lying: (A) side-lying, trunk supported, roll between thighs to stabilise the position; (B) supine lying, feet supported, using a T-roll to stabilise position (Pope 1992).

ment regime. The supported positions illustrated in Figures 9.24A and B offer a simple and effective means of posture control (Pope 1992).

Corrective positioning to control posture in lying should be immediate in the acute stage of any disease or injury which threatens to incapacitate motor or posture ability, and certainly before any support for the sitting posture is considered. Appropriate action at this stage will considerably lessen the problems associated with seating at a later time.

CONCLUSIONS

Successful outcome in terms of matching posture needs with lifestyle is dependent upon an understanding of problem causation, comprehensive assessment, accurate problem identification, cooperative discussion and effort, judicious compromise and compliance with recommendations.

Appropriate and consistent posture management can reduce or prevent secondary complications associated with posture impairment and do much to contribute to 'quality of life' (Pope 1994). Although initial outlay in terms of available resources may be comparatively large, effective intervention can reduce the cost and effort of care in the long term. In addition, effect-

ive posture management can enhance and reinforce recovery of function in those with potential. In fact, it provides the 'platform' from which movement is encouraged and facilitated.

As a final word, problems presenting in the seated posture should not be treated in isolation. Consideration must be given to the management of body posture in all other positions and situations. However complex and diffuse the pathology, there are few, if any, who do not benefit from appropriate management.

ACKNOWLEDGEMENTS

The author wishes to thank Gavin Jenkins, previously of Mary Marlborough Centre, Oxford, for the initial drawings; the Medical Illustrations Department of the John Radcliffe Infirmary, Oxford, for completion of the diagrams; the people with disabilities from whom I have learnt so much; and family and colleagues for their comments during preparation of the manuscript.

The statement attributed to Deane on page 197 was made by Mr G Deane, Consultant Orthopaedic Surgeon, during a lecture at the University of Surrey in 1982, and confirmed in discussion with me thereafter.

REFERENCES

Bartelink D L 1957 The role of abdominal pressure in relieving the pressure on the lumbar intervertebral disc. Journal of Bone and Joint Surgery 39B: 718–725

Condie E 1991 A therapeutic approach to physical disability. Physiotherapy 77(2): 72–77

Edelman G M 1993 Neural Darwinism: selection and reentrant signalling in higher brain function. Neuron 10(2): 115–125

Fulford G E, Brown J K 1976 Position as a cause of deformity in children with cerebral palsy. Developmental Medicine and Child Neurology 18: 305–314

Fulford G E, Cairns T P, Sloan Y 1982 Sitting problems of children with cerebral palsy. Developmental Medicine and Child Neurology 24: 48–53

Glazer R M, Sawka M N, Brukne M F, Wilde S W 1980 Applied physiology for wheelchair design. Journal of Applied Physiology 1: 41–44

Hallett R, Hare N, Milner A D 1987 Description and evaluation of an assessment form. Physiotherapy 73(5): 220–225

Hare N 1990 The analysis and measurement of physical ability – the human sandwich factor. Book 1: Proceedings of meeting November 10th. Hare Association for Physical Ability. Available from HAFPA, 3 Melton Grove, West Bridgford, Nottingham, England

Karni A, Meyer G, Re-Hipolito C et al 1998 Acquisition of skilled motor performance: fast and slow experience-driven changes in primary motor cortex. Proceedings of the National Academy of Sciences of the USA 95: 861–868

Kelly E D 1949 Teaching posture and body mechanics. Barnes, New York

Kidd G L, Brodie P 1980 The motor unit: a review. Physiotherapy 66(5): 146–152

Koreska J, Robertson D, Mills R H, Gibson D A, Albisser A M 1977 Biomechanics of the lumbar spine and its clinical significance. Orthopedic Clinics of North America 8: 121–133

Latash M L, Anson J G 1996 What are normal movements in atypical populations. Behavioural and Brain Science 19: 55–106

Latash M L, Nicholas J J 1996 Motor control research in rehabilitation medicine. Disability and Rehab 18(6): 293–299

Letts M R 1992 Principles of seating the disabled. CRC Press, Florida

Massion J 1992 Movement, posture and equilibrium: interaction and co-ordination. Progress in Neurology 38: 35–56

Massion J, Gahery Y 1978 The reflex control of posture and movement. Proceedings of IBRO Conference, Pisa, Italy 50: 219–226

Morris J M, Lucas D B, Bresler B 1961 Role of the trunk in stability of the spine. Journal of Bone and Joint Surgery 43A: 327–351

Mulcahy C M, Pountney T E, Nelham R L, Green E, Billington G D 1988 Adaptive seating for motor handicap: problems, a solution, assessment and prescription. Physiotherapy 74(7): 531–536

Murphy W 1999 The caring experience – a qualitative study of carers of people with complex disability. MSc thesis, Oxford University, England

Norris C M 1995 Spinal stabilisation. Physiotherapy 81(2): 64–79

Oda I, Abani K, Lu D, Shono Y, Kaneda K 1996 Biomechanical role of posterior elements of the costovertebral joints and rib cage in the stability of the thoracic spine. Spine 21(12): 1423–1429

Onan O A, Heggeness M H, Hipp J A 1998 A motion analysis of cervical facet joints. Spine 23(4): 430–439

Pope P M 1985 A study of postural instability in relation to posture in the wheelchair. Physiotherapy 71(3): 127–129

Pope P M 1992 Management of the physical condition in patients with chronic and severe neurological pathologies. Physiotherapy 78(12): 896–903

Pope P M 1993 Measurement of postural competency in the severely disabled patient. Book 5: Proceedings of meeting May 17th, Hare Association for Physical Ability. Available from HAFPA, 3 Melton Grove, West Bridgford, Nottingham, England

Pope P M 1994 Advances in seating the severely disabled neurological patient. Physiotherapy Ireland 15(1): 9–14

Pope P M 1997a Management of the physical condition in people with chronic and severe neurological disabilities living in the community. Physiotherapy 83(3): 116–122

Pope P M 1997b Assessment of people with severe and complex physical disability. Paper presented at the Congress of the Chartered Society of Physiotherapy, September

Pope P M, Booth E, Gosling G 1988 The development of alternative seating and mobility systems. Physiotherapy Practice 4: 78–93

Pope P M, Bowes C E, Tudor M, Andrews B 1991 Surgery combined with continued post-operative stretching and management of knee flexion contractures in cases of multiple sclerosis. A report of six cases. Clinical Rehabilitation 5: 15–23

Pope P M, Bowes C E, Booth E 1994 Postural control in sitting, the SAM system: evaluation of use over three years. Developmental Medicine and Child Neurology 36: 241–252

Pountney T E, Mulcahy C M, Green E 1990 Early development of postural control. Physiotherapy 76(12): 799–802

Putz R L, Muller-Gerbl M 1996 The vertebral column – a phylogenetic failure? A theory explaining the function and vulnerability of the human spine. Clinical Anatomy 9(3): 205–212

Quint U, Wilke H J, Shirazi-Adl A, Parnianpour M, Loer F, Claes L E 1998 Importance of the intersegmental trunk muscles in the stability of the lumbar spine. A biomechanical study in vitro. Spine 23(18): 1937–1945

Reynolds H 1978 The inertial properties of the body and its segments. NASA Reference Publication 1024. Anthropometric Source Book IV: 1–55

Shadmehr R, Holcomb H H 1997 Neural correlates of motor memory consolidation. Science 277(8): 821–825

Shirazi-Adl A, Ahmed A M, Shrivastava S C 1986 Mechanical response of a lumbar motion segment in axial torque alone and combined with compression. Spine 11: 914–927

Son K, Miller J A, Schultz A B 1988 The mechanical role of the trunk and lower extremities in a seated weight moving task in the sagittal plane. Journal of Biomechanical Engineering 110(2): 97–103

Whitman A 1924 Postural deformities in children. New York State Journal of Medicine 24: 871–874

Zacharkow D J 1988 Posture sitting and standing, chair design and exercise. Charles C Thomas, Springfield, Ill

10

Splinting and the use of orthoses in the management of patients with neurological disorders

Susan Edwards, Paul T. Charlton

INTRODUCTION

The use of different types of splints and orthoses in the management of patients with neurological disorders has been, and remains, somewhat controversial, particularly for patients with hypertonus. As with all interventions, splints and/or orthoses should only be used after detailed assessment of the patient's problems, taking into consideration the effect that their application may have holistically.

An orthosis or splint is an external device designed to apply, distribute or remove forces to or from the body in a controlled manner to perform one or both of the basic functions of:

- control of body motion
- an alteration or prevention of alteration in the shape of body tissues (Rose 1986).

They may be used to compensate for weak or absent muscle function or to resist the unopposed action of hypertonic muscles (Fyfe et al 1993).

Throughout this chapter, the term orthosis is used to describe the more permanent devices either 'off the peg' or 'made to measure' by an orthotist, and the terms 'splinting' or 'casting' are used to describe the more temporary devices usually made by physiotherapists or occupational therapists.

PHYSICAL PRINCIPLES

It is important to understand a number of physical principles when considering splinting for

219

patients either as an aid to function or as an adjunct to treatment.

Forces

A force has magnitude and direction and when applied to a mass tends to result in movement in the direction the force is applied. Force may be defined as a physical action that always acts along a straight line and may be represented by a line, the length of which is proportional to the magnitude of the force, the beginning of which represents the point of application of the force and the direction of which corresponds to the direction of the force (Rose et al 1982). The graphical representation of force is known as a vector.

Ground reaction force

This is the force exerted by the ground to counteract:

- the vertical force of body weight
- the horizontal force in the line of propulsion
- the lateral force exerted as the body moves forward during the gait cycle.

These forces may be represented as a resultant vector which describes magnitude and direction. Its origin is the point of application of the resultant forces.

Moments

When a force acts on a body, the effect of the force is dependent upon the distance from application to the turning point or joint. This effect is the moment of force which is equal to the magnitude of the force multiplied by the perpendicular distance of the force from the joint axis (Galley & Forster 1987).

Pressure

This is the intensity of the force applied to a particular area and is the force per unit area. Pressure may be reduced by increasing the surface area over which the force acts.

Clinical application

Motion may be caused or prevented by forces which, in the human body, are produced by muscle contractions. Patients with neurological disability often demonstrate abnormal tone and movement that may lead to insufficient and/or inappropriate forces being generated. Those with low tone are unable to generate sufficient force to maintain stability or produce movement. In this instance, the orthosis is merely required to oppose the weight of the limb and stabilise the joint(s), allowing use of any residual, purposeful movement. Those with hypertonus may also have difficulty in generating sufficient force to counteract what may be both neural and non-neural contributions to shortening of the antagonist muscle groups. In this situation the orthosis is required to resist a much higher force and must be rigid to prevent unwanted movement by the pull of hypertonic muscles. In both instances, extrinsic support in the form of an orthosis may be required to facilitate stability and/or movement and thereby function.

The problem of an unstable knee illustrates the importance of these physical principles. In standing, the knee may be maintained in a position of extension in spite of minimal activity of the quadriceps muscle group, providing that the ground reaction force passes in front of the knee joint. In effect, the knee can be 'locked' in extension, often in association with flexion of the hip. The knee is protected in part by the anterior cruciate ligament and the posterior capsule of the joint, but if this posture is maintained over a protracted period of time, these structures become lax, causing the knee to move further into a position of hyperextension.

In this situation an orthosis may be recommended to provide stability and protect the integrity of the joint. The caliper is designed so that the line of force passes directly through the knee joint, thereby minimising the moment arm. Applied in this manner, the orthosis acts as a stabilising device with only small forces acting between the leg and the caliper.

Where there is a knee flexion deformity, the ground reaction force passes behind the knee

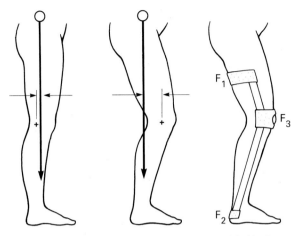

Figure 10.1   Three-point force application provided by long leg caliper (after Rose et al 1982).

joint. A flexion moment is produced, the magnitude of which rises as the degree of flexion increases. An orthosis may resist this moment by producing an equal and opposite moment through three-point fixation (Fig. 10.1).

The pressure exerted by this resistance is determined by the length of the moment arm and the surface area over which it acts. For this reason the caliper should extend the full length of the leg, with a broad thigh band at the line of the hip joint, and attach into the shoe (Fig. 10.2).

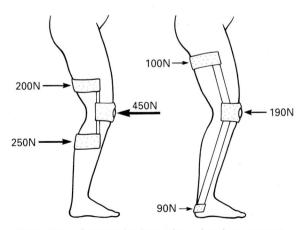

Figure 10.2   Comparative forces for a short knee support and a long leg caliper (after Rose et al 1982).

CLASSIFICATION OF ORTHOSES

Orthoses are classified in relation to the parts of the body over which they act. Below-knee calipers or drop-foot splints are referred to as ankle–foot orthoses (AFOs), full leg calipers as knee–ankle–foot orthoses (KAFOs) and, if extending above the hip, as hip–knee–ankle–foot orthoses (HKAFO) (Training Council for Orthotists 1980).

LOWER LIMB ORTHOSES

FOOT INSOLES

Paralysis or an imbalance of muscular activity at the foot will compromise the normal transition of weight during the gait cycle.

Insoles may be used for two main purposes:

- to realign the foot by means of wedges and/or medial and lateral arch supports to provide a more even weight-bearing surface
- to unload painful areas.

There have been tremendous advances in the availability of moulded insoles which may be adapted to provide the total contact support required to ensure a more appropriate weight dispersal during walking. The texture of these supports varies, the more pliable being used for improved comfort whereas the more rigid give greater control. Factors to consider include:

1. *The height of the heel.* This should be low to provide greater stability. However, if there is shortening of the Achilles tendon (TA), this may be accommodated by increasing the heel height of either the insole or the shoe. Where the objective of treatment is to regain loss of range at the TA, gradual reduction in the height of the heel may facilitate this process. The width of the heel may be increased to improve either medial or lateral stability.
2. *Lack of mobility in the forefoot.* This may be compensated for by incorporating a raise at the level of the metatarsal heads. This will allow

the patient to roll from heel to toe-off, with reduced movement necessary at the meta-tarsalphalangeal joints.

3. *Muscle imbalance.* This may be either the primary or secondary problem in respect to foot deformity. In conditions such as heredit-ary motor and sensory neuropathy, the disease process affects the distal musculature and the muscle imbalance at the feet and ankles is therefore the primary problem. The foot may be pulled into inversion with the weight being taken predominantly over the lateral border. Provision of an insole with a lateral wedge lifting the outer border and/or a post under the fifth metatarsal head may assist in the redistribution of weight over the full surface of the foot. However, the changes which occur at the foot may be caused by muscle imbal-ance and malalignment of joints proximally, and as such are secondary complications. An example of this may be observed in the cere-bral palsy patient with a spastic gait. The pre-dominant flexed posture of the hips and knees and plantar flexion of the feet may lead to collapse of the medial arch and plantar fas-cia with resultant painful, pronated feet (Fig. 10.3).

Foot insoles may still be of value but it is important to recognise the primary problem and take steps to address this.

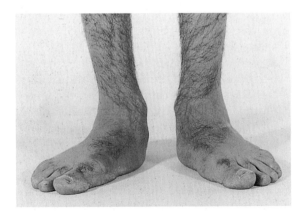

Figure 10.3 Pronated feet.

ANKLE–FOOT ORTHOSES (AFOS)

The purpose of the AFO is to effect control of the ankle and subtalar joints and maintain the foot in a degree of slight dorsiflexion. In this way, the AFO has a direct influence on:

- the quality of the gait pattern
- the maintenance of range of the triceps surae and of the TA.

A patient with weakness or flaccid paralysis requires a less supportive device to maintain the foot in slight dorsiflexion, whereas a patient with hypertonus pulling the foot into plantar flexion and inversion requires more rigid control.

Posterior leaf AFO

This is the most common type of AFO, made from plastic material which extends over the pos-

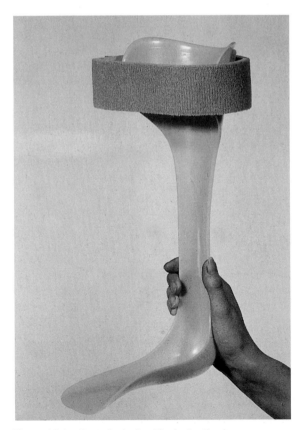

Figure 10.4 Posterior leaf ankle–foot orthosis.

terior aspect of the calf from below the fibula head to the metatarsal heads (Fig. 10.4).

Temporary stock AFOs are available in different materials and sizes and provide varying degrees of rigidity. Unless there is a significant deformity of the foot or excessive hypertonus, they may continue to be used by the patient in the longer term or until such time as adequate control of the plantargrade position is regained.

Temporary AFOs may be used to control the position of the foot when there is weakness or a flaccid paralysis of the foot and ankle musculature. If the patient has insufficient dorsiflexion, the walking pattern is altered, with compensatory strategies adopted to counteract this inadequacy. Hip hitching or a high-stepping gait may be used in order to ensure clearance of the ground when stepping through. Application of an AFO controls the foot position and enables a more efficient and effective gait pattern.

For patients with increased tone where the foot is pulled into plantar flexion and inversion, the compensations are more complex due to the overall effects of this hypertonus. Where there is predominant extensor tone of the lower limb, the patient may attempt to hitch the leg through with overactivity of the trunk side flexors, there being inadequate release of the knee into flexion. Temporary AFOs are often ineffective in controlling the position of the foot and may worsen the hypertonus with the pressure under the metatarsal heads. In this situation a more rigid, made-to-measure, polypropylene AFO may be required, extending under the toes, to incorporate the whole foot.

Transposition of weight during the gait cycle produces movement at the ankle joint into both plantar and dorsiflexion. However, in the event of fixation at the ankle joint, providing this is the only determinant of gait that is affected, increased flexion of the knee during the swing phase maintains the smoothness of the path of translation of the centre of gravity (Saunders et al 1953). This may be observed in a patient with an L4–5 or L5–S1 root lesion affecting the anterior tibial muscle group. The dropped foot corrected with a posterior leaf AFO can be compensated for by increased flexion of the knee with little effect on the efficiency of the gait pattern. However, for many patients with neurological disability, the problem is rarely confined to the ankle joint and the compensatory strategies adopted are, of necessity, more extensive and diverse.

Considerations when prescribing AFOs

Splint flexibility. A more rigid AFO may be required for patients with severe hypertonus or when there is already an established deformity. The degree of rigidity is dependent upon the type and extent of the plastic material. For example, in patients with marked plantar flexion and inversion hypertonus, the foot may be supported with a rigid polypropylene AFO extending to include the toes and encasing the malleoli. A strap over the line of the ankle joint helps to ensure correct positioning of the heel in the splint (Fig. 10.5).

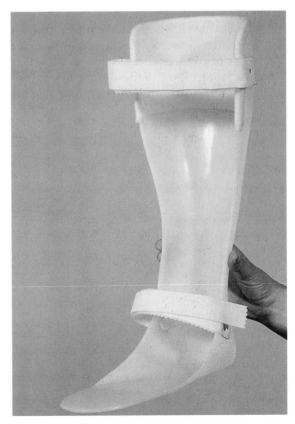

Figure 10.5 Rigid ankle–foot orthosis.

Established or predicted inversion deformity. A similar design is advocated for patients with established deformity, most commonly into inversion. Patients with hereditary motor and sensory neuropathy may develop such deformity unless there is appropriate, early intervention. The relative unopposed action of tibialis posterior will cause inversion of the foot, which in severe cases can create a deformity that resembles a club foot. A similar AFO to that described for the patient with hypertonus is required to prevent further deterioration. Here, the purpose of the AFO is to exert pressure to prevent increasing inversion, and it is important that this pressure is dissipated away from the bony lateral malleolus. For this reason, the lateral border of the AFO from below the fibula head to just above the lateral malleolus is moulded inwards during the splint manufacture to redistribute pressure to this more fleshy part of the leg rather than over the more vulnerable malleolus.

The fixed position as provided by the posterior leaf AFO has both advantages and disadvantages.

Advantages

1. The fixed position into slight dorsiflexion will facilitate the transference of weight over the full surface of the foot. (Where the initial contact is made with the forefoot, the weight tends to remain over the heel, which may result in compensatory flexion at the hips and hyperextension of the knees.)
2. More even transference of weight over the full surface of the foot tends to stimulate extension and abduction at the hips during stance phase of gait with the more forward placement of the centre of gravity.
3. With the foot positioned in slight dorsiflexion, this tends to introduce an element of flexion at the knee through the mechanical stretch of gastrocnemius and thereby prevents or reduces hyperextension at this joint.
4. Forced maintenance of a hypertonic foot in dorsiflexion can be effective in decreasing extensor tone proximally to enable a more fluent swing phase of gait.

Disadvantages

1. The posterior leaf AFO prevents movement into dorsiflexion and plantar flexion. Many patients complain of difficulty in negotiating stairs due to the rigid position at the ankle joint. If only one foot is splinted, the patient may compensate by always stepping down with the supported leg, but where two AFOs are required, going downstairs may be impossible without assistance.
2. Patients with hypertonus tend to be dominated by stereotyped postures and movements. Immobilisation of the foot and ankle will restrict potential postural adaptation within the foot and ankle and may lead to increased immobility of the intrinsic foot musculature. When used for patients with weakness, the support provided by the splint may discourage return of function due to the lack of stimulation of muscle activity within the foot and of the muscles acting over the ankle and subtalar joints.
3. Where there is excessive hypertonus, the foot may resist the splint, thereby exacerbating the increased tone. Splints that terminate at the metatarsal heads may stimulate a positive support response, but those which extend to include the toes may restrict movement at the metatarsalphalangeal joints.
4. Forced maintenance of a hypertonic foot in dorsiflexion may lead to increased flexion proximally and increasing difficulty in attaining extension during stance phase of gait.
5. This device is unsuitable for patients with oedema of the legs.

The hinged AFO

A hinge mechanism may be incorporated at the ankle joint to allow for dorsiflexion (Fig. 10.6).

This is an obvious advantage during the gait cycle and in negotiating stairs, and is beneficial for most patients with flaccid paralysis. Those with hypertonus often require the more rigid splint to eliminate the potential for clonus which may be stimulated by the movement.

Cusick (1988) advocates the use of a hinged 'crouch-control' ankle–foot splint whereby the

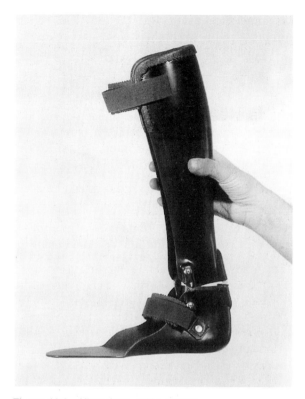

Figure 10.6 Hinged toe–ankle orthosis.

patient is able to plantarflex the ankle but dorsiflexion is restricted. This splint is recommended for children with excessive flexion of the lower limbs, this being the position referred to as 'crouch'. Although this relates to the management of foot deformity in children, the same principles may apply for adults. The most common cause of this posture is surgical overlengthening of the Achilles tendons (Sutherland & Cooper 1978).

Below-knee calipers

Although now less frequently used, these calipers may be the support of choice when:

- There is oedema of the leg.
- The foot is unable to conform to the rigid support of the posterior leaf AFO and resists the controlling force, thereby exacerbating the increased tone.

- The predominant deformity of the foot is into inversion. A below-knee iron with an outside T- or Y-strap to control the foot in a neutral alignment may prove to be more effective than a posterior leaf AFO. The pressure exerted by the strap is often more tolerable than that provided by a rigid AFO.

It is important to ensure that the foot does not rotate within the shoe. It is not uncommon to find that the shoe itself deforms due to continued dominance of the hypertonic muscle groups.

These iron calipers with the socket fitted into the heel of the shoe are undoubtedly heavier than the plastic AFOs and this must be taken into consideration in respect of the effects on increased tone. In general, it would seem that most people prefer the appearance of the plastic AFOs, often referred to as cosmetic devices, rather than the metal irons.

Anterior shell AFO

This extends from an anterior band at the level of the patella tendon, laterally and downwards to terminate in a foot support similar to that of the posterior leaf AFO (Fig. 10.7). Carbon reinforce-

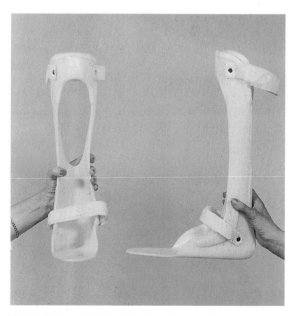

Figure 10.7 Anterior shell ankle–foot orthosis.

ments may be required at the ankle to ensure adequate rigidity and a calf strap may be needed to prevent hyperextension of the knee.

The anterior shell AFO is of benefit for patients with weakness of the knee extensors but sufficient strength of the hip extensors to transfer the body weight forwards during stance phase of gait. The orthosis stabilises the knee in extension through the rigidity at the ankle and the anterior band prevents knee flexion as the hip extends.

It is important to monitor the efficacy of this splint when supplied to patients with progressive neurological disorders. The anterior shell AFO becomes ineffective without the sustained control of the hip extensors.

Toe-off orthosis

This AFO is made of carbon fibre and Kevlar to produce a design which 'loads' the material as the ankle dorsiflexes over it during mid to late stance (Fig. 10.8). This energy is then released,

assisting propulsion and toe off. This effect combined with the light weight and relatively unobtrusive design has been extremely popular with patients without excessive hypertonus using this device thus far. Unfortunately, to date, there appears to be a design flaw causing the orthosis to delaminate at the junction of the foot and ankle in patients who exhibit a large range of movement into plantar and dorsiflexion. Hopefully, this will be rectified in the near future.

Dorsiflexion bandage

A crepe bandage may be used as a temporary means of supporting the foot in dorsiflexion or the plantigrade position (Fig. 10.9).

Advantages

1. It enables movement into dorsiflexion while limiting plantar flexion.

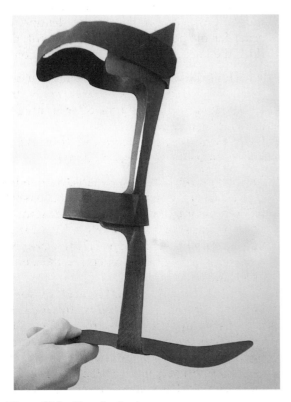

Figure 10.8   Toe-off orthosis.

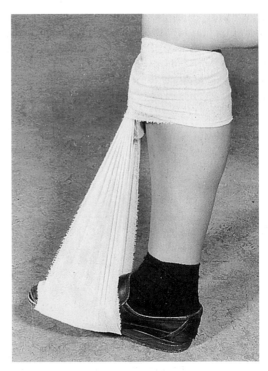

Figure 10.9   Application of bandage to hold foot in dorsiflexion and eversion. (Reproduced from Bromley 1998 with kind permission.).

2. For patients with hypertonus affecting the plantar flexors and invertors it may be applied with increased eversion to inhibit this increased tone.
3. It improves stability, particularly where there is flaccid paralysis, in that it restricts posterior displacement of body weight. It also facilitates more normal alignment of the centre of gravity through the foot rather than through the heel during stance phase or when standing with the feet astride.
4. The foot itself maintains a greater degree of flexibility than with the more rigid AFO.
5. It serves as a means of evaluating the effects of a more permanent device.

Disadvantages

The main disadvantage of the dorsiflexion bandage is that it can only be used on a temporary basis due to the potential restriction to the circulation. A piece of foam circumventing the leg just below the fibula head goes some way to minimising the pressure applied around the leg and thus the circulatory effects. When used to control a flail foot, little pressure is required to maintain the plantigrade position. However, when it is used to inhibit strong plantar flexion and inversion hypertonus, greater pressure is required to obtain the desired positioning with an increase in the potential risk of circulatory impairment. When this bandage is used in conjunction with a back slab, the effects on the circulation are minimised due to the hard shell reducing the constricting effect.

KNEE–ANKLE–FOOT ORTHOSES (KAFOS)

In normal stance, the line of force of the body weight passes in front of the knee (Rose et al 1982, Galley & Forster 1987), and minimal quadriceps activity is required to maintain the upright position. In the event of neurological impairment resulting in impaired lower limb control, various types of support need to be considered if the patient is to maintain or regain an independent gait.

The KAFO applies a three-point leverage system about the knee to support the leg in extension (see p. 221). It may be used to control either hyperextension or flexion of the limb.

Hyperextension of the knee

The knee may become hyperextended for several reasons which include:

1. To gain stability by 'locking' against the posterior structures of the knee if there is insufficient quadriceps activity to maintain normal stance.
2. Abnormal muscle tone whereby the quadriceps muscle group forces the knee into hyperextension.
3. Weakness of the hip extensors whereby the hip is flexed with subsequent hyperextension of the knee.
4. Weakness of the hamstring muscle group allowing unopposed action of quadriceps.
5. Mechanical shortening of the triceps surae muscle group and of the Achilles tendon. In order for the heel to achieve contact with the floor, the knee is forced into hyperextension.

In each of these examples, the hyperextended position of the knee creates tension on the posterior structures of the joint, often leading to overstretching and pain.

The management and control of knee hyperextension varies, depending on the cause.

1. The patient with weak and ineffective quadriceps control may benefit from an anterior shell AFO, providing there is adequate activity of the hip extensors. Alternatively, a KAFO may be required if there is more diffuse weakness preventing effective alignment of the pelvis and trunk.
2. A rigid AFO with the ankle held in dorsiflexion affects the knee position by virtue of the stretch applied to gastrocnemius. The greater the angle of dorsiflexion the greater the influence of flexion at the knee joint. It is important to recognise that the effect of this increase of flexion may render the quadriceps ineffective, in which case a KAFO may be

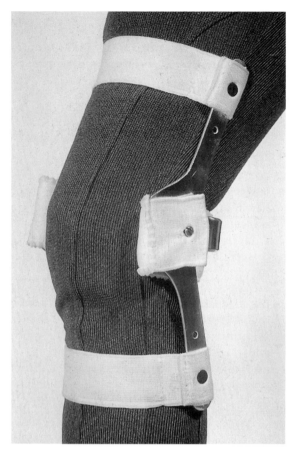

Figure 10.10 Swedish knee cage.

required. The use of a bandage, holding the foot in dorsiflexion, is of particular value to assess the most appropriate orthosis.

3. A Swedish knee cage may prove effective in preventing hyperextension as a result of weakness or paralysis of the hamstrings (Fig. 10.10). This should be used with caution as the imposition of flexion at the knee may prevent full extension at the hip during stance phase of gait. This may lead to the development of hip flexor contracture.

4. Mechanical shortening of the calf muscles and Achilles tendon may be accommodated for by provision of a heel raise, thereby reducing the tension of gastrocnemius. This maintains alignment of the body by preventing the otherwise necessary compensation of flexion at the hips to keep the centre of gravity within

the base of support. Again there must be sufficient control of the quadriceps muscle group to stabilise the knee once forward from the hyperextended position.

Flexor hypertonus of the lower limbs

This can severely impair or prevent an upright stance. Patients may stabilise using adduction and medial rotation at the hips, often with plantar flexion at the ankles. The consequence of this activity is usually that of increased extension at the lumbar and thoracic spine with retraction of the shoulders to generate sufficient anti-gravity control. Those with long-standing problems of flexor hypertonus may walk in this way for many years. However, over time, the mechanical deficiencies of this means of ambulation may lead to joint damage and ultimately wheelchair dependence.

From a biomechanical viewpoint, early provision of KAFOs may be considered appropriate. However, maintenance of range of movement of the flexor muscle groups enables patients to use their extensor muscles more effectively and may prevent the need for such intervention. In this way, the compensations described above may be minimised.

Inevitably there are some patients with flexor hypertonus of the lower limbs who have inadequate underlying extensor activity to maintain themselves upright against gravity without excessive use of trunk and head extension. In this instance, the patient must be given the choice of continuing to walk in the way described above, with the possible long-term consequences of muscle and joint problems, or using KAFOs.

Patients with a more acute onset of flexor hypertonus of the legs should be encouraged to use mechanical support to effect extension of the knees and to maximise recovery of the extensor muscle groups. The severity of hypertonus will dictate the intervention. If the patient has severe flexor hypertonus, mechanical support should be used with caution in that forcing the legs into extension may exacerbate this tone. Tone-reducing techniques such as mobilisation of the trunk and pelvis and controlled stretching of the affected muscle groups may prove effective in enabling the patient to accommodate to the support.

It is important that the patient is able to accept the support. If there is ongoing resistance, the flexor hypertonus may manifest itself in other areas of the body. For example, if the knee is held rigidly in extension but the flexor hypertonus persists, it may shunt into the hip flexors and abdominal muscle groups, preventing normal alignment of the body in standing.

Patients with paralysis or weakness of the lower limbs

Standing patients with insufficient extensor activity of the lower limbs has been discussed in Chapter 6. The use of various standing frames and standing the patient between two or more therapists relates to the unconscious or more severely disabled patient. Patients with persistent or progressive weakness may require a KAFO to enable them to become or remain ambulant. For example, a patient with a low thoracic or lumbar spinal cord lesion and complete paralysis of the legs requires full leg support to stand and walk using a four-point or swing-through gait (Bromley 1998).

There are various types of KAFO, which differ primarily in the material from which they are made and the locking mechanism of the knee. The KAFOs made from plastic materials are generally lighter in weight and are moulded to the contour of the leg. They terminate in a plastic foot piece which inserts into the patient's shoe. The metal KAFOs are not as close fitting and are therefore preferred where there is oedema or potential changes in muscle girth. A socket is inserted into the heel of the patient's shoe (Fig. 10.11).

For patients who hyperextend but are stable in flexion, with good quadriceps activity, a free knee joint with an extension stop is required. This allows for full range of movement at the knee joint throughout the gait cycle while preventing hyperextension of the joint.

If the knee is unstable in flexion, with inadequate quadriceps activity, the knee must be

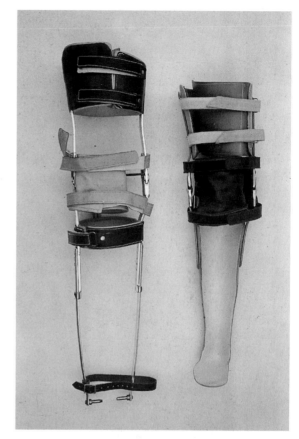

Figure 10.11   Knee–ankle–foot orthoses.

locked into extension to effect weight-bearing. There are two main types of locking mechanisms:

- manual, where the patient must lock and unlock the device by hand with the knee in the extended position
- semi-automatic, where the KAFO locks automatically by means of a spring device when the leg is fully extended but which requires manual release into flexion.

Determining factors in the choice of locking mechanism include hand function and the ease of knee extension.

SUMMARY

There appears to be a growing acceptance of the use of orthoses to control abnormal movement or deficits at the foot and ankle to produce more normal alignment and recruitment proximally.

The orthoses described above are by no means exclusive. Patients with more extensive paralysis or movement impairment may require additional control extending above the hip. Examples of what may be considered 'walking systems' include the 'para-walker' (hip guidance orthosis) (Nene & Patrick 1990) and the reciprocal gait orthosis (Beckman 1987). Details of these more complex orthoses are to be found in Bromley (1998).

Temporary orthoses are useful in assessing their effect and patient tolerance and compliance before proceeding to a definitive orthosis. The patient must be fully involved in the assessment procedure. The most mechanically appropriate orthosis may, for some patients, be cosmetically unacceptable and it is essential to establish that the splint will be worn before embarking on what is a costly intervention.

SPLINTING AND CASTING

Throughout this section the terms splinting and casting are used interchangeably.

General principles

Casts may be used as a prophylactic measure, to maintain range of movement and to prevent the development of muscle and tendon shortening, or as a corrective device, to regain range of movement where shortening has already become established.

The Association of Chartered Physiotherapists Interested in Neurology (ACPIN) have prepared guidelines for splinting adults with neurological dysfunction (ACPIN 1998). These provide detailed information regarding the assessment procedure, risk factors and protocols for casting. However, in spite of the increasing use of casting in the management of patients with neurological disability, there is very little scientific evidence to support its use. The literature review, conducted by ACPIN, in the preparation of the splinting

guidelines, highlighted both the paucity of clinically based research studies and the lack of knowledge about when to splint, for how long, using what materials and for which type of patient?

Various materials are available for use in casting. Plaster of Paris (POP) is often recommended as it moulds more readily to the contour of the limb (Booth et al 1983, Sullivan et al 1988). Fibreglass casting tape with polyurethane resin sets more quickly than POP and is increasingly being used in the management of fractures. Thermoplastic materials are often preferred, particularly for hand and wrist splints.

More recently, a combination of Soft Cast and Scotch Cast Plus, a fibreglass material (available from 3M, Loughborough, Leicestershire), has been used in clinical practice. These combination splints, which are described below, may be removed, using scissors as opposed to a plaster saw, within 15 min of application and then re-applied with Velcro or straps, to be worn on either a constant or an intermittent basis. One of the main benefits of using these combination casts is that they may be removed during physiotherapy to enable mobilisation of the affected muscles and soft tissues.

The choice of material is very much a matter of personal preference and experience. The rigid support provided by POP or fibreglass may be preferred when the cast is made for constant use, for example to maintain range of movement at the ankle joint for patients following head injury (Conine et al 1990, Moseley 1993, 1997), and the lightweight fibreglass splint is often useful for patients who use this as a walking cast. However, in the opinion of the authors, the combination splints have been shown to be as effective in providing support and stability as the rigid non-removable casts, and these are now the materials of choice.

Principles of application

Two people are required to apply the cast: ideally, a therapist to hold the limb in the optimum position and a technician or therapist experienced in the use and application of the chosen materials. The illustrations below show the application of the combination casts made on unimpaired, adult subjects.

When making these casts, a protective cover over the working area, aprons for the therapists applying the cast, *blunt-ended* scissors and a bowl of tepid water are required. *Rubber gloves are essential when working with synthetic materials.* Routine monitoring must be carried out to ensure that there are no pressure or circulatory problems. If there is any suspicion that the cast may be causing such problems, it must be removed immediately.

The use of Soft Cast in combination with Scotch Cast Plus is described for each of the following casts. These synthetic materials are impregnated with a polyurethane resin which sets on exposure to water or air (Schuren 1994). Soft Cast is a flexible material which can be used to produce casts of varying degrees of rigidity. In contrast, Scotch Cast Plus is a rigid fibreglass material which may be used to provide specific control across a joint as the clinical presentation dictates. The setting time of these casting tapes is determined by the amount of water added and its temperature. More water added to the bandage will shorten the setting time as will the use of higher-temperature water. Applying the bandages dry gives a longer setting time and thus more time for moulding, whereas soaking in warmer water speeds up the setting process and reduces the applicators' working time. A combination of the first Soft Cast bandage and the Scotch Cast Plus used dry, with the final Soft Cast soaked in tepid water, is the recommended mode of application.

BELOW-KNEE CASTS

Patients with hypertonus, pulling the foot into plantar flexion and inversion, are in danger of developing shortening of the triceps surae and of the Achilles tendon. This is a recognised complication following head injury where hypertonus may become a dominant feature (Yarkony & Sahgal 1987, Kent et al 1990). The early use of casting as a prophylactic measure, to maintain the plantigrade position of the foot and ankle, is recommended (Sullivan et al 1988, Conine et al 1990).

Casting may also be of benefit for those with established shortening of the triceps surae to maintain the shortened muscles in a stretched position. Casts are changed on a regular basis, approximately every 7–10 days. This type of serial casting, used in conjunction with stretching, has been shown to be effective in regaining range of movement (Moseley 1997).

Below-knee casts are useful to control excessive plantar flexion, which may be a compensatory mechanism for patients with poor hip, pelvic and trunk control. By correcting the position of the foot and ankle and preventing plantar flexion, the primary problem is exposed. For some people, there is insufficient underlying proximal activity to maintain an upright stance, indicating that they are dependent on the compensatory plantar flexion. However, for others, preventing plantar flexion facilitates proximal activity and enables the patient to strengthen the proximal musculature and develop a more effective balance mechanism and improved walking pattern.

Application

The cast should be applied with the knee flexed, which allows for maximum dorsiflexion by stretching soleus while relieving pressure on the gastrocnemius component of the triceps surae.

The position of the patient when the cast is being applied will depend upon the medical status. The patient with acute brain injury may need to have the cast applied in supine lying, whereas patients who are medically stable may sit, with or without support, or have the cast applied in prone lying.

More recently, two types of combination casts have been used to control the position of the foot and ankle: the posterior support cast is based on the principles of the posterior leaf AFO, with the fibreglass material supporting under the foot and over the calf muscles; the anterior support cast is based on the principles of the anterior shell AFO, with the fibreglass material supporting under the foot and extending over the front of the tibia. In both types of splints, the medial arch of the foot should be supported and the cast moulded around the contour of the leg to prevent movement within the cast. This is particularly relevant at the Achilles tendon with the posterior support cast. If the plantigrade position is not achievable, the heel is built up to ensure even weight-bearing over the full surface of the foot. This is particularly important when standing the patient to prevent hyperextension of the knee.

The materials which are required for both the posterior and anterior below-knee (BK) casts are:

- two layers of 3-inch stockinet with an additional piece of stockinet (sausage stockinet) between the two layers
- microfoam padding over the medial and lateral malleoli and over the anterior aspect of the ankle joint

- 2 × 3 inch (7.5 cm) Soft Cast bandages
- 1 × 4 inch (10 cm) Scotch Cast Plus bandage
- 1 wet cotton bandage to ensure lamination of the layers of casting tape
- zinc oxide tape
- Velcro fastening.

The posterior BK combination cast

The application of the cast is illustrated in Figure 10.12. Two layers of stockinet are applied from the knee line to include and extend beyond the toes. A sausage stockinet is positioned longitudinally between the two layers of stockinet, over the muscle belly of the anterior tibial muscle group. The two layers of stockinet are cut in front of the ankle joint and overlapped to prevent creasing. Microfoam tape is applied over the

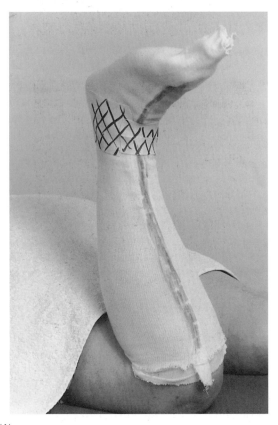

(A)

(B)

Figure 10.12   (A–B) Posterior support below knee cast.

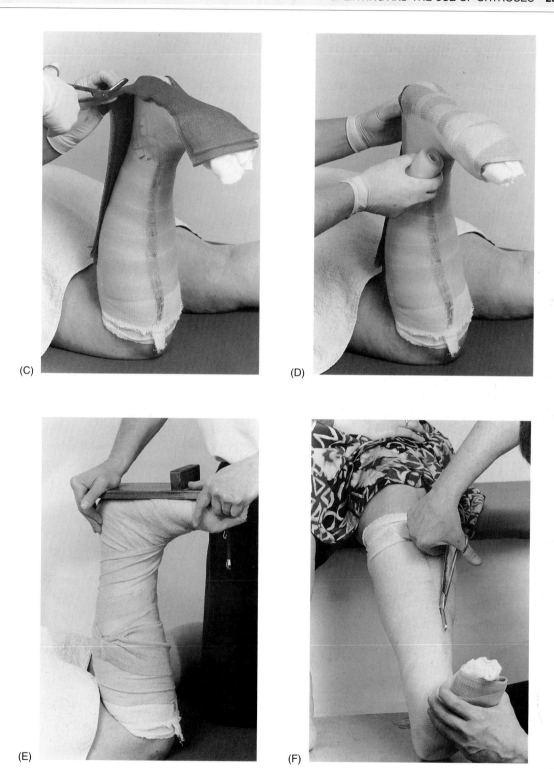

(C)

(D)

(E)

(F)

Figure 10.12 (C–F) Posterior support below knee cast.

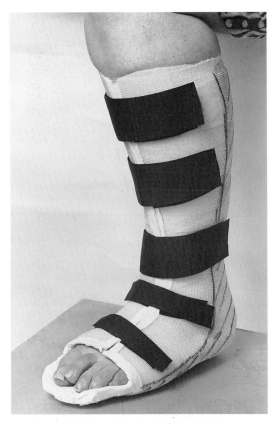

Figure 10.12 (G) Posterior support below knee cast.

malleoli and across the anterior aspect of the ankle joint.

A Soft Cast bandage is applied, extending from just below the head of fibula to the end of the toes, with each turn of the bandage covering half of the preceding one. A slab of five layers of Scotch Cast Plus is placed over the calf and under the foot including the toes. A section is cut out around the heel to encase the ankle joint. The second Soft Cast bandage is immersed in water and then applied in the same way as the first to secure the slab in place. The Scotch Cast Plus should be trimmed around the toes before hardening and before overwrapping with the wet cotton bandage. The wet cotton bandage should be applied with slight tension to enhance lamination between the layers of casting tape.

The Scotch Cast Plus slab becomes rigid within approximately 10 minutes, at which time the wet cotton bandage and sausage stockinet are removed. The purpose of this additional piece of stockinet is to give a little more room when removing the cast, which is of particular relevance when cutting around the front of the ankle joint. The cast should be removed with the blunt-ended scissors, cutting vertically over the anterior tibial muscle group, just lateral to the midline at the ankle joint and over the fourth metatarsal. The section of Soft Cast over the toes is then cut away, the cast is trimmed and the edges secured with zinc oxide tape. Velcro fastenings are attached when the cast is dry to enable reapplication.

The anterior BK combination cast

The application of the cast is illustrated in Figure 10.13. The two layers of stockinet, the cut across the front of the ankle to prevent creasing, and the microfoam tape are applied in the same way as with the posterior BK combination cast. For this cast, the sausage stockinet is placed longitudinally down the middle of the calf to the point of the heel and extending along the lateral border of the foot.

The first Soft Cast bandage is applied as above, but the Scotch Cast Plus slab for this cast consists of two separate sections each of five layers.

- The first section extends from just below the tibial tubercle, over the anterior aspect of the leg, to the end of the toes. The section which lies across the front of the foot is then cut vertically as far as the ankle joint, creating two stirrups.
- The second part is the foot piece which extends from the point of the heel to beyond the toes. It is essential that the posterior end of the foot piece does not extend up behind the heel as this will make removal of the cast very difficult.

These two slabs of Scotch Cast Plus are then joined by the medial and lateral stirrups of the shin section attaching under the foot, but not overlapping, to secure the foot piece. The second

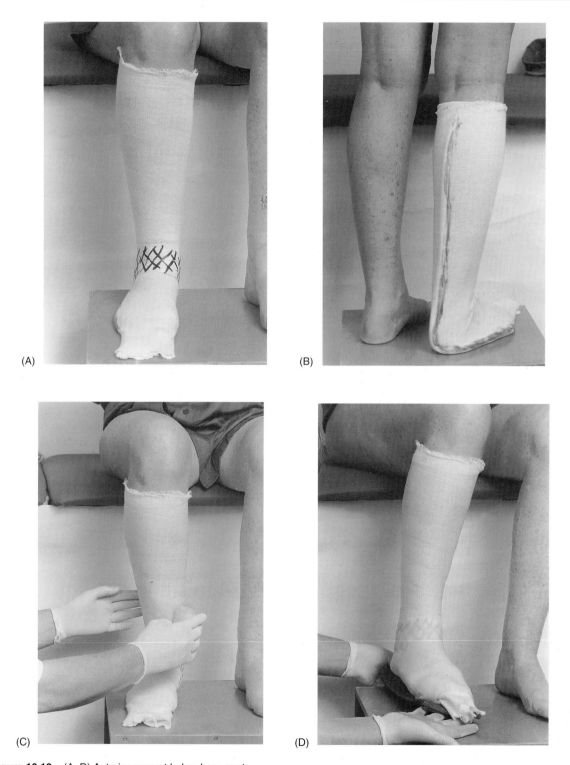

Figure 10.13   (A–D) Anterior support below knee cast.

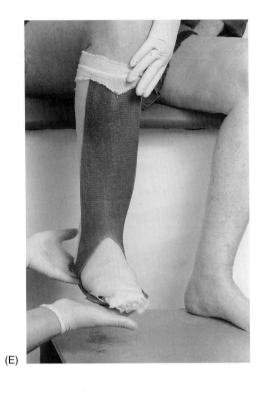

(E)

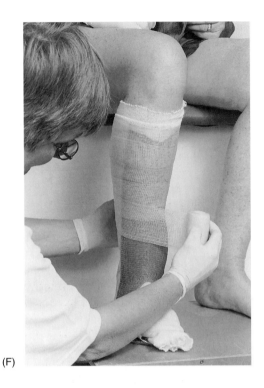

(F)

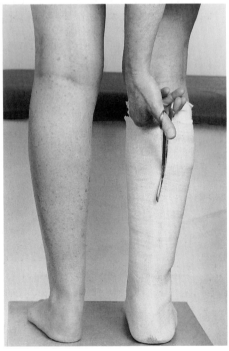

(G)

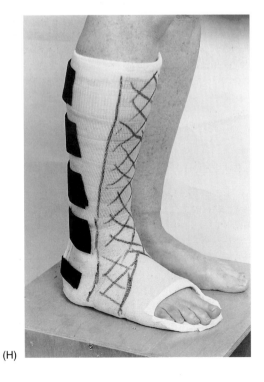

(H)

Figure 10.13 (E–H) Anterior support below knee cast.

Soft Cast bandage is then applied, following immersion in water, to secure the Scotch Cast Plus in position. Again, the Scotch Cast Plus should be trimmed around the toes before hardening and prior to application of the wet cotton bandage.

After 10 minutes, the wet cotton bandage and the sausage stockinet are removed. This cast is cut, using the blunt-ended scissors, by cutting the Soft Cast vertically down the centre of the back of the calf, to the point of the heel. Where the Soft Cast meets the Scotch Cast Plus, at the heel, the Soft Cast is cut horizontally to approximately 1 inch (2.5 cm) to allow removal of the cast. The Soft Cast section is removed to expose the toes and the cast is then trimmed and the edges secured with zinc oxide tape. Velcro straps are then attached to enable reapplication of the splint.

With the anterior BK combination cast, the foot piece remains intact save for the area over the toes. The longitudinal piece of stockinet is of particular value in giving a little more room within this foot section to facilitate putting on and taking off cast. The intact foot piece can be very useful when using this cast for patients with resistance to dorsiflexion in that the foot can be placed within the cast with plantar flexion at the ankle. The calf muscles may then be mobilised and, with gradual stretching, the cast brought into contact with the shin, securing the foot in a position of dorsiflexion.

Serial casting of the foot and ankle

Where there is established shortening of the posterior crural muscle group and of the Achilles tendon, serial casting using only fibreglass materials may be preferred. These rigid casts follow the same principles with regard to maintaining the optimal joint position but, *because only fibreglass is used, undercast padding must be applied between a single layer of stockinet and the casting tape. A plaster saw is required for removal of this rigid cast.*

LONG LEG CASTS

Back slabs to support the lower limbs in extension

The advantages and disadvantages of back slabs to secure the knees in extension have been discussed in Chapter 6 in relation to patients with varying levels of disability. They may be used for patients with either flexor or extensor hypertonus or for those with inadequate extensor activity to maintain the legs in extension. They are invariably a temporary measure and may be used:

- to determine the patient's ability to utilise this support in a functional way prior to supplying more permanent KAFOs
- to achieve a more normal alignment in standing with improved pelvic, trunk and head control
- to stimulate extensor activity of the hips
- to maintain or regain range of movement of the hip flexors
- to attain a plantigrade position of the feet by controlling the position of the knees and mobilising the patient over the base of support.

Application

The patient is positioned in prone lying with the feet extended over the end of the bed. This is to ensure that the bulk of the triceps surae is arranged similarly to when the patient is standing. If the feet are in plantar flexion, the contour of the leg is significantly altered. The legs are positioned in neutral or slight lateral rotation. For those patients with complete flaccid paralysis, a small bandage may need to be positioned under the ankle to prevent hyperextension of the knee. The back slab extends from the line of the hip joint, on a diagonal plane, to at least 2 cm above the malleoli. The slab provides a shell which extends laterally to encompass just less than 180 degrees of the leg circumference to enable the splint to be put on and taken off.

The materials required to make the back slabs are:

- 4 inch (10 cm) stockinet
- 2 × 5 inch (12.5 cm) Scotch Cast Plus
- 2 wet cotton bandages
- zinc oxide tape.

The application of back slabs is illustrated in Figure 10.14. The stockinet extends from above the line of the hip joint to below the heel. The length of the leg is measured and the dry bandages unwound to make the back slab with a minimum of seven layers. The slab is fanned out over the hamstrings to accommodate the increased girth of the thigh. Each alternate layer at the lower end of the slab stops at mid-calf to prevent excessive thickness of the cast around the ankle joint.

The slab is applied following immersion in tepid water and moulded around the contour of the leg. The material is trimmed while still wet and malleable to follow the line of the hip joint and to ensure a uniform edge above the malleoli. The wet cotton bandages are applied to laminate the material and to secure the slab in place. Alternatively, a wet towel may be placed over the cast. The fibreglass hardens sufficiently to remove the splint after 10 minutes.

Rough edges are sanded down and zinc oxide tape applied around the borders of the splint to provide greater comfort. The splint may be used within 30 minutes of being made.

The important aspects of the back slab are that:

- It extends up to and follows the line of the hip joint to enable extension of the hip with slight posterior tilt of the pelvis. This allows for full range of movement of the iliopsoas muscle and of the iliofemoral ligament.
- It finishes at least 2 cm above the malleoli to prevent pressure over these bony prominences.
- It maintains the knee in full, but not hyper-extension.

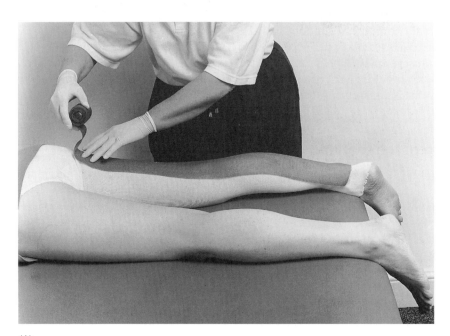

(A)

Figure 10.14   (A) Back slabs.

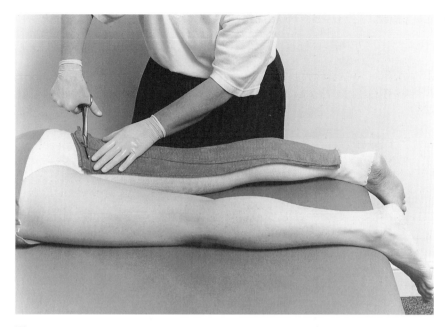

(B)

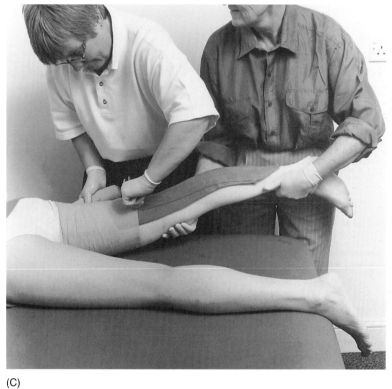

(C)

Figure 10.14   (B–C) Back slabs.

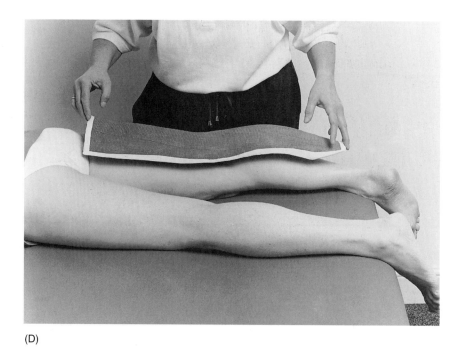

(D)

Figure 10.14 (D) Back slabs.

CASTING TO CORRECT KNEE FLEXION DEFORMITY

This has been advocated as a means of regaining range of movement at the knee (Booth et al 1983, Davies 1994). These casts may be either a full cylinder or a drop-out cast where the section over the tibial shaft is removed (Fig. 10.15). The principles underlying the use of drop-out casts and their application are provided on page 245.

UPPER LIMB ORTHOSES

Upper limb supports or casts may be of value in the management and treatment of upper limb dysfunction, particularly in improving joint alignment and in preventing trauma. This section considers different types of splints and materials which may prove effective in achieving these objectives.

SHOULDER SUPPORTS

The mechanics of the shoulder joint and subsequent problems which may arise following neurological impairment have been discussed in previous chapters. This section considers the different supports which may prove of benefit to patients where there is either insufficient tone, or increased tone affecting the shoulder musculature.

Subluxation of the shoulder is a common sequel to changes of tone affecting the muscles that provide stability around the shoulder joint (Davies 1985, Williams et al 1988, Bobath 1990) and it has been reported that, immediately following an upper motor neurone lesion such as stroke, the affected extremities become flaccid in approximately 90% of patients (Griffen & Reddin 1981, Faghri et al 1994). Depending on the prevailing abnormal tone, the patient with severe weakness or hypotonia may demonstrate extreme subluxation, whereas those with hyper-

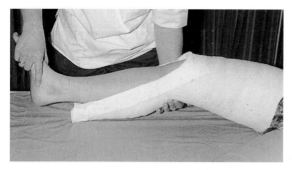

(A)

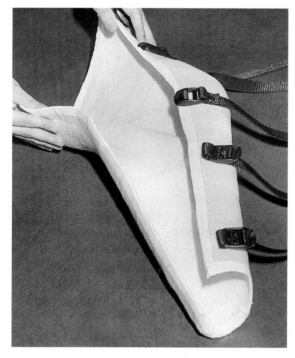

(B)

Figure 10.15   (A) Drop out cast and (B) long leg cylinder.

tonus may retain some, if inadequate, control. The different types of support which are available for the shoulder include:

- the collar and cuff
- cuff support
- the abduction roll or wedge
- strapping
- support using pillows or a tray/table.

The collar and cuff

This may be used to support the arm at the elbow and the hand. It passes around the shoulder as opposed to round the neck and is fitted so as to maintain alignment of the glenohumeral joint with the elbow at 90 degrees or slightly less.

Advantages

- This provides full support for the limb and therefore protects against overstretching of the structures around the shoulder. The conventional sling has been found to be effective in controlling shoulder subluxation (Buccholz-Moodie et al 1986) although these authors are quick to highlight the disadvantages of this support and do not advocate its use.
- The hand is supported level with the elbow and there is therefore less likelihood of the limb swelling.

Disadvantages

- The fully supported, flexed position discourages active movement and, for those patients with increased tone, this posturing tends to reinforce the flexor hypertonus and may lead to contractures.
- This positioning does not allow for any potential balance response of the upper limb and therefore affects postural adjustments within the trunk.
- Patients with sensory problems or neglect of the affected side have less stimulation to use the arm if it is fully supported.

Cuff support

This support is advocated particularly in the management of patients with hemiplegia where the disadvantages of the collar and cuff are most relevant (Williams et al 1988, Bobath 1990). The cuff support is attached around the upper arm and attached by means of a sheepskin-lined strap in a figure of eight around the other shoulder (Fig. 10.16). The weak or flaccid arm tends to

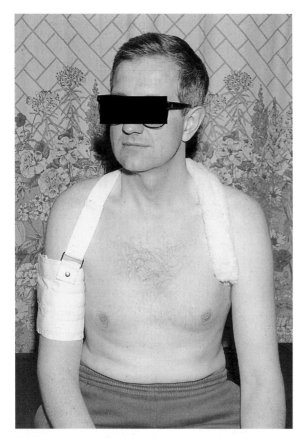

Figure 10.16 Cuff support.

hang in adduction and medial rotation and the hypertonic limb is often pulled into this position. For this reason, the strap should be secured anteriorly to encourage lateral rotation.

Advantages

- Williams et al (1988) noted a significant reduction in the degree of inferior subluxation. However, there is some debate in clinical practice as to whether the cuff does in fact achieve this.
- The support around the upper arm does not interfere with distal movements and potential return of active movement.
- The arm is able to respond more appropriately to postural adjustments occurring in the trunk and in the maintenance of balance.

- The patient and all personnel involved in the care of the patient are constantly reminded that this is a vulnerable joint if the cuff is worn over clothing.

Disadvantages

- The flaccid arm hangs dependently by the side and is prone to swelling.
- It is difficult for the patient to apply this support unaided.
- If it is applied tightly enough to correct the subluxation, it may affect the circulation.
- If the cuff is worn over clothing, the patient may find this stigmatising and degrading.

The abduction roll or wedge

This is used for patients with increased tone and was first advocated by Bobath (1978). Following a cerebrovascular accident (CVA), the pattern of hypertonus affecting the upper limb is usually one of predominant flexion (Rothwell 1994). The roll/wedge is placed in the axilla, attached by means of a strap passing across the back and around the opposite shoulder in a figure of eight (Fig. 10.17).

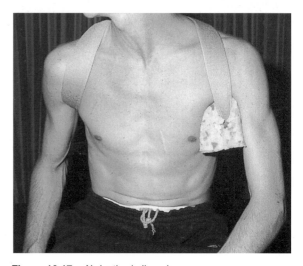

Figure 10.17 Abduction/roll wedge.

Advantages

- The bulk afforded by the roll/wedge brings the arm away from the body. This places the arm in a position of slight abduction, thereby inhibiting the dominance of adduction, flexion and medial rotation.
- Placing the roll/wedge in the axilla and removing it ensures that the upper limb is moved away from the body on a regular basis and thus improves hygiene. All personnel involved in this procedure should be trained to handle the limb with care to prevent traumatising the joint.

Disadvantages

- Positioning the arm in slight abduction may create greater mechanical instability due to the effect on the locking mechanism (see Ch. 6).

- Movement of the arm into abduction by untrained personnel may traumatise this vulnerable joint.
- It is difficult for the patient to position the roll independently.

Strapping

Strapping or taping the shoulder girdle is often used in the management of patients with orthopaedic conditions and much of the literature regarding this treatment technique relates to this field of practice (Host 1995). A commonly used technique is to apply three straps from the insertion of deltoid to pass anterior, central and posterior to the acromion process with a lateral strap from in front of the humeral head extending laterally to the spine (Fig. 10.18).

In a pilot study of eight patients, strapping the affected shoulder following stroke delayed the

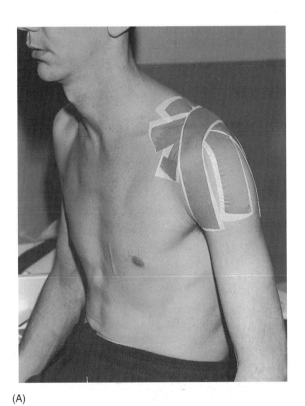

(A)

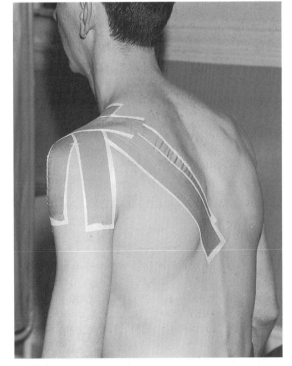

(B)

Figure 10.18   (A) and (B) Strapping for the shoulder.

onset of shoulder pain (Ancliffe 1992). Not only did the strapping promote an improved alignment and delay the onset of pain but also physiotherapists reported an increased awareness of the affected shoulder from both patients and staff. The main disadvantages are the potential for an adverse skin reaction and the need for regular reapplication.

Support using pillows or a tray/table

The chair-bound patient may have the shoulder joint supported by means of pillows or resting the arms forwards on a table or on a tray attached to the wheelchair. Attention must be paid to the arrangement of the pillows and the alignment of the shoulder girdle, particularly in terms of protraction. Many patients utilise this means of support but, in some instances, the pillows are inappropriately positioned and serve more as 'leg warmers' than as support and protection for the shoulder joint.

Summary

The benefit of these various supports with regard to correcting shoulder subluxation is questionable. In a recent study comparing four different supports used to correct shoulder subluxation there was no evidence to show that the use of these supports prevented or reduced long-term subluxation (Zorowitz et al 1995). Based on these findings, Jackson (1998) has suggested 'that until evidence is provided to the contrary, there is little justification for their use'.

ELBOW CASTS

Contracture of the elbow joint is a not uncommon sequel of increased tone affecting the flexor muscle groups. Flexor hypertonus of the upper limb is the most prevalent synergy following CVA and is frequently observed in patients following traumatic brain injury or disease. Other patients who are susceptible to flexor contracture of the elbow joint are those with cervical cord lesions where biceps is unopposed by triceps.

Various types of splints made from different materials may be utilised to prevent or correct these contractures.

Drop-out casts

The principle of regaining range of movement is to apply stretch to the shortened structures, and a full cylinder may be used to this effect. However, it is the opinion of these authors that the drop-out cast provides a more dynamic and less forceful means of regaining range of movement. The arm is extended to its maximum range and the cast is then applied with the elbow at 5 or 10 degrees less than the full available range. This reduces the stress on the shortened structures but, at the same time, prevents further flexion of the elbow and enables either passive or active movement into extension.

This type of cast is only effective if the available range is greater than 70 degrees of full extension. If the elbow cannot be extended to this range, the forces are such as to cause the elbow to pull backwards out of the splint. For this reason, serial casting using full cylinders is recommended until such time as 70 degrees is attainable.

The cast extends the length of the arm from just below the axilla to include the wrist and hand up to just below the palmar crease. The arm is extended to 5 or 10 degrees less than the maximum available range of elbow extension with the forearm in neutral. The position of the wrist is determined by the degree of flexion or extension, pronation and supination and ulnar or radial deviation, the mid-position being optimal. The section over triceps is cut away to allow for extension at the elbow.

Application

The cast is applied with the patient in supine or in sitting, depending upon the medical status. The materials required are:

- 2 or 3 inch (5 or 7.5 cm) stockinet
- microfoam tape
- 2 × 3 inch (7.5 cm) Soft Cast bandages
- 1 × 3 inch (7.5 cm) Scotch Cast Plus bandage

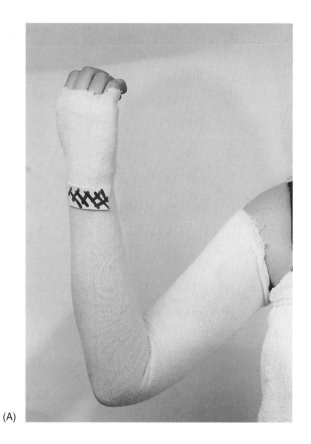

(A)

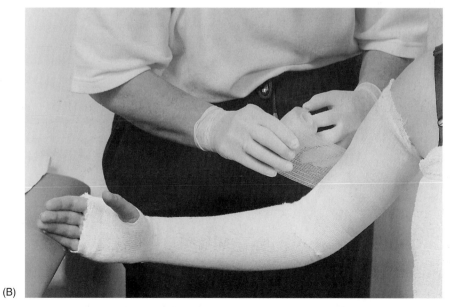

(B)

Figure 10.19 (A–B) Drop-out elbow cast.

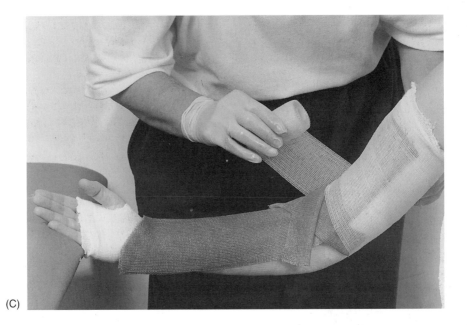

(C)

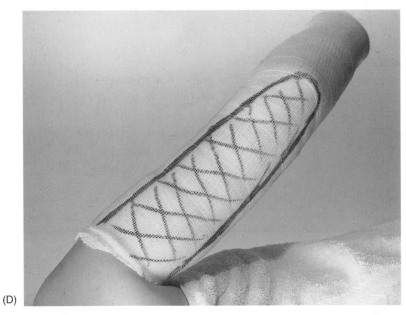

(D)

Figure 10.19   (C–D) Drop-out elbow cast.

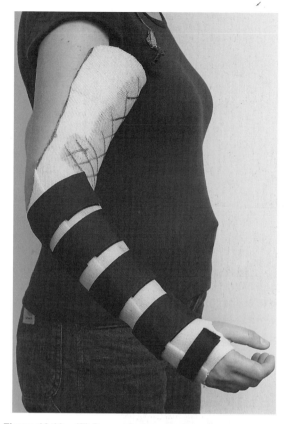

Figure 10.19   (E) Drop-out elbow cast.

- 1 wet cotton bandage
- zinc oxide tape
- Velcro fastening.

The method of application is illustrated in Figure 10.19. The two layers of stockinet extend from just below the acromion process to below the metacarpal heads. The stockinet is cut to free the thumb. Microfoam tape is applied over the ulnar styloid.

The first Soft Cast bandage is applied dry from just below the axilla extending down to the metacarpalphalangeal joints, cutting the casting tape as required to prevent creasing as the bandage passes around the base of the thumb.

A dry slab of five layers of Scotch Cast Plus is positioned longitudinally over the flexor aspect of the arm with two small two-layer strips crossing at the elbow joint. This slab is cut at the lower end to avoid the thenar eminence and remain below the palmar crease.

The second Soft Cast bandage is then used to secure the slab and cross in place following immersion in tepid water. The wet cotton bandage is applied over the·cast to laminate the materials.

Once the Scotch Cast Plus slab has hardened, the wet cotton bandage is removed. The U-shaped section over triceps is marked with a felt tip pen, ensuring the lower part of the U is over the olecranon process. Using the blunt-ended scissors, this section of Soft Cast is cut away. The forearm section of the cast is cut longitudinally from the lateral epicondyle and over the extensor forearm muscles.

The cast may then be removed and, when the cast is dry, zinc oxide tape is placed over the edges of the cast. Velcro fastening is attached to the forearm section of the cast, leaving the humeral section free to enable the arm to 'drop-out' into extension when the patient is up against gravity.

Cautionary note

Some patients with severe flexor hypertonus affecting the arm may have relatively low tone proximally at the shoulder. For this reason, *POP is not recommended for casting of the upper limb* as it tends to be very heavy. Patients are usually encouraged to stand and, with POP splints, the excessive weight applied to the arm may contribute to subluxation of the shoulder.

Myositis ossificans or heterotopic ossification is a complication which may affect various soft tissues and joints of the body, particularly following head injury (Garland & Keenan 1983, Wildburger et al 1994). The elbow joint is often affected, and splinting for these patients should be used with caution. Forcing of range may lead to an increase in the severity of symptoms and must be avoided (Ada et al 1990). For this reason the drop-out cast is preferred in that it does not need to be applied with the arm in its maximally extended position.

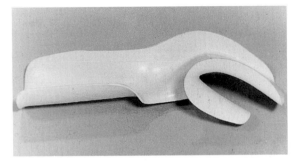

Figure 10.20 Volar splint.

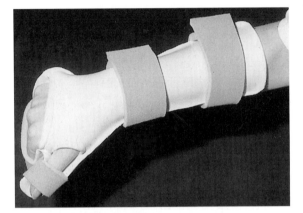

Figure 10.21 Dorsal splint.

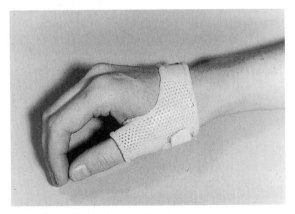

Figure 10.22 Thumb opposition splint.

WRIST AND HAND SPLINTS

Splinting of the wrist and hand is often deemed to be the remit of the occupational therapist and details of the different types of thermoplastic splints that may be used to maintain or improve

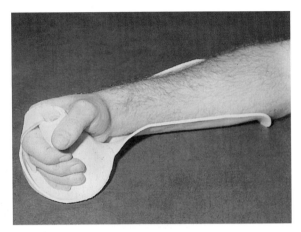

Figure 10.23 Cone/volar splint.

hand function are to be found in Malick (1982, 1985). Examples of some of these splints are shown in Figures 10.20–10.22.

Other types of splints are available which include the cone (Fig. 10.23) which was first introduced by Rood (1954 as cited by Stockmeyer 1967) and the boxing glove splint (Fig. 10.24, Bromley 1998) for use with spinal cord injured patients.

Hand splinting is a specialised area of treatment. The splints illustrated above are only a small selection of those which may be utilised in the management of the many and varied hand deformities which may arise as a result of neurological damage.

Combination cast

Although thermoplastic materials remain the most commonly used materials for wrist and hand splints, the combination casts using Soft Cast and Scotch Cast Plus may also be effective.

The materials required are:

- 2 inch (5 cm) and 1 inch (2.5 cm) stockinet
- microfoam tape
- 2 × 2 inch (5 cm) Soft Cast
- 1 × 2 inch (5 cm) Scotch Cast Plus
- 1 wet cotton bandage
- zinc oxide tape
- Velcro fastening.

The method of application is illustrated in Fig. 10.25. The two layers of 2 inch (5 cm) stockinet

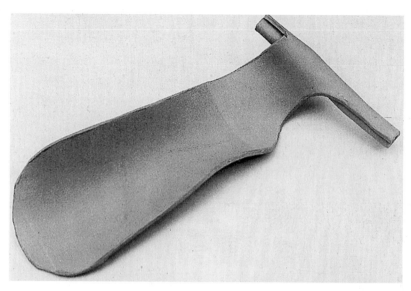

Figure 10.24 Unpadded cock-up support for the boxing glove splint. (Reproduced from Bromley 1998 with kind permission.)

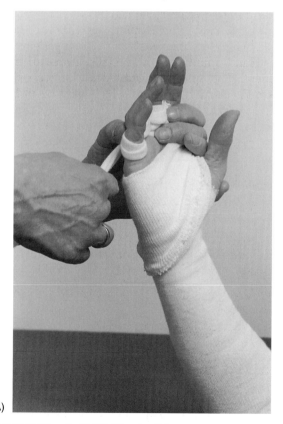

(A)

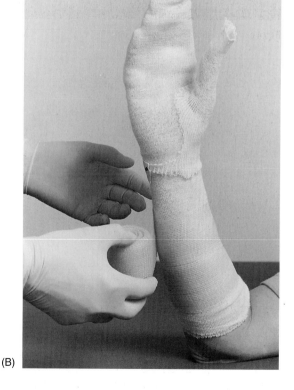

(B)

Figure 10.25 (A–B) Wrist/hand splint.

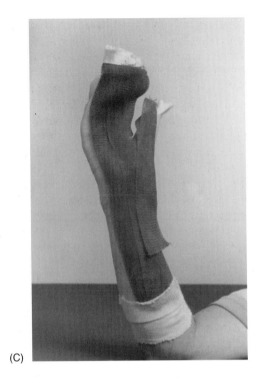
(C)

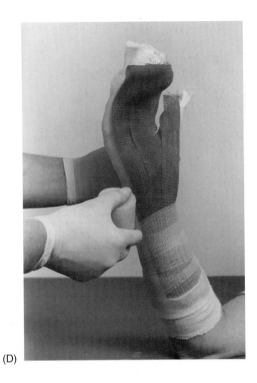
(D)

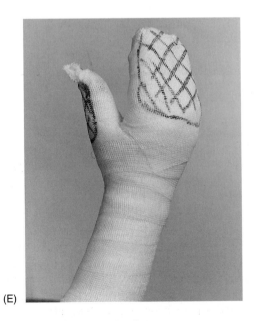
(E)

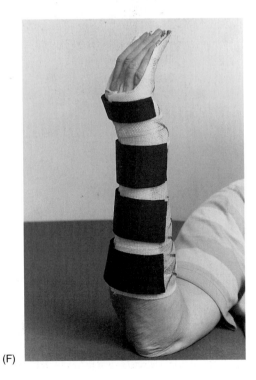
(F)

Figure 10.25   (C–F) Wrist/hand splint.

are applied from just below the elbow, extending down to and including the fingers. A piece of 1 inch (2.5 cm) stockinet is placed between the fingers to prevent them being squeezed together as the splint is made and another piece of 1 inch (2.5 cm) stockinet is placed over the thumb. Microfoam tape is placed over the ulnar styloid.

The first Soft Cast bandage is applied dry from 2 inches (5 cm) below the elbow down to the hand to include the thumb and fingers. The scissors are required to cut the bandage as required to ensure a smooth fit around the wrist and thumb.

A dry slab of four-layer Scotch Cast Plus is placed over the flexor aspect of the forearm to beyond the tips of the fingers. An additional piece of Scotch Cast Plus, doubled over and approximately 4 inches (10 cm) in length is applied from the tip of the thumb to the mid-forearm over the flexor aspect.

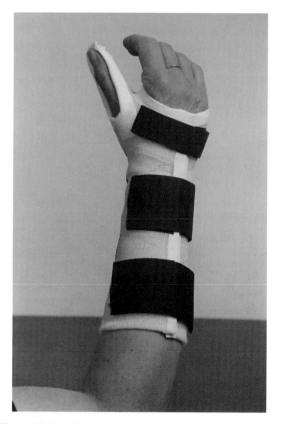

Figure 10.26   Wrist and thumb splint.

The second Soft Cast bandage is applied to secure these slabs in place following immersion in tepid water and then the wet cotton bandage to ensure lamination of the layers.

When the Scotch Cast Plus is hard, the splint is removed by cutting longitudinally over the forearm extensor muscles and down the back of the hand. The section over the extensor aspect of the fingers and thumb is cut away to the meta-carpalphalangeal joints. This is particularly important at the thumb as patients with flexor hypertonus will be unable to place the thumb in a spica without assistance.

The edges of the cast are secured with zinc oxide tape and Velcro fastening attached for reapplication.

This cast may also be used purely to support the wrist and thumb, leaving the fingers free (Fig. 10.26). In this case, the splint must finish below the palmar crease to prevent the metacarpalphalangeal joints being held in extension.

In summary, it is important to discuss the proposed splinting intervention with the occupational therapist. Modifications and new materials continue to be developed and, in clinical practice, it is often a case of trial and error to determine the most effective splint for management of hand dysfunction. Investigations to date do not indicate for whom hand splints may produce beneficial effects in reducing or limiting the effects of hypertonus (Langlois et al 1989).

SUMMARY

The use of casts in the management of patients with neurological dysfunction should always be considered an adjunct to treatment as opposed to a treatment in its own right. Careful assessment is essential to determine the most effective intervention and to ensure that the patient is able to accommodate to the support provided by the splint.

Jackson (1998) commented that physiotherapists are often reluctant to use splints in the management of patients with spasticity as some practitioners believe that the restraint imposed by the cast can further exacerbate this hypertonus. However, there is no scientific evidence to support this assumption, and reduction in contracture with no adverse effects on muscle tone has been reported (Mills 1984).

In some instances, splinting may be used after injection of botulinum toxin (see Ch. 7). It is suggested that the weakening effect of the toxin provides the multidisciplinary team with 'a window of opportunity' to make changes in patterns of movement, antagonistic control, muscle length and function (Richardson et al 1997). Splinting may be considered as an adjunct to treatment in achieving these goals (Richardson & Thompson 1999).

There are many different types of splints and orthoses which may be used to obtain the desired support or maintenance of range of movement of a limb. Plaster of Paris has long been the casting material of choice for patients with neurological dysfunction. Sullivan et al (1988) consider plaster to be the preferred material in that 'it is strong, inexpensive, easily moulded, reinforced or repaired once dry, and does not splinter leaving sharp edges, as may occur with fibreglass'.

Moseley (1997) advocates the use of fibreglass casting tape when using casts in combination with stretching to regain dorsiflexion range of movement at the ankle of patients following head injury. Fibreglass is strong, slightly more expensive than POP (on average half the quantity of fibreglass is required to that of POP), easily moulded, rarely needs reinforcement, and sharp edges may be avoided with appropriate use of padding. An additional advantage of the fibreglass materials, including the combination casts, is that there is considerably less mess and therefore reduced time spent clearing up.

As new materials, such as Soft Cast, are developed, clinicians will invariably alter their practice. There will almost inevitably be a disparity of views with regard to the most effective casting regime and choice of materials but, in the opinion of these authors, the combination of Soft Cast and Scotch Cast Plus can be used in most situations where splinting is indicated.

Whichever materials are chosen, the therapist must follow the manufacturer's guidelines, and practice is recommended on normal subjects prior to attempting this intervention on patients.

The use of orthoses and casts can prove beneficial in the management of patients with neurological dysfunction. However, this is a complex speciality and, in order to avoid adverse effects, advice should be sought from staff experienced in this field.

REFERENCES

Ada L, Canning C, Paratz J 1990 Care of the unconscious head injured patient. In: Ada L, Canning C (eds) Key issues in neurological physiotherapy. Butterworth-Heinemann, London

Ancliffe J 1992 Strapping the shoulder in patients following a cerebral vascular accident (CVA): a pilot study. Australian Physiotherapy Journal 38: 37–40

Association of Chartered Physiotherapists Interested in Neurology (ACPIN) 1998 Clinical practice guidelines on splinting adults with neurological dysfunction. Chartered Society of Physiotherapy, London

Beckman J 1987 The Louisiana State University reciprocating gait orthosis. Physiotherapy 73(8): 386–392

Bobath B 1978 Adult hemiplegia: evaluation and treatment, 2nd edn. Heinemann Medical Books, London

Bobath B 1990 Adult hemiplegia: evaluation and treatment, 3rd edn. Heinemann Medical Books, London

Booth B J, Doyle M, Montgomery J 1983 Serial casting for the management of spasticity in the head injured adult. Physical Therapy 63(12): 1960–1966

Bromley I 1998 Tetraplegia and paraplegia: a guide for physiotherapists, 5th edn. Churchill Livingstone, Edinburgh

Buccholz-Moodie N, Brisbin J, Morgan A 1986 Subluxation of the glenohumeral joint in hemiplegia: evaluation of supportive devises. Physiotherapy Canada 38: 151–157

Conine T, Sullivan T, Mackie T, Goodman M 1990 Effect of serial casting for the prevention of equinus in patients with acute head injury. Archives of Physical Medicine and Rehabilitation 71(5): 310–312

Cusick B D 1988 Splints and casts: managing foot deformity in children with neuromotor disorders. Physical Therapy 68(12): 1903–1912

Davies P M 1985 Steps to follow: a guide to the treatment of adult hemiplegia. Springer-Verlag, Berlin

Davies P M 1994 Starting again. Springer-Verlag, Berlin

Faghri P D, Rodgers M M, Glaser R M, Bors J G, Akuthota P 1994 The effects of functional electrical stimulation on shoulder subluxation, arm function recovery and shoulder pain in hemiplegic stroke patients. Archives of Physical Medicine and Rehabilitation 75: 73–79

Fyfe N, Goodwill J, Hoyle E, Sandles L 1993 Orthoses, mobility and environmental control systems. In: Greenwood R, Barnes M P, McMillan T M, Ward C D (eds) Neurological rehabilitation. Churchill Livingstone, London

Galley P M, Forster A L 1987 Human movement: an introductory text for physiotherapy students, 2nd edn. Churchill Livingstone, London

Garland D E, Keenan M-A E 1983 Orthopaedic strategies in the management of the adult head-injured patient. Physical Therapy 63(12): 2004–2009

Griffen J, Reddin G 1981 Shoulder pain in patients with hemiplegia: a literature review. Physical Therapy 61: 1041–1045

Host H H 1995 Scapular taping in the treatment of anterior shoulder impingement. Physical Therapy 75: 803–812

Jackson J 1998 Specific treatment techniques. In: Stokes M (ed) Neurological physiotherapy. Mosby, London

Kent H, Hershler C, Conine T A, Hershler R 1990 Case control study of lower extremity serial casting in adult patients with head injury. Physiotherapy Canada 42(4): 189–191

Langlois S, MacKinnon J, Pederson L 1989 Hand splints and cerebral spasticity: a review of the literature. Canadian Journal of Occupational Therapy 56(3): 113–119

Malick M H 1982 Manual on dynamic hand splinting with thermoplastic materials. Am Rehab Ed. Newark (AREN) Publications, USA

Malick M H 1985 Manual on static hand splinting. New materials and techniques. Am Rehab Ed. Newark (AREN) Publications, USA

Mills V 1984 Electromyographic results of inhibitory splinting. Physical Therapy 64: 190–193

Moseley A M 1993 The effect of a regimen of casting and prolonged stretching on passive ankle dorsiflexion in traumatic head-injured adults. Physiotherapy Theory and Practice 9(4): 215–221

Moseley A M 1997 The effect of casting combined with stretching on passive ankle dorsiflexion in adults with traumatic head injuries. Physical Therapy 77: 240–247

Nene A V, Patrick J H 1990 Energy cost of paraplegic locomotion using the Parawalker – electrical stimulation 'hybrid orthosis'. Archives of Physical Medicine and Rehabilitation 71: 116–120

Richardson D, Thompson A J 1999 Botulinum toxin. Its use in the treatment of acquired spasticity in adults. Physiotherapy 85: 541–551

Richardson D, Edwards S, Sheean G L, Greenwood R J, Thompson A J 1997 The effect of botulinum toxin on hand function after incomplete spinal cord injury at the level of C5/6: a case report. Clinical Rehabilitation 11: 288–292

Rood M 1954 Neurophysiological reactions as a basis for physical therapy. Physical Therapy Review 34: 444–449

Rose G 1986 Orthotics: principles and practice. Heinemann, London

Rose G K, Butler P, Stallard J 1982 Gait: principles, biomechanics and assessment. Orlau Publishing, Oswestry

Rothwell J 1994 Control of human voluntary movement, 2nd edn. Chapman and Hall, London

Saunders J B, Inman V T, Eberhart H D 1953 The major determinants in normal and pathological gait. Journal of Bone and Joint Surgery 35A(3): 543–558

Schuren J 1994 Working with soft cast. 3M Minnesota Mining and Manufacturing, Germany

Stockmeyer S A 1967 An interpretation of the approach of Rood to the neuromuscular dysfunction. American Journal of Physical Therapy 46: 900–961

Sullivan T, Conine T, Goodman M, Mackie T 1988 Serial casting to prevent equinus in acute traumatic head injury. Physiotherapy Canada 40(6): 346–350

Sutherland D H, Cooper L 1978 The pathomechanics of progressive crouch gait in spastic diplegia. Orthopedic Clinics of North America 9(1): 143–154

Training Council for Orthotists 1980 Classification of orthoses. Department of Health and Social Security. HMSO, London

Wildburger R, Zarkovic N, Egger G, Petek W, Zarkovic K, Hofer H P 1994 Basic fibroblast growth factor (BFGF) immunoreactivity as a possible link between head injury and impaired bone fracture healing. Bone & Mineral 27: 183–192

Williams R, Taffs L, Minuk T 1988 Evaluation of two support methods for the subluxated shoulder of hemiplegic patients. Physical Therapy 68: 1209–1214

Yarkony G M, Sahgal V 1987 Contractures: a major complication of craniocerebral trauma. Clinical Orthopaedics and Related Research 219: 93–96

Zorowitz R D, Idank D, Ikai T, Hughes M B, Johnstone V 1995 Shoulder subluxation after stroke: a comparison of four supports. Archives of Physical Medicine and Rehabilitation 76: 763–771

11

Longer-term management for patients with residual or progressive disability

Susan Edwards

INTRODUCTION

There is little dispute that people sustaining neurological damage or disease with resultant disability should receive a period of physical treatment and management following the initial onset of that impairment. The duration and timing of interventions vary considerably and are determined not only by the prognosis and perception of need but to an increasing extent by the resources available to support health care. The purpose of this chapter is to discuss the level of care which is necessary to maintain optimum physical status in people with residual or progressive disability and handicap and to consider those factors which relate to management.

The main emphasis for patients with chronic and progressive conditions, where functional recovery is limited, is twofold: to prevent secondary complications and to maintain function at an optimal level. Compensation for neurological disability is often considered to be undesirable, the aim of treatment being to 'restore normal movement'. However, where there is diffuse, irreversible damage to the central nervous system or progressive deterioration, this aim may not be realistic and compensatory strategies which are appropriate for the patient should be encouraged in order to maximise function.

The population comprises two categories of patients when considering long-term management:

- non-progressive impairment
- progressive impairment.

The first category includes patients following cerebrovascular accident (CVA), head or spinal injury and those with cerebral palsy. For these patients, although the impairment itself is non-progressive, the disability and subsequent handicap may increase over time (Bax et al 1988).

The second category of progressive impairment includes patients with a wide range of conditions such as multiple sclerosis, Parkinson's disease, cerebellar degeneration and neuromuscular disorders.

PRINCIPLES OF MANAGEMENT

With the number of people with more severe neurological impairments surviving trauma, together with the increased longevity, due to medical and technological advancements, of those with deteriorating conditions the level of residual disability is increasing. In consequence, already overtaxed resources are being further stretched.

Currently, physiotherapeutic intervention for people with residual or potentially progressive disability does not differ significantly from that provided in the acute care setting. In the case of injury or exacerbation of disease, the patient is discharged home or into residential care after a varying period of time in an acute hospital and/or rehabilitation unit at a time when most recovery is deemed to have taken place. While continuation of intensive therapy, such as that advocated in the acute condition, is inappropriate, ongoing management is essential to maintain and possibly regain optimum function. Part of this management process is to monitor for change in the level of disability, at which juncture a period of more intensive therapy may be instigated. For example, despite unchanging impairment, improvements in the level of disability were demonstrated following inpatient rehabilitation for patients with multiple sclerosis (Freeman et al 1997, 1999, Solari et al 1999).

In order to deal with complex and long-term conditions it is important to clarify the terms 'management' and 'treatment':

- *Management* is primarily concerned with 'the maintenance of the optimal physical condition through control of posture, movement and handling techniques. It is primarily preventative in nature (of secondary problems), but may be corrective if such problems have already occurred'.
- *Treatment* is 'a technique or modality used or monitored by a physiotherapist for the purpose of enhancing motor performance, reducing the impairments and symptoms of the pathology' (Pope 1997).

There is obvious overlap in that appropriate management of the patient forms the basis of any recovery of functional ability and, therefore, although it is possible to have management without treatment, the reverse is not the case. Management of the physical condition should underpin all forms of therapeutic intervention and should be ongoing for as long as is necessary. Treatment may be considered to be complementary to the underlying management and is usually not ongoing.

To illustrate the problems encountered by patients and their long-term management, two examples from each category will be discussed:

- In the non-progressive category: the vegetative state following head injury; and cerebral palsy in adulthood.
- In the progressive category: multiple sclerosis; and hereditary motor and sensory neuropathy.

NON-PROGRESSIVE IMPAIRMENT
The vegetative state

Introduction

Severe brain injury or disease may result in such irrevocable damage to the central nervous system that functional recovery becomes an unattainable goal and patients remain dependent on others for the rest of their lives. This condition was referred to as persistent or permanent vegetative state (Jennett & Plum 1972). However, it is now recommended that the terms 'persistent' and 'permanent' be dropped from the diagnosis of 'vegetative state' as these confuse prognosis with diagnosis (International Working Party 1996).

There are three prime features of the vegetative state:

- the patient has sleep–wake cycles
- all responses can be identified as reflex patterns
- the patient makes no meaningful responses and has no awareness (Andrews 1999).

The term 'silent epidemic' has been used to describe people who survive brain injury in a vegetative state (Klein 1982, Freeman 1992). Andrews (1999) highlights the difficulty with diagnosis in that 'the only way anyone can demonstrate their awareness is through a motor function, that is, speech, facial expression, or physical gesture. In the presence of severe spasticity, muscle inactivity and dysphasia it is extremely difficult for even an aware person to demonstrate their awareness'. Childs et al (1993) and Andrews et al (1996) have shown that misdiagnosis is not uncommon.

Although a high proportion of people in a vegetative state die during the first 6 months, a life expectancy of at least 15 years is not uncommon (International Working Party 1996). It is therefore essential for all staff to ensure that the optimal level of care is provided to maintain the patient's dignity and hygiene.

The management of these patients offers the sternest challenge to all personnel involved in their care and there is a lack of agreement of the focus that long-term management should take. Vogenthaler (1987) stated that 'obviously living and vocational rehabilitation are not relevant' but Pope (1988) asks the question 'if not, then what is?'. The main criterion for determining a successful outcome is the promotion of both physical and mental recovery but, for those in a vegetative state, this will never be realised. For these patients, it is inappropriate to evaluate success or failure using these performance indicators. The patient who remains free from contracture and pressure sores, and with the positive release phenomena under control, can be considered as a static success (Pope 1988).

In some instances, it may be possible for a patient to be cared for at home, provided adequate support is available from the community services. In others, long-term management of the patient in some form of institution where constant nursing care is available is necessary. Irrespective of the ultimate placement, the immediate family and friends must be considered as part of the team and be involved in the decision-making process at all stages of the patient's management.

Ethical considerations

Advances in medical science and technology are enabling many more people to survive even the most severe trauma, which may lead to the vegetative state. The British Medical Association (BMA) Medical Ethics Committee states that treatment can only be justified if 'it makes possible a decent life in which a patient can reasonably be thought to have continued interest'. However, in the immediate aftermath of severe brain damage, it is often difficult for medical staff to assess the probability of meaningful recovery. It is debatable what a meaningful recovery is. Whatever the satisfaction it may bring to family and friends, the recovery of a limited degree of awareness may be worse than total loss of cognitive function for the patient.

There have been a number of legal cases regarding the cessation of treatment of patients in a vegetative state. Initially these were requests to withdraw ventilation as in the Quinlan case of 1976 (Hannan et al 1994) but, more recently, actions have been brought to stop nasogastric tube feeding (Tribe & Korgaonkar 1992). The findings in these cases have confirmed that these are legitimate and ethically acceptable options that the family and doctors of some patients may consider (Jennett 1992).

For patients in a vegetative state, where there is little or no hope of functional recovery, it may be recommended that all active treatment should cease. The implications of such a decision may have a devastating effect on patients and their carers. Optimal care may be considered to be the maintenance of the patient's bodily functions, joint and muscle range of movement, tissue viability, and stimulation of cognitive awareness. Withdrawal of active treatment usually refers to the more dynamic intervention such as that which may be carried out by the physiotherapist. Maintenance of joint and muscle range, considered by many to be the remit of the physiotherapist, is difficult and potentially damaging where there is excessive hypertonus (Ada et al 1990). Changes of position are frequently utilised to minimise or control the effects of this stereotyped posturing. The provision of appropriate support in sitting and when standing the patient may prove effective in reducing the influence of hypertonus. This type of intervention may be considered inappropriate by the medical staff where there is little hope of functional recovery. However, if outcome is measured by the prevention of deterioration as opposed to the attainment of function, active treatment can be viewed as a key component within the management process rather than as a waste of resources on a patient who may be considered to be a hopeless case (Fig. 11.1). It must be recognised that this dynamic intervention may make the difference between the patient being 'manageable' and the patient deteriorating with the development of gross contracture leading to deformity. The patient is likely to be dominated by positive neurological signs and at high risk of tissue breakdown (Pope 1988).

A diagnosis of the vegetative state should be used with caution. Applied too soon following trauma, it may lead to the denial of further therapy and appropriate management. The effect can be catastrophic for the patient, emotionally devastating for the family and financially demanding for the community (Freeman 1992).

Most importantly, the person in a vegetative state must be recognised as an individual, albeit with little or no cognitive awareness. Communication is a two-way process and where there is no response or recognition from one party, inevitably this will affect the approach of the other. Where there is little or no response over a protracted period of time, it is often difficult for carers, be they professional staff, family or friends, to remain positive in their approach towards that person. It is all too easy to treat patients in a vegetative state on a routine basis with little thought as to how a particular intervention may affect them.

Physiotherapy intervention

The diagnosis of the vegetative state should not preclude treatment. Prevention of secondary complications is essential to optimise potential function and management. The principles of treatment as described in Chapter 6 are of as great an importance to this patient group as to those with a more optimistic prognosis. The majority of patients will demonstrate hypertonus, the extent, severity and distribution being dependent upon the site and extent of the area of damage and on the environmental influences to which the patient is subjected (Finger & Almli 1985, Bach-y-Rita 1990).

The speed at which therapy intervention is carried out is of vital importance; these patients often have difficulty in accommodating to change in respect of movement or position. The proprioceptive input provided by the physiotherapist should ensure appropriate support to facilitate a feeling of stability and security, allowing time for the patient to respond to the movement. Sudden movements, for example attempting to stand the patient without adequate preparation, may lead to an increase in tone which may preclude attainment of this position.

Physiotherapy for people with severe brain injury is part of a 24-hour management process and cannot be viewed in isolation. The remit of the physiotherapist caring for patients in a vege-

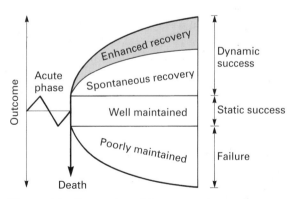

Figure 11.1 Range of possible outcomes following brain trauma (reproduced from Pope 1988 with kind permission).

tative state is to maintain and, where appropriate, increase range of movement to enable the optimal level of care. Orofacial treatment as advocated in Chapter 6, in conjunction with the speech and language therapist, is of particular value for these patients. Full or improved range of movement throughout the body will enable more appropriate seating, positioning in bed, washing, dressing and, perhaps, the ability to stand the person with suitable support. It is only by constant reinforcement of correct positioning and handling that deterioration may be prevented.

Positioning should be considered a dynamic aspect of treatment. Prior to moving the patient from one position to another, an explanation should be given of the proposed manoeuvre. Staff and/or carers should inform the patient that, for example, the pillows are going to be removed and request assistance from the patient to accomplish the movement. Mobilisation of the trunk on the pelvis may be used to influence the prevailing tone in an attempt to facilitate the change of position (Davies 1994). At all times, patients must be stimulated to maximise any recovery in both their physical and cognitive status.

The use of splinting for maintaining and regaining joint range is of great value in the management of patients in a vegetative state. For patients with severe hypertonus it is often difficult to maintain full muscle and joint range without using some form of splintage. The types of splints which may be used and the situations in which to use them are described in detail in Chapter 10. However, splinting should not be viewed as a static intervention replacing the need for physiotherapy, but as a dynamic adjunct to treatment. The splinted part must accommodate to the cast in order for it to be effective. Any evidence of increased tone or agitation may be indicative of discomfort and potential pressure sores. In this situation, the splint must be removed without delay in case it is the splint that is giving rise to these adverse symptoms.

Summary

Many patients may be diagnosed as being in a vegetative state, often only a short time after their injury or illness. Jennett & Plum (1972) describe the clinical features: '[patients] have periods of wakefulness when their eyes are open and move, their responsiveness is limited to primitive postural and reflex movements of the limbs, and they never speak …. Few would dispute that in this condition the cerebral cortex is out of action'. This state may prevail for years with no tangible change in the patient's condition but Berroll (1986; cited by Freeman 1992) found that a significant number of patients diagnosed as vegetative became conscious within 12 months of trauma.

Every effort should be made to ensure that each patient receives appropriate stimulation to maximise recovery. Many patients diagnosed as being in a vegetative state are often maintained in a state of gross sensory deprivation with the utilisation of scarce resources on active treatment being considered inappropriate. The brain is exquisitely responsive to the environment (Delgado 1977; cited by Freeman 1992) and as such is dependent upon the management and variety offered by the environment for any positive change in outcome. The use of a gastrostomy as opposed to a nasogastric tube and a leg bag for urine collection as opposed to a mounted catheter bag are examples of sensitive management, respecting patients' dignity in spite of their lack of awareness.

Active intervention such as that described above need not necessarily mean a great increase in expenditure. Education and involvement of family and friends and other health care workers in patient management promotes stimulation of both cognitive and physical function. Prevention of loss of joint and muscle range provides not only easier nursing care but also greater comfort for the patient. The management of complications such as pressure sores and contractures, which may arise following severe brain injury, may prove to be expensive; prevention of these complications inevitably reduces the ultimate cost of care.

Cerebral palsy in adulthood

Introduction

Cerebral palsy is the result of a lesion or maldevelopment of the brain; it is non-progressive in character and exists from earliest childhood (Bobath 1974). The management of children with cerebral palsy is generally recognised as an ongoing process from birth, or when the condition is first diagnosed, to adulthood. By this time the individuals should be fully equipped for their needs in life, with equipment such as communication aids, wheelchairs and splints. Physiotherapy for those with physical disabilities is an accepted part of management. However, for many people with cerebral palsy, problems may intensify over time when, in many instances, physiotherapy is no longer available. Poor quality of management and treatment becomes increasingly widespread when considering patients who have chronic, often more severe, disabilities. These patients may not experience an acute episode which would, at least, bring them into contact with the existing services (Condie 1991).

The paediatric services are used to dealing with what are often diverse and complex problems. Maintenance of range of movement and prevention of postural deformity are recognised as key principles of physiotherapy throughout the period of growth. While at school, regular standing, ongoing review of seating and postural supports, and provision of appropriate footwear are examples of components of a physiotherapy programme which is supported by all personnel. However, when the child becomes an adult, such intervention often ceases in spite of the fact that many people show signs of physical deterioration when routine care is withdrawn (Bax et al 1988).

The term 'management' can be used to refer to the entire process whereby patients' problems are identified and their needs analysed, as a result of which they are subsequently admitted to an individually tailored programme of treatment and review which continues for as long as their disability persists (Condie 1991). Unfortunately, this is rarely the case, in spite of people with physical disability being designated a priority group in *Care in Action*, the Government's 1981 handbook of policies and priorities for health and social services in the UK. Services for disabled people remain confused and extremely variable with a distinct lack of good practice (Beardshaw 1988).

In a study looking into the health care of handicapped adults (Bax et al 1988), many subjects with cerebral palsy reported that their physical condition had deteriorated after leaving school; they had become less mobile and their contractures more fixed.

Where there is diffuse brain damage, the whole body may be involved. Symptoms may include quadriplegia, visual and hearing deficits and intellectual dysfunction. The inability to communicate needs, thoughts and feelings is perhaps the most serious defect and one which may lead to an individual being labelled mentally retarded. Many people who were unable to communicate verbally were found to have normal intelligence once taught alternative means of communication (McNaughton 1975; cited by Bleck 1987). 'Because these persons present an almost overwhelming number of problems, efforts toward rehabilitation are apt to be truncated, individuals relegated to the waste-basket category of medical care and their potential as persons neglected' (Bleck 1987). It is essential to make resources available which enable the individual to achieve an optimal level of functional independence consistent with the limitations imposed by the neurological and musculoskeletal impairment.

Physiotherapy intervention

Many people with cerebral palsy maintain an independent lifestyle and do not want or need regular therapy intervention. They may be wheelchair dependent or ambulant, albeit with an abnormal gait, but they cope with their disability and are content with their situation. Indeed, professional overtreatment and striving to remedy deficits rather than compensate for them may be the cause of 'mental distress', which was identified as a predominant disability in adolescents and adults with spastic diplegia (Bleck 1987).

Many people with spastic diplegia walk independently, often with flexion, adduction and medial rotation of the hips, flexion of the knees and plantar flexion and equinus of the feet. The pelvis is usually anteriorly tilted with a marked lumbar lordosis. The arms, which often have minor motor deficits, are constantly active in maintaining balance. The abnormal stresses and strains imposed on the musculoskeletal system by this posture may lead to arthritic changes in joints. Some of the problems which may arise include:

- Poor alignment of the hip joint during stance phase of gait results in damage to the joint surfaces. The constant pull into adduction and medial rotation may, in severe cases, cause displacement of the joint (Bleck 1987).
- The constant flexion of the knees causes 'alta patella' through overstretching of the patella ligament (Sutherland & Cooper 1978). Effective action of the quadriceps muscle group is never developed and, as the child becomes older and heavier, joint changes are almost inevitable.
- The feet may be severely deformed with breakdown of the medial arch and plantar fascia through the constant forces imposed on these structures with toe walking (Fig. 11.2).
- The anterior tilt of the pelvis may lead to contracture of the psoas muscle, further increasing the lumbar lordosis.

These problems may increase in severity over the years and yet, at the most vulnerable time of adolescence and early adulthood, when increased weight and reduced mobility increase disability, therapy is withdrawn. It is at this time that, in more severe cases, the individual may become wheelchair dependent. This is obviously a critical time from both a physical and an emotional perspective. Provision of a wheelchair should not only involve a thorough assessment as to the most appropriate chair but should also include physiotherapy to advise and instigate an exercise programme to prevent physical deterioration. In many cases there will already be some shortening of the flexor muscles, and prolonged sitting will exacerbate this problem. A regimen of standing and appropriate stretches should be devised for the individual, to guard against this possibility.

The structural and functional problems of people with cerebral palsy are often neglected and viewed as an integral part of the condition. This is not always the case. For example, pain, which may result from musculoskeletal changes arising from the abnormal postures and movements, requires treatment just as it does in the able-bodied population. A detailed assessment may be able to identify a specific cause of the pain, which may respond to treatment.

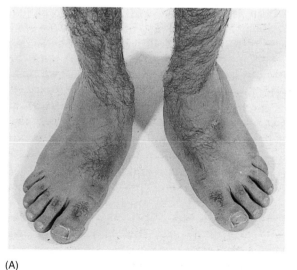

(A)

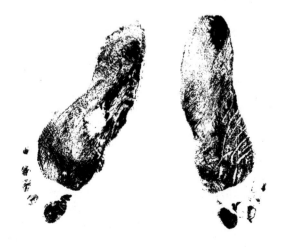

(B)

Figure 11.2   (A) Collapse of the medial arch in an adult with cerebral palsy; (B) weight-bearing surface.

Summary

For those with chronic residual physical disability, the danger of secondary complications, such as respiratory problems, contracture and postural deformity, remains throughout the course of their lives. The more severe the abnormal postures and movements, the greater is the danger. Regular assessment and treatment intervention as indicated is essential to prevent their occurrence. However, it must be recognised that many people cope adequately, even with gross disability and deformity, and do not desire ongoing therapy.

Currently, very few specialist health and co-ordinated services are organised for people who are only physically disabled, and the development of such services is recommended in each district health authority (Bax et al 1988).

PROGRESSIVE NEUROLOGICAL AND NEUROMUSCULAR DISORDERS

Introduction

Patients with progressive neurological and neuro-muscular disorders will require ongoing treatment and management appropriate to the stage of the disease process for the purpose of ensuring optimum function and the prevention of secondary complications. Regular reviews should be arranged in order to monitor the condition.

Examples of these disorders include multiple sclerosis, muscular dystrophy, Friedreich's ataxia, spinocerebellar degeneration and the hereditary motor sensory neuropathies (HMSN). The changing neurological and/or muscular status usually affects the clinical signs and symptoms and thereby the patient's functional capability. These conditions are often associated with a multiplicity of symptoms, the management of which requires a coordinated, multidisciplinary intervention.

Some people, for example those with multiple sclerosis, may experience exacerbations and remissions as part of the disease process, whereas others, such as those with muscular dystrophy, show a steady deterioration of varying severity. The aim of physiotherapy is to maxi-

mise function and prevent secondary complications. To date, there is little that can be done to halt the progression of many of these diseases, but an understanding of the expected complications and compensations from the primary impairment will enable the physiotherapist to intervene more appropriately.

Multiple sclerosis (MS)

Multiple sclerosis is an inflammatory, demyelinating disorder which is the most common cause of neurological disability in young adults (Thompson & McDonald 1992, Barnes 1993). A relapsing and remitting course is common but the condition may subsequently become progressive, when it is termed 'secondary progressive'. Between 15 and 20% of all MS patients have benign MS where there are few attacks early on and little if any residual disability (Weinshenker 1994). Less than 10% show a primary progressive course (Thompson & McDonald 1992). Over the past decade there has been a significant increase in the survival time, resulting in an almost normal life expectancy for the 'average person' with MS (Mertin 1994).

A diagnosis of MS is dependent upon the clinical demonstration of lesions disseminated in time and space and the exclusion of other conditions which may produce the same clinical picture (Thompson & McDonald 1992). Magnetic resonance imaging (MRI) may support the clinical diagnosis by identifying multiple lesions which indicate dissemination in space, but these do not always correlate with the clinical status (Thompson et al 1991).

The disease is characterised by multiple lesions (plaques) of demyelination with differing degrees of inflammation. There is a predilection for the optic nerve, periventricular areas and the cervical cord but all parts of the brain and spinal cord may be involved. The functional deficit is ultimately due to abnormalities in conduction. Demyelination causes a slowing or impairment of the ability of the nerve fibres to transmit impulses. Both demyelination and inflammation contribute to the conduction block and clinical deficit (Thompson & McDonald 1992).

The outstanding characteristic in the early stages is the patient's capacity for clinical recovery from individual episodes, primarily through the resolution of oedema and inflammation with some remyelination. With partial demyelination, some functional recovery takes place. This is mediated by the surviving fibres, either of the same system, or of other systems, that permit learning of new strategies to compensate for the deficit. However, compensation for progressive axonal loss continues to become less effective as more fibres subserving a particular function are impaired, leading to permanent disability (Thompson & McDonald 1992).

The clinical manifestations of the disease are varied but often include optic neuritis, sensory and motor disturbance of the limbs and symptoms relating to brain stem and cerebellar dysfunction (Thompson & McDonald 1992). Cognitive disturbances and emotional problems are prevalent (Poser 1980, Minden & Schiffer 1990). Psychiatric disturbance is seen in 40–50% of patients and there is a greater incidence of suicide in the MS population (Weinshenker 1994). Fatigue is common and frequently disabling (Krupp et al 1988). Pain is often associated with MS (Barnes 1993) and bladder symptoms occur in between 50 and 75% of patients (Thompson & McDonald 1992).

Pseudobulbar and respiratory symptoms may occur and respiratory muscle weakness, particularly of the diaphragm, is the most common cause of respiratory distress (Howard et al 1992). Bronchopneumonia is the leading cause of death in MS and may be related to swallowing difficulties with resultant aspiration (Barnes 1993).

The course of MS is extremely variable in terms of the frequency and severity of attacks, the degree of recovery and the development of progressive disability. Progressive onset of symptoms, secondary progression after a remitting phase, older age of onset and motor symptoms at onset generally indicate a poor prognosis (Miller et al 1992, Weinshenker 1994).

Physiotherapy intervention

Given the complexity and variability of the clinical signs and symptoms which may present in MS, a full and accurate assessment is essential to determine the primary problems resulting from the disease pathology. Compensatory strategies, adopted by the patient in an attempt to achieve function, may then be analysed as to their effectiveness, not only in the short term but also over a protracted period of time.

The initial interview between the patient and the physiotherapist must be handled with great sensitivity. It is essential that the physiotherapist is fully aware of information already given to the patient. Has the patient been told of the diagnosis? The majority of people with MS wish to know their diagnosis at an early stage, wish their family to be informed at the same time and wish to be given adequate background information on the disease and a chance to ask their own questions (Barnes 1993). However, in spite of this, doctors occasionally delay giving a definitive diagnosis and patients may learn of their diagnosis in an inappropriate manner.

Referral to physiotherapy in the early stages of disability can be of great benefit, both in planning a long-term management strategy and for instigating preventive therapeutic regimens. Continued monitoring with intervention as required is essential to cater for the changing needs of the patient (DeSouza 1990, Mertin & Paeth 1994). Unfortunately, many patients do not receive this ongoing care, and additional problems arising, either from the disease pathology or secondary to imposed abnormal movement strategies, are not addressed. An exercise programme that was designed in the early stages may, over time, become not only ineffective but possibly detrimental.

The patient must be an active participant in the planning of treatment. The patient's priorities may differ from those of the therapist, and discussion is essential to determine effective intervention which meets the requirements of both parties (DeSouza 1990). Multidisciplinary clinics are recommended which facilitate interdisciplinary cooperation (Fig. 11.3). This professional cooperation is of benefit to all personnel, not least the patients and their relatives (Barnes 1993, Mertin 1994). The aim should be to ensure that there is consistency in approach to treatment and mutually agreed goals.

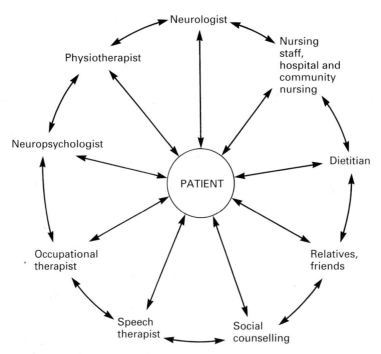

Figure 11.3 The interdisciplinary rehabilitation team (adapted from Mertin 1994).

Although the physiotherapist is often the key player in the management of motor disorders, the management of motor problems cannot be viewed in isolation from the other aspects of disability which may prevail. It is important that the physiotherapist has an understanding of the pathophysiology of MS in that the prognosis is so variable. Physiotherapists may themselves view MS as a progressive disease which ultimately leads to wheelchair dependence and perhaps death. This pessimistic attitude is not generally appropriate. Although consideration must be given to the mode of onset and type of MS, physiotherapy intervention should be geared towards the presenting signs and symptoms.

In many instances, a period of rehabilitation may be of value in ensuring optimal function following any change in the level of disability (Freeman et al 1997). Not only is this beneficial in terms of reassessment and restructuring of therapy intervention, but of equal importance is the often dramatic remission after hospitalisation. However, it must be recognised that psychological factors such as anxiety over financial difficulties, marital discord and academic pressures play an important role in the patient's ability to cope with the disease. When the patient is removed from his normal, possibly stressful environment, this in itself may have a therapeutic effect (Poser 1980).

Treatment of patients with MS is determined by the presenting signs and symptoms, those affecting posture and movement being of greatest relevance to the physiotherapist. The most common forms of movement deficit are associated with hypertonus and/or ataxia along with the secondary effects of fatigue, disuse, pain and sensory impairment (Barnes 1993). The primary aims of physiotherapy are to:

- maintain and increase range of movement
- encourage postural stability
- prevent contractures
- maintain and encourage weight-bearing (Ashburn & DeSouza 1988).

To this end, therapy should not be restricted to passive interventions such as stretching and mobilisation of specific parts. The patient must be involved as an active participant in the promotion of purposeful movements which are part of everyday function (Mertin & Paeth 1994). Exercise programmes are particularly useful in enabling patients to take responsibility for their own management and are often effective in maintaining range of movement and maximising muscle power.

Mertin & Paeth (1994) advocate approaches that differ according to the patient's level of impairment/disability as measured on the Kurtzke Disability Status Scale (DSS). Patients are stratified as having mild (DSS grade 0–2), moderate (DSS grade 3–5) or severe (DSS grade 6–9) disability (Miller et al 1992).

For those with a score of less than 5, the emphasis should be on the normalisation of postural control and inhibition of compensatory strategies. Facilitation of more normal movement patterns, particularly those of standing and gait, and an individual home programme of exercises are recommended. For those with increasing levels of impairment/disability, with a DSS score of greater than 6, compensatory strategies should be utilised and refined to improve functional independence with appropriate selection of aids and training in their usage. Maintenance of muscle and joint range, improving postural control, facilitation of normal movement patterns as appropriate, and maintenance of standing posture should be continued as before. Adaptation of the home exercise programme and the training of carers are necessary to respond to the changing functional status of the patient (Mertin & Paeth 1994).

Difficulty in walking is one of the most frequent symptoms of MS, and analysis and treatment of mobility problems provides perhaps the greatest challenge in MS management (Barnes 1993). Standing is of value for virtually all patients with abnormal tone and movement. This is effective in both maintaining and regaining range of movement, stimulating extensor activity (Brown 1994) and in improving the body's spatial orientation. Assessment of the primary cause of the gait impairment is essential in determining the most appropriate intervention. For those who are mobile without aids, facilitation of

a normal gait pattern is recommended. Those requiring mobility aids should receive appropriate training to ensure that these aids are used effectively.

For example, an ankle–foot orthosis (AFO) to control loss of adequate dorsiflexion may assist in the prevention of unnecessary proximal compensation. Without such support, the patient must inevitably use excessive knee flexion or circumduction at the hip to clear the foot during swing phase of gait. The AFO may allow for a more fluid and efficient walking cycle. For those with ataxia, the use of a rollator walking frame may prove of benefit in enabling the patient to gain improved stability. However, it is important that the patient uses this aid as a means of balance as opposed to fixation (see Ch. 5).

Hydrotherapy is considered to be effective for patients with MS (Barnes 1993) but treatment in a hydrotherapy pool, where the temperature of the water is often quite high, may increase fatigue. The temperature of the water is important, with increased temperatures potentially slowing nerve conduction (Poser 1980). Patients who enjoy exercise in water may derive more benefit from the cooler temperatures of general swimming pools.

Weights are considered to be effective in the management of ataxia (Morgan et al 1975), but these may cause fatigue and often do not have a lasting effect. The patient may accommodate to the weights over a period of time with the ataxia remaining relatively unaltered. Following removal of the weight, the ataxia may be greater than before and postural stability further compromised (DeSouza 1990). Weights may be of value as a temporary aid to compensate or dampen tremor, prior to or during performance of a functional task.

Appropriate seating, particularly for those with severe neurological deficit who are wheelchair dependent, is essential. Detailed description of postural control and specialised seating is provided in Chapter 9.

Splinting may be effective in maintaining range of movement, or can be used as a corrective measure for regaining range (Barnes 1993, Mertin 1994).

The management of respiratory complications, particularly in the advanced stages of MS, raises ethical issues. It is important that patients who are at risk of acute respiratory complications, associated with bulbar and spinal cord relapses, are identified early; provision of appropriate support during the period of respiratory insufficiency reduces the incidence of sudden death and reduces distress (Howard et al 1992). Some patients were found to improve significantly with remission and not all required continued mechanical assistance.

Summary

The likely progressive nature of the disease makes it imperative that regular multidisciplinary assessment, including physiotherapy, continues for so long as patients demonstrate changes in their clinical signs and symptoms. Wherever possible, this monitoring should be undertaken by staff who are familiar with the patient. All too frequently, patients with MS whose condition is being regularly reviewed are seen by different therapists at each assessment. This makes it very difficult to plan and monitor long-term treatment strategies and to evaluate the functional consequences of the changing neurological status. It is inevitable, however, where staff are on rotation through different specialities and spend only a limited period of time in any one department.

Standardised testing with the use of appropriate outcome measures, as advocated in Chapter 2, is essential to monitor any change in function and effectiveness of intervention.

Hereditary motor and sensory neuropathy (HMSN)

Introduction

This term is used to describe a group of conditions which give rise to progressive weakness and wasting of the distal muscles of the legs and of the hands (Harding 1993). Other names which may be used to describe HMSN include Charcot–Marie–Tooth disease, after the three neurologists who first described the condition, and peroneal muscular atrophy. Most people with HMSN have a dominantly inherited disorder associated with a duplication of chromosome 17 (Malcolm 1993).

There are many different types of HMSN, the most common forms being referred to as types I and II (Geurts et al 1992a). Type I is characterised by a demyelinating neuropathy causing slow nerve conduction, whereas type II is the result of axonal degeneration. The clinical signs and symptoms are similar in both type I and type II, the main difference being the age of onset. Type I usually produces symptoms earlier, most commonly between the ages of 5 and 15. In type II, although symptoms may develop in childhood they occur more commonly between the ages of 10 and 20 and often not until much later (Harding 1993).

The sensory symptoms are usually less severe than the motor and generally occur later in life (Medhat & Krantz 1988). However, impaired proprioception is seen in many older patients and may contribute to the balance problems associated with HMSN (Harding & Thomas 1980, Geurts et al 1992b). Postural and intention tremor may be associated with type I HMSN (Harding 1984).

Clinical signs and symptoms

Hereditary motor and sensory neuropathy, although showing great variability in the severity of symptoms, has a predictable course, affecting the feet and legs and much later the hands and forearms (Harding & Thomas 1980).

Lower limb muscle impairment and functional deficit. The lower limb weakness initially affects the intrinsic foot musculature and peroneus brevis, followed by tibialis anterior, peroneus longus and the long toe extensors, later progressing to affect the plantar flexors (Mann & Missirian 1988, Geurts et al 1992a). This creates an imbalance of activity at the foot and ankle that may result in deformed, unstable and often painful feet, which interferes with gait (Wetmore & Drennan 1989). Pes cavus, equinus and clawing of the toes are typical aspects of the foot deformity (Medhat & Krantz 1988). Contracture of the triceps surae is common (Mann &

Missirian 1988) and ankle sprains are frequently reported (Barcardi & Alm 1986).

The progressive atrophy and the resulting deformity and functional loss are described by Mann & Missirian (1988):

The weakness of the tibialis anterior permits the peroneus longus to function relatively unopposed, which accounts for most of the marked plantar flexion of the medial side of the foot. The lack of function of peroneus brevis permits the tibialis posterior to function without significant opposition, which results in the hind foot being brought into inversion (varus) and the forefoot into a certain degree of adduction. The deformity is further enhanced by the progressive contracture of the intrinsic muscles and plantar aponeurosis, which further brings the forefoot into an adducted and plantar-flexed position. The normal long toe flexors contribute to the adduction of the forefoot because their normal antagonists, i.e., the extensor digitorum longus and the extensor hallucis longus muscles, are weakened by the disease process.

Geurts et al (1992b) demonstrated a decreased postural control in patients with HMSN, even when there was full perceptual information. This was attributed to the lower limb paralysis and the ankle–foot deformities impairing postural sway. For those with no restriction of range of movement of the plantar flexors, a few degrees of forward body inclination was noted.

Difficulties with walking arising from the progressive muscle imbalance are typically those of a high-stepping gait to compensate for the lack of dorsiflexion (Geurts et al 1992a), weight-bearing over the lateral border of the foot (Bacardi & Alm 1986) and lateral instability of the ankle (Wukich et al 1989).

Upper limb problems associated with HMSN. The weakness of the hands is characterised by wasting of the intrinsic hand muscles, which may progress to the forearms (Harding 1984). Sensory impairment is variable but in severe cases the numbness of the hands may result in injury such as burns to the hands (Harding 1993).

The thenar and hypothenar muscles become progressively weaker and opposition of the thumb to the fingers is impaired. Functionally, these people adapt by using gross flexion for tasks requiring a pinch grip. This is illustrated by the manner in which they write (Fig. 11.4).

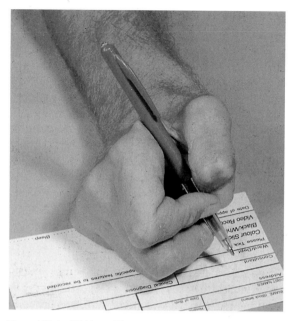

Figure 11.4 Writing without splint.

Overuse of the affected muscle groups seems to compound the weakness, many people giving personal accounts of how they have never recovered from a bout of strenuous exercise such as painting and decorating. Being so dependent on the hands for function, it is unrealistic to expect people not to use them.

Physiotherapy intervention

Assessment and appropriate intervention by a physiotherapist is of vital importance for patients with HMSN. One of the major problems is that the insidious onset of the disease is often missed by both the patient and the clinician (Geurts et al 1992b) and, unless there is a family history of the disease, patients may not present for treatment before symptoms become established.

Harding (1993) stresses the importance of suitable footwear and, particularly for those with sensory impairment, the need to examine both the feet and the inside of the shoes on a regular basis to reduce the risk of ulceration. Splints are advocated to control the foot in the plantigrade position to reduce ankle instability and to allow for a more economic gait pattern (Medhat & Krantz 1988, Geurts et al 1992a, Harding 1993).

There is little literature regarding specific physiotherapy intervention. However, with the relatively stereotyped picture which emerges as a result of the disease process, physiotherapy treatment and management can be instrumental in preventing or minimising the expected deformity. For example, the progressive contracture of the intrinsic foot musculature and the plantar fascia may be reduced by an early programme of massage and mobilisation of the feet to maintain flexibility within these structures. This intervention may also prove effective in maintaining range of movement within other muscles affected in the disease process.

The relatively unopposed action of the gastrocnemius has particular consequences which may be managed effectively with appropriate physiotherapy intervention. Shortening of gastrocnemius restricts dorsiflexion and may cause hyperextension of the knee in standing and walking, due to its action over the two joints – the ankle and the knee. The weight tends to be displaced backwards, due to the inability to transfer the weight over the full surface of the foot during stance phase of gait. Maintenance of the centre of gravity within the base of support can only be effected by flexion at the hips. Flexion at the hips produces an anterior tilt of the pelvis, creating an excessive lordosis if the individual is to maintain an upright posture.

Regular stretching of gastrocnemius and other affected muscle groups may go some way towards preventing the onset of contracture. However, stretching must be used with caution, particularly where there is substantial somatosensory impairment, with special attention paid to the correct alignment of bony structures.

The imbalance of muscle activity caused by the progressive weakness can be best managed by earlier rather than later use of insoles and AFOs. Insoles may prove effective in the redistribution of weight across the full surface of the foot (see Ch. 10).

The main advantage of the polypropylene AFO is that it is moulded to each individual's foot. It therefore supports the medial arch and the toes, in addition to maintaining the foot in a plantigrade position and preventing lateral instability. The disadvantage of this type of splint is that it does not permit talocrural mobility, particularly dorsiflexion which would redress the varus deviation (Geurts et al 1992a). The use of a hinged AFO may be of benefit to allow this movement into dorsiflexion, but the bulk of these splints often makes them aesthetically unacceptable. A below-knee caliper with heel socket and outside T-strap may be more effective, but these are more obtrusive. The choice of orthosis should be discussed between the patient, the physiotherapist and the orthotist. Whichever type of orthosis is provided, it is essential that the patient be given a structured programme of stance and gait training (Geurts et al 1992a). Monitoring the continued efficacy of the splint or insoles should be carried out on a regular basis and, where the patient is dependent on the splints for ambulation, an additional pair should be provided in case of breakage. The different types of orthoses are described in Chapter 10.

Documented treatment of the foot deformities usually relates to surgery, particularly that of tendon transfer (Medhat & Krantz 1988, Wetmore & Drennan 1989). This would still appear to be appropriate early intervention in redressing the muscular imbalance (Mann & Missirian 1988). Triple arthrodesis was commonly carried out in the past but is now considered to be a 'salvage' procedure limited to those with severe rigid deformity (Wetmore & Drennan 1989, Wukich et al 1989).

The use of a thumb opposition splint may serve to maintain more normal function of the hand by facilitating opposition of the fingers to the thumb without overuse of opponens pollicis. This splint is compact, easy to make and readily applied or removed as the situation demands. People with early signs of hand weakness should be encouraged to use this support to maintain normal hand function with opposition of the thumb to the fingers. Its use is illustrated in Figure 11.5 as a means of improving writing.

Patients with more severe weakness may demonstrate signs of diaphragmatic weakness. This is often characterised by the patient com-

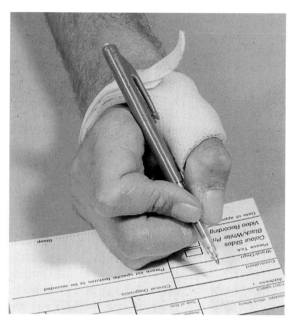

Figure 11.5 Writing with splint.

plaining of morning headaches, interrupted sleep and daytime somnolence. The physiotherapist should be aware of this complication and, if it appears to be a problem, check the patient's vital capacity in both sitting and supine positions. Sleep studies may be necessary to determine the extent of the problem, and ventilatory support may be required.

Summary

The fairly clear-cut and progressive nature of this disease makes its course relatively easy to predict, and thus appropriate interventions can be instigated.

One of the major problems facing this group of patients is the comparative rarity of the disease. Many therapists, particularly those working in neurology, may have heard of Charcot–Marie–Tooth disease or HMSN but see very few people with this condition. The literature is scarce regarding physiotherapy intervention. Provision of splints is often delayed until there is established deformity and, when provided, they are ill-fitting, causing additional problems of pressure and skin breakdown (CMT International,

HMSN Self-Help Group 1995, personal communication).

By identifying the potential problems, appropriate stretching to maintain range of movement, exercise to improve postural alignment and provision of suitable orthoses may markedly reduce the onset of structural deformity. Early and continuing management of these patients may substantially reduce the need for what is often painful, expensive and, in many cases, preventable surgical intervention. If surgery is deemed necessary, physiotherapy is essential postoperatively to ensure a good functional outcome.

DISCUSSION

The management of these patient groups raises several issues that relate to many with chronic or progressive disability:

- the timing, extent and duration of therapy
- surgical intervention
- the most effective use of finite resources.

The timing, extent and duration of physiotherapy intervention

This is of particular concern, especially for those with severe residual disability such as may arise following severe head injury. These patients may require physiotherapy over a period of many years in order to achieve and maintain the optimal level of function.

Early treatment and management is rarely disputed, but the duration of this intervention is increasingly questioned (Bax et al 1988, Condie 1991). Adults with cerebral palsy illustrate this point. These people may receive ongoing care throughout childhood and adolescence but, on leaving school, the therapy input is reduced, and this may lead to a deterioration in their condition with resultant loss of function.

The prevention of secondary complications, such as contracture, and maximising function is the main remit of the physiotherapist (Pope 1992). Treatment to this effect should be instigated in the immediate aftermath of injury or at the onset of disease. This may involve a period of intensive rehabilitation or merely advice to the patient regarding appropriate maintenance. The timing and duration of rehabilitation is of special concern.

For example, some patients such as those with cervical cord injuries may benefit from an interim period, to come to terms with their disability, prior to undertaking intensive rehabilitation. Their time in hospital may be affected by problems such as respiratory tract infections and autonomic dysfunction. This affects their ability to participate in an intensive rehabilitation programme and, in some cases, they may not realise their full potential prior to discharge from hospital. In the majority of cases, the level of function attained by discharge is that which is assumed to be optimum. Patients who have been managed in a spinal injuries unit will usually be 'followed up' on a regular basis to ensure there are no medical complications. However, it is rare for patients to be offered an additional period of rehabilitation even though their capability to benefit from this may have significantly improved.

The timing of physiotherapy intervention has been questioned in the management of stroke (Partridge 1994). Providing the patient is not at risk of deterioration, consideration should be given to delaying intensive rehabilitation following sudden onset of disability. Although it is crucial to ensure correct maintenance by instructing carers in appropriate methods of positioning, handling and exercise, patients must be assessed individually to determine the most appropriate timing for intensive rehabilitation.

Surgical intervention

With some conditions, surgical intervention may be necessary to restore range of movement in a contracted limb, stabilise a joint or transfer a tendon to improve function.

The risk of contracture is greatest for those with impaired cognition and hypertonus (Ough et al 1981) and increases with prolonged duration of coma (Yarkony & Sahgal 1987). Contractures are best treated by prevention (Cherry 1980, Frank et al 1984), and joint management should

be based on the assumption that the patient will make a good neurological recovery (Yarkony & Sahgal 1987).

It is important to distinguish between neural and non-neural components that contribute to changes in muscle and joint contracture (Ough et al 1981, Garland & Keenan 1983). Treatment using temporary paralysing agents such as phenol or botulinum toxin may be effective in determining the extent of contracture as opposed to the effects of hypertonus. These agents may also be of value in determining the effects of surgical intervention. For example, children with spastic diplegia characteristically demonstrate predominant flexion of the lower limbs. Plantar flexion at the ankle provides an extensor component which may be essential to keep them upright against gravity. Surgery to elongate the Achilles tendon may permanently take away this extensor component, and further flexion may ensue, which can lead to progressive crouch gait (Sutherland & Cooper 1978).

Extensive procedures have been described for the management of residual limb deformities following head injury (Ough et al 1981, Garland & Keenan 1983). Surgical intervention should be considered on a holistic basis and not purely in respect of elongating a contracted muscle or decreasing muscular activity. The functional implications of surgery, particularly of muscles acting over more than one joint, must be considered. It is important to remember that surgical procedures are a means to an end and not the end in itself. Postoperative management is mandatory if a successful outcome is to be achieved and must continue until such time as is necessary to prevent reversal (Pope et al 1991).

Heterotopic ossification is a recognised complication in patients following spinal cord injury (Silver 1969, Daud et al 1993) or head injury (Garland & Keenan 1983, Yarkony & Sahgal 1987, Davies 1994). It occurs predominantly around proximal joints. Surgical excision of heterotopic bone has had variable results (Garland & Keenan 1983) and conservative management is recommended (Andrews & Greenwood 1993). The incidence of recurrence following surgery is high, particularly in patients with hypertonus.

Perioperative radiotherapy may be useful in inhibiting the recurrence of heterotopic ossification following surgical excision (International Working Party 1996). Surgical excision should not be performed until at least 1½ years after injury, when calcification is no longer an active process. A bone scan should demonstrate a decrease in activity (Garland & Keenan 1983).

The surgical management, such as tendon transfer and joint stabilisation, for patients with progressive neuromuscular disorders has been discussed in relation to patients with HMSN. Similar principles apply for others with muscle imbalance. In all instances, if surgery is deemed necessary, physiotherapy is essential post-operatively to ensure a good functional outcome (Pope 1992).

The most effective use of finite resources

Resources for health care provision are finite and it is therefore essential that further research is undertaken in the field of chronic neurological disability to ensure that there is appropriate use of these resources. There is an approximate ratio of 1 chartered physiotherapist to 86 severely disabled people in the United Kingdom (Condie 1991) and clearly, no matter how well man-power resources are deployed, there will be a continuing problem.

Prevention of secondary complications is of primary concern and physiotherapy may be required for an indefinite period of time to ensure optimal function. Ongoing assessment for people with progressive neurological disorders is essential to contend with any deterioration in their physical status. However, those with non-progressive impairment, such as patients with cerebral palsy or following stroke, brain damage or spinal cord injury, may also deteriorate over time. Abnormal tone may lead to progressive disability due to the impoverishment of movement. People who are restricted to a limited array of postures and movements are as vulnerable to the development of secondary complications as are those with progressive disorders.

Therapists must produce evidence that on-going treatment for the more severely disabled may significantly improve their level of function, with a consequent reduction in resources being required in the longer term. Given that these resources are limited, the timing of intervention as discussed above is of primary concern. This is an issue of great importance and demands the urgent attention of physiotherapy researchers, as recommended in Chapter 12.

REFERENCES

Ada L, Canning C, Paratz J 1990 Care of the unconscious head-injured patient. In: Ada L, Canning C (eds) Key issues in neurological physiotherapy: physiotherapy foundations for practice. Butterworth-Heinemann, Oxford

Andrews K 1999 The vegetative state – clinical diagnosis. Postgraduate Medical Journal 75: 321–324

Andrews K, Greenwood R 1993 Physical consequences of neurological disablement. In: Greenwood R, Barnes M P, McMillan T M, Ward C D (eds) Neurological rehabilitation. Churchill Livingstone, London

Andrews K, Murphy L, Munday R, Littlewood C 1996 Misdiagnosis of the vegetative state: retrospective study in a rehabilitation unit. British Medical Journal 313: 13–16

Ashburn A, DeSouza L H 1988 An approach to the management of multiple sclerosis. Physiotherapy Practice 4: 139–145

Bacardi B E, Alm W A 1986 Modification of the Gould operation for cavovarus reconstruction of the foot. Journal of Foot Surgery 25: 181–187

Bach-y-Rita P 1990 Brain plasticity as a basis for recovery of function in humans. Neuropsychologia 28: 547–554

Barnes M 1993 Multiple sclerosis. In: Greenwood R, Barnes M P, McMillan T M, Ward C D (eds) Neurological rehabilitation. Churchill Livingstone, London

Bax M C O, Smyth D P, Thomas A P 1988 Health care of physically handicapped young adults. British Medical Journal 296: 1153–1155

Beardshaw V 1988 Last on the list: community services for people with physical disabilities. King's Fund Centre, London

Bleck E E 1987 Orthopaedic management in cerebral palsy. Blackwell Scientific Publications, Oxford

Bobath K 1974 The motor deficit in patients with cerebral palsy. Clinics in Developmental Medicine. No. 23. Spastics International Medical Publications, William Heinemann Medical Books, London

Brown P 1994 Pathophysiology of spasticity. Journal of Neurology, Neurosurgery and Psychiatry 57: 773–777

Cherry D B 1980 Review of physical therapy alternatives for reducing muscle contracture. Physical Therapy 60: 877–881

Childs N L, Mercer W N, Childs H W 1993 Accuracy of diagnosis of persistent vegetative state. Neurology 43: 1465–1467

Condie E 1991 A therapeutic approach to physical disability. Physiotherapy 77: 72–77

Daud O, Sett P, Burr R G, Silver J R 1993 The relationship of heterotopic ossification to passive movement in paraplegic patients. Disability and Rehabilitation 15: 114–118

Davies P M 1994 Starting again. Springer-Verlag, London

DeSouza L 1990 Multiple sclerosis: approaches to management. Chapman and Hall, London

Finger S, Almli C R 1985 Brain damage and neuroplasticity: mechanisms of recovery or development? Brain Research Reviews 10: 177–186

Frank C, Akeson W H, Woo S L-Y, Amiel D, Coutts R D 1984 Physiology and therapeutic value of passive joint motion. Clinical Orthopaedics and Related Research 185: 113–125

Freeman E A 1992 The persistent vegetative state: a 'fate worse than death'. Clinical Rehabilitation 6: 159–165

Freeman J A, Langdon D W, Hobart J C, Thompson A J 1997 The impact of inpatient rehabilitation on progressive multiple sclerosis. Annals of Neurology 43: 236–244

Freeman J A, Langdon D W, Hobart J C, Thompson A J 1999 Inpatient rehabilitation in multiple sclerosis. Do the benefits carry over into the community? Neurology 52: 50–56

Garland D E, Keenan M-A E 1983 Orthopaedic strategies in the management of the adult head-injured patient. Physical Therapy 63: 2004–2009

Geurts A C H, Mulder T W, Nienhuis B, Rijken R A J 1992a Influence of orthopaedic footwear on postural control in patients with hereditary motor and sensory neuropathy. Journal of Rehabilitation Sciences 5: 3–9

Geurts A C H, Mulder T W, Nienhuis B, Mars P, Rijken R A J 1992b Postural organisation in patients with hereditary motor and sensory neuropathy. Archives of Physical Medicine and Rehabilitation 73: 569–572

Hannan C, Korien J, Panigraphy A, Dikkes P, Goode R 1994 Neuropathic findings in the brain of Karen Ann Quinlan – the role of the thalamus in the persistent vegetative state. New England Journal of Medicine 330: 1469–1475

Harding A E 1984 The hereditary ataxias and related disorders. Churchill Livingstone, London

Harding A E 1993 Hereditary motor and sensory neuropathies (HMSN). Fact Sheet HE1. Muscular Dystrophy Group of Great Britain and Northern Ireland, London

Harding A E, Thomas P K 1980 The clinical features of hereditary and motor sensory neuropathy types I and II. Brain 103: 259–280

Howard R S, Wiles C M, Hirsch N P, Loh L, Spencer G T, Newsom-Davis J 1992 Respiratory involvement in multiple sclerosis. Brain 115: 479–494

International Working Party 1996 Report on the Vegetative State. The Royal Hospital for Neuro-disability, London

Jennett B 1992 Letting vegetative patients die. British Medical Journal 305: 1305–1306

Jennett B, Plum J 1972 Persistent vegetative state after brain damage – a syndrome in search of a name. Lancet i: 734–737

Klein F C 1982 The silent epidemic. Wall Street Journal 24 November

Krupp L B, Alvarez L A, La Rocca N G, Scheinberg L C 1988 Fatigue in multiple sclerosis. Archives of Neurology 45: 435–437

Malcolm S 1993 CMT: clearing up a mystery. Muscular Dystrophy Group of Great Britain and Northern Ireland, London

Mann R A, Missirian J 1988 Pathophysiology of Charcot–Marie–Tooth disease. Clinical Orthopaedics and Related Research 234: 221–228

Medhat M A, Krantz H 1988 Neuropathic ankle joint in Charcot–Marie–Tooth disease after triple arthrodesis of the foot. Orthopaedic Review XVII(9): 873–880

Mertin J 1994 Rehabilitation in multiple sclerosis. Annals of Neurology 35(S): 130–133

Mertin J, Paeth B 1994 Physiotherapy and multiple sclerosis: application of the Bobath concept. MS Management 1(1): 10–13

Miller D H, Hornabrook R W, Purdie G 1992 The natural history of multiple sclerosis: a regional study with some longitudinal data. Journal of Neurology, Neurosurgery and Psychiatry 55: 341–346

Minden S L, Schiffer R B 1990 Affective disorders in multiple sclerosis. Review and recommendations for clinical research. Archives of Neurology 47: 98–104

Morgan M H, Langton Hewer R, Cooper R 1975 Application of an objective method of assessing intention tremor: a further study on the use of weights to reduce intention tremor. Journal of Neurology, Neurosurgery and Psychiatry 38: 259–264

Ough J L, Garland D E, Jordan C, Waters R L 1981 Treatment of spastic joint contractures in mentally disabled adults. Orthopedic Clinics of North America 12: 143–151

Partridge C J 1994 Evaluation of physiotherapy for people with stroke. King's Fund Centre, London

Pope P M 1988 A model for evaluation of input in relation to outcome in severely brain damaged patients. Physiotherapy 74: 647–650

Pope P M 1992 Management of the physical condition in patients with chronic and severe neurological pathologies. Physiotherapy 78: 896–903

Pope P M 1997 Management of the physical condition in people with chronic and severe neurological disabilities living in the community. Physiotherapy 83: 116–122

Pope P M, Bowes C E, Tudor M, Andrews B 1991 Surgery combined with continued post-operative stretching and management of knee flexion contractures in cases of MS. A report of six cases. Clinical Rehabilitation 5: 15–23

Poser C M 1980 Exacerbations, activity and progression in multiple sclerosis. Archives of Neurology 37: 471–474

Silver J R 1969 Heterotopic ossification: a clinical study of its possible relationship to trauma. Paraplegia 7: 220–230

Solari A, Filippini G, Gasco P et al 1999 Physical rehabilitation has a positive effect on disability in multiple sclerosis patients. Neurology 52: 57–63

Sutherland D H, Cooper L 1978 The pathomechanics of progressive crouch gait in spastic diplegia. Orthopedic Clinics of North America 9: 143–154

Thompson A J, McDonald W I 1992 Multiple sclerosis and its pathophysiology. In: Asbury A K, McKhann G M, McDonald W I (eds) Diseases of the nervous system, clinical neurobiology, 2nd edn. W B Saunders, Philadelphia, vol 2: 1209–1228

Thompson A J, Kermode A G, Wicks D et al 1991 Major differences in the dynamics of primary and secondary progressive multiple sclerosis. Annals of Neurology 29: 53–62

Tribe D, Korgaonkar G 1992 Withdrawing medical treatment: implications of the Bland case. British Journal of Hospital Medicine 48: 754–756

Vogenthaler D R 1987 An overview of head injury – its consequences and rehabilitation. Brain Injury 1: 113–127

Weinshenker B G 1994 Natural history of multiple sclerosis. Annals of Neurology 36: S6–S11

Wetmore R S, Drennan J C 1989 Long-term results of triple arthrodesis in Charcot–Marie–Tooth disease. Journal of Bone and Joint Surgery 71-A(3): 417–422

Wukich D K, Usar M C, Bowen J R 1989 A long-term study of triple arthrodesis for correction of pes cavovarus in Charcot–Marie–Tooth disease. Journal of Paediatric Orthopaedics 9: 433–437

Yarkony G M, Sahgal V 1987 Contractures: a major complication of craniocerebral trauma. Clinical Orthopaedics and Related Research 219: 93–96

12

The way forward

Cecily Partridge

INTRODUCTION

This book provides physiotherapists with an in-depth understanding of many of the problems encountered by patients with neurological conditions and demonstrates ways of solving them. The emphasis is on the analysis of abnormal pathology and determining appropriate treatment interventions. Problem solving is the key to this approach not only on the part of the therapist but also by encouraging the patient's own problem-solving abilities. Treatment of neurological disorders takes place within the wider context of the delivery of health services and, here too, there are many problems to be solved to ensure patients are able to have access to optimal care. What I propose to do is to look at some of these broader issues that currently impinge on the provision of treatment for neurological patients.

There will be a number of major influences on the delivery of health services in the next decade that are common to most countries in the Western world, and probably elsewhere. They include the overall increase in the demand for health services, exacerbated by the increasing proportion of elderly people in the population, the recent availability of expensive super drugs and the overall scarcity of financial resources to meet these demands. The current emphasis on evidence-based practice and the overall scarcity of research in physiotherapy are also key issues, as are the patterns of delivery of services and information about the actual content of treatment.

FINANCIAL RESOURCES FOR HEALTH

Because of recent advances in medicine over the last 50 years or so, many more conditions can now be successfully treated and, for others, symptoms can be relieved or life prolonged by the use of medication, which is sometimes extremely expensive. Increasing longevity brings an added burden, as the elderly consume a disproportionate amount of health services. As there will never be unlimited resources, some form of rationing will always be necessary, although health agencies are often reluctant to use the term. The percentage of the gross domestic product (GDP) spent on health differs between countries; in the Western world, for example, Britain is one of the lowest at under 6%, Denmark 8%, Australia 8.4%, France 9.6%, Germany 14%, with the USA as the highest at 16%, but even those countries with high percentages still report problems in deciding on priorities and meeting demands.

Difficult choices must be made between funding treatment for (a) different groups of people, such as children, the active work force and the elderly; (b) different conditions, such as mental health, cancer or cardiac conditions; (c) prevention and medication which will relieve symptoms but not cure; and (d) treatments for which there is little evidence of efficacy but a high demand, such as the use of hyperbaric oxygen for patients with multiple sclerosis. There is also, in some countries such as the UK, an ideological problem over state versus private funding for health services, which is a further complication.

Where services are provided is also an issue. There has been a move to more provision of services in the community, but there is some controversy about where provision is most economic; in general, it is seen to be more expensive in hospitals. However, moving services into the community can mean that instead of receiving treatment from an experienced neurological therapist in the clinic or hospital, patients may be seen by therapists who do not have comparable skills.

National health services and health insurance agencies have to make major decisions about priorities and then use different ways of allocating limited resources. These include selection by choosing to restrict funding to specific services, or limiting the number and type of treatments that will be funded for specified conditions. Neurological physiotherapy is vulnerable to both of these models: if in competition with, say pathology or surgery, or with funding for cardiac services, it does not have the same immediate life-saving image and is likely to lose out. Limiting the number of treatments for patients with long-term conditions such as Parkinson's disease, multiple sclerosis or head injury, who are likely to require treatment over a prolonged period, presents a problem. The therapy sessions themselves are usually on a one-to-one basis with fairly lengthy treatment sessions, and are therefore relatively expensive.

Health care agencies are used to funding treatment at the level of diagnostic categories, where the pathology and the likely outcomes of treatment are well recognised. Because the focus of physiotherapy for neurological conditions is on treating and managing the *consequences* of disease, rather than the pathology itself, the results of treatment are likely to be more individual, less clear cut and less familiar to administrative managers. This again mitigates against easy allocation of resources.

All this places a new urgency on physiotherapists to demonstrate exactly what their treatments can achieve with different patient groups, to clarify the implications of treatment given in different settings and to justify the need for specialist staff. It will also mean admitting what cannot be achieved. If it can be demonstrated that patients actually deteriorate without treatment, this too will strengthen the case for physiotherapy. Services which can demonstrate their effectiveness are clearly likely to get priority and be funded. If it can be clearly demonstrated that physiotherapy has a real-life value for these patients, the case could be made that, as lifelong treatment for something like diabetes is widely accepted, lifelong treatment for some neurological conditions can be justified if it saves money by keeping patients more able and independent and increasing their overall quality of life.

TREATMENT

Although textbooks contain detailed explanations of different methods of physiotherapy treatment, little clear information is available about what physiotherapists actually do in practice, even when working within the framework of a particular named approach. Because neurological patients are treated on the basis of the results of an individual assessment and progression based on the response to that intervention, the scope for variability is considerable. Some therapists may be 'disciples' of a given approach and follow texts fairly rigorously, yet there is little evidence to date that even when working within a named approach similar treatments are given (Partridge & De Weerdt 1995). Other therapists may take a more eclectic approach, using all their clinical skills, often gleaned from a number of different sources. The diversity here is likely to be even greater.

A complicating factor here is the lack of an agreed language for describing patient symptoms or physiotherapy interventions. Harms Ringdahl (1998) stresses the importance of describing practice in sufficient detail. She discusses the current problems by highlighting the frequent use of terms such as *conventional* and *standard* in relation to physiotherapy, whereas no one would think of describing any treatment as 'standard *psychology*', or conventional '*physician treatment*'. This highlights the lack of appropriate and agreed terminology.

A situation, somewhat similar to that of physiotherapy, occurred in the field of rehabilitation in the late 1970s when it was realised that there was considerable semantic confusion in describing the consequences of disease. The language for disease pathology for acute conditions was well established but was not appropriate for describing longer-term conditions where cure was unlikely. This resulted in the World Health Organisation (WHO) developing the International Classification of Impairments, Disabilities and Handicaps (ICIDH 1980). This was updated after wide consultation with both professionals and patients and published as the Classification of Functioning and Disability (ICIDH 1999). The definition of *impairment* remains similar and is at the level of systems and structures, but both the terms and the underlying concepts for *disability* and *handicap* have changed. Disability is altered to restrictions of *activity*, and handicap to restrictions of *participation* in everyday life. Both these underlying concepts and the terms used are more patient friendly and more appropriate for neurological therapists, who usually operate at the level of activity and the facilitation of participation in everyday life. Work similar to this needs to be undertaken in physiotherapy. As a profession, we have started to recognise this problem but, as Stephenson et al (1998) found on discussing associated reactions, it can arouse strong feelings and great controversy. Consultation to arrive at a consensus is clearly necessary but does present a formidable challenge.

There are many anomalies in describing treatment and management by neurological physiotherapists. First, there is considerable heterogeneity in the conditions treated themselves. They may be single incidents such as stroke, spinal cord or head injury where there is damage to the nervous system which does not of itself progress, but where there may be secondary changes resulting from dysfunction and inactivity. Some natural resolution is expected to occur in the early stages. The manifestation of similar conditions may vary widely between patients, and in the same patient over time, as will their individual response to their condition. Because of this diversity, the same treatment for the same condition cannot be prescribed. For those with progressive conditions, the aims of treatment may be more to do with maintaining levels of activity, or slowing the progressive loss of activity despite increasing neurological deterioration. This is an area which may make a big difference to the patient concerned but clearly, successful outcomes are much more difficult to demonstrate.

The first challenge is to tackle the problem of describing what physiotherapists do in their work with patients. Because of the great diversity it may be necessary to classify types of treatment in terms of their similarity. In a recent trial of physiotherapy for patients with stroke, Partridge et al (in preparation) used *aims* of treatment to describe the type of treatment given to patients. It was found that therapists working within the Bobath approach used similar methods of treatment under a given aim. Aims were much fewer in number than the potential number of treatments.

In the Bobath approach to treatment, quality of normal movement is a key aim of many of the techniques used. It is an elusive phenomenon which is difficult to describe and quantify. Quality usually refers to the extent to which movement follows normal patterns. These patterns are familiar to those following the Bobath (1990) approach but they are less clear to others. Even within the Bobath approach, therapists may not be using the terms in the same way, as there is no agreed written language. Terms such as specific inhibitory mobilisation of muscle (SIMS) are frequently used to describe a treatment technique, yet there appears to be no reference to the term in the literature. This situation presents two major problems: first, without clear definitions of terms used it is difficult to explain what treatment was given; and, secondly, it is almost impossible at present to measure or monitor 'quality' of movement in any reliable or objective way. We need to demonstrate clearly the value, and indeed the possibility, of more normal movement in someone with a damaged nervous system.

Another major question which remains to be answered is how long do treatment effects last, and what is the extent of transfer to everyday life? Remarkable changes can be achieved by physiotherapists with specialised neurological skills in demonstration sessions and in practice in the clinic, but the extent to which these gains are maintained and transferred to activity in daily life is not known.

How does the patient who can walk with an even balanced gait under supervision in the treatment gym, walk when he is about his daily business in everyday life? Getting to the shops or office may take priority over maintaining a more normal gait; speed and function are surely of the essence here. In the problem-solving approach adopted in this book, the authors clearly accept that not all patients will achieve completely

normal movement and feel that compensatory strategies may need to be adopted and sometimes actively encouraged. It requires great clinical skill and judgement to know when a patient's optimal level of normal movement has been reached and that compensation is now the best strategy: too soon, and true gains may be missed and the patient left with movements which will encourage future secondary complications; too late, and the patient may lose motivation to continue striving, as their efforts appear to produce no practical benefits. It is common practice for some therapists not to allow patients to stand or walk until they have achieved a level of 'normality' in the walking, but is there evidence to support this and what about the psychological effect of being held back? All these questions need to be addressed without delay.

EVIDENCE-BASED PRACTICE

The importance of evidence-based practice (EBP) is presented as somewhat novel at the beginning of the 21st century, yet the desire to know what effect treatments have, and the search for evidence of success of treatment have a long history, going back as far as 300 BC (Lloyd 1996). The recent emphasis is perhaps more related to the vast range of treatments that have been developed over the last decade and the limited finance available to purchase them from health insurance or national health services. There is also the increased expectations of the general population about provision of health services. Evidence-based practice will certainly influence provision of physiotherapy services in the future.

Much more has been written about evidence-based medicine (EBM) than about evidence-based physiotherapy, although its important relationship to physiotherapy has recently been highlighted by Bithell (2000). The medical literature provides a good starting point as there are many similarities, though some clear differences. One definition widely quoted by major British proponents of EBM is 'integrating individual clinical experience with the best available external evidence from systematic research' (Sackett et al 1996). Others consider objective evidence to

---

Box 12.1 Other 'hierarchies' of evidence (Source: Centre for Reviews and Dissemination, University of York)

Clinical trials
I Well-designed randomised controlled trials
II-1a Well-designed controlled trial with pseudo-randomisation
II-1b Well-designed controlled trial with no randomisation

Cohort studies
II-2a Well-designed cohort (prospective) study with concurrent controls
II-2b Well-designed cohort (prospective) study with historical controls
II-2c Well-designed cohort (retrospective) study with concurrent controls
II-3 Well-designed case-control (retrospective) study
III Large differences from comparisons between times and/or places with and without intervention (in some circumstances these may be equivalent to level II-1)
IV Opinions of respected authorities based on clinical experience: descriptive studies and

---

be the only real evidence and this is shown in the various hierarchies that have been developed. In medicine the gold standard, the double-blind randomised controlled clinical trial, is seen as the pinnacle of excellence (Box 12.1). In this schema, the least valued is clinical opinion and the new 'authority' is seen as the empirical evidence. Individual clinical experience of the treating clinician is not even mentioned.

The same is also true for the hierarchy devised by Hadorn (1996), given below, where the categories are somewhat similar and clinical opinion is rated the lowest. Supportive evidence from well conducted:

1. randomised controlled trials that include 100 patients or more
2. randomised controlled trials with less than 100 patients
3. cohort studies
4. case-control study
5. supportive evidence from poorly controlled or uncontrolled studies
6. conflicting evidence, with the weight of evidence supporting the recommendation
7. expert opinion.

However, clinical opinion is the basis of practice in both medicine and physiotherapy. It seems rather like throwing the baby out with the bath water to disregard the importance of clinical experience. It should probably not even be included in these empirical lists as it is, of its nature, in a different category, and indeed may vary between experts. One problem is the importance of well-conducted and well-designed studies, as it is not always easy for a clinician to decide on the rigorousness of the methods used. It does raise the important fact that no one method per se is sound unless well designed and carried out.

There tend to be two extremes of thinking in the field of EBM:

1. Where the proponents feel that experiential knowledge lacks legitimacy for guiding medical decision making (Hadorn 1996). From this point of view, the value of expert opinion lasts only until such time as the data to make EBP becomes available. Relying on expert opinion is regarded as an 'unfortunate' feature of modern medical practice.
2. For others, the whole topic is perceived differently. Grimley Evans (1995), a geriatrician, suggests a major fear for unconvinced clinicians is that the development of mandatory guidelines will be for the treatment of *diseases* rather than for the treatment of *patients*. Tonelli (1990) regards 'reliance on expert opinion' not as an unfortunate consequence of an underdeveloped evidence base in medicine but a necessary requirement for optimal practice of clinical medicine'. Bithell (2000) also supports the importance of experiential evidence in physiotherapy.

Though the hierarchies of evidence provided in the medical literature are not directly applicable to physiotherapy, evidence does come into different categories, and is at different levels. The well-conducted randomised controlled trial (RCT) does contain elements which will control for bias and produce reliable results if rigorously conducted. In interpreting the results, however, it is important to recognise that these studies usually seek to recruit homogenous groups of subjects, which means that the results need not necessarily be directly applicable to an individual patient who may have a number of additional complications.

Randomisation is a process which seeks to smooth out the effect of individual differences by ensuring they are equally distributed between the treatment groups, but it is often those very individual differences which will be of importance to the treating clinician. Questions that need to be asked about an RCT should include: Are the patients in this study similar to my patient in terms of age, stage of disease, and other complicating factors? Do I know what treatment the patients in the study received? Are the outcome measures used valid for the purpose and reliably administered, and are they related to the aims of treatment? It is essential that evidence be considered at the appropriate level and in an appropriate way with different criteria being used to examine quantitative and qualitative research. Elimination of bias is essential in clinical trials, yet when we want to know what patients' views are about their treatment or condition, it is that very 'bias', their personal viewpoint, that is of interest.

Many papers are published, even in learned journals, that are seriously flawed, and therapists must be prepared to challenge them when necessary. One such example was published in the *British Medical Journal* by Brocklehurst et al (1978) entitled 'How much physiotherapy for patients with stroke?'. It was described as a comparative study of physiotherapy, occupational therapy and speech therapy. Although it looked like a trial and had a statistician listed as an author, on reading the paper it was clear that the authors had described practice in their own hospital rather than conducting a trial; there was no random allocation of patients. The authors showed a correlation between depression and the amount of occupational therapy, and between shoulder pain and physiotherapy. In their discussion they made the assumption that depression was caused by occupational therapy and shoulder pain by physiotherapy. Equally valid alternative explanations for these results include the fact that depressed patients may have

been referred for occupational therapy, and those with shoulder pain for physiotherapy; hence, the link. It is also impossible to compare physiotherapy, occupational therapy and speech therapy as they have such very different aims and deal with different aspects of the stroke patient's problems.

It is important for physiotherapists not to feel constrained by the comparison between the evidence base for medicine and that for physiotherapy. Physiotherapy is not doing too badly at this stage of its professional development. Despite at least 100 years of scientific medicine, at present only around 20% of medical practice is said to be evidence based (USA Office of Technology 1995). Medicine's claim to scientific status is also still tenuous (Munson 1981). It is extremely important not to be misled by the popularity of current buzz words but to ask common-sense questions.

Evidence for the effectiveness of different forms of physiotherapy treatment is essential for a number of reasons. Clinicians need the information to enable them to provide optimal treatment. It is also important for patients to be able to make informed decisions and to do this they need to be given information when entering a treatment programme to enable them to assess the costs and likely benefits for themselves. This is of course a continuing process, as new information will constantly be arriving.

Administrators and managers are interested in making the best use of resources, although what is considered 'best' will vary from different perspectives. Patients treated by physiotherapists are categorised by their diagnoses but the results of physiotherapy are likely to be at the level of influencing the consequences of the disease at the levels of activity restriction and participation (ICIDH 1999). In acute medicine, diseases can be 'cured' and an absence of symptoms demonstrated. In physiotherapy, changes achieved tend to be more ordinal in nature: for example, patients may achieve more activity, or feel less pain, which are more difficult to demonstrate clearly.

It is a great challenge for therapists to start this new century with a fresh outlook: not disregarding the value of clinical experience and the views of authority figures, but critically assessing them; not being afraid to challenge established practice, but using all evidence as it becomes available to make decisions about the treatment needed for each individual patient. This will inevitably be a continually changing process, taking on board new evidence and new insights as they become available.

RESEARCH

It is well recognised that overall there is a scarcity of research in physiotherapy. This is well demonstrated in a meta-analysis of treatment for stroke. Langhorne et al (1996) could only find *seven* trials which met their criteria for producing reliable results. Also in many databases such as MEDLINE, physiotherapy references are relatively sparse in contrast to medicine references on the same subject.

The scarcity of research in neurological physiotherapy is not altogether surprising. This is a relatively young profession and the speciality of neurological physiotherapy is even younger, as is described in the first chapter of this book. As newcomers to research, we suffer from a lack of appropriate methodologies to use in investigations and so have borrowed from disciplines such as neurophysiology, biomechanics and the social sciences. In the 1940s authors cited earlier work as a physiological basis for the phenomena they observed. For example, Brunström (1970) relied on the laboratory work of Riddock & Buzzard (1921) on reflex movements and postural reactions, and Magnus (1926) on tonic neck reflexes. Bobath (1970, 1990) cites Sherrington (1931) on reflex inhibition and Magoun & Rhines (1948) on spasticity. Later work by Carr & Shepherd (1998) cites Rosner (1970) on redundancy theory and Luria (1963) on behavioural strategy change. Affolter (1980) cites Piaget (1936) and Chomsky (1969).

While providing possible explanations for the phenomena observed, these do not in general provide hard evidence to explain the mechanisms involved in patients or the effects of treatment: rather, they pose questions which need

to be answered, and provide hypotheses to be tested. Citing work that seems to explain mechanisms was an important stage in our development, but we now need to test theories and hypotheses in direct relation to physiotherapy in the clinical situation. Until we do, the link remains unproven.

More recent laboratory work has been helped by the advances in technology such as positron emission tomography (PET) and functional magnetic resonance imaging (fMRI). These techniques have great possibilities in terms of increasing our understanding of movement and recovery. There is, however, still a quantum leap between the results of laboratory investigations and clinical practice and it is important not to try to extrapolate these results directly to practice. They provide useful insights into cerebral mechanisms and help to formulate hypotheses to be tested in further work. Other forms of laboratory work include research on normal subjects such as reliability and validity of active knee measurement in healthy subjects, by Brosseau et al (1997), and Haas & Whitmarsh (1998) on the reliability of the balance performance monitor. Again, these provide useful information but may not be applicable for patient populations.

The key issue in sound research is asking the right questions that are answerable within the time and resources available and where the answers will be applicable to practice. There are a number of hurdles for all researchers; they must fit their proposals to the interests of those with finance available, and try to relate to topics of current interest. Physiotherapy is rarely a top priority among major funding agencies and its profile needs to be raised.

Many important questions remain to be answered in neurological physiotherapy at a clinical level. We cling to our different treatment approaches yet, to date, we have been unable to demonstrate, in studies comparing different treatments, that there is a clear advantage of any one method over the others (Logigian et al 1983, Partridge & De Weerdt 1995). Is this because of lack of information about the content of treatment and therefore the possibility of a lack of mutual exclusiveness between the treatment received by patients in the two groups? Is the problem the use of inappropriate or insensitive outcome measures that do not relate directly to the aims of treatment, or is it that the use of named 'approaches' is not the critical factor in success? Clinical skills will vary but this is rarely taken into account in clinical trials and we do not yet know, except intuitively and at an anecdotal level, that skilled therapists achieve better results. These are really crucial questions for the future of neurological physiotherapy.

Another factor that makes clinical evaluations more difficult is that because physiotherapy is now a routine part of practice, treatment/no treatment group comparisons are considered unethical. Therefore, all patients in any trial will receive their usual treatment with the experimental treatment given in addition to the experimental group. This diminishes the likelihood of obtaining clear differences between the treatment groups, if they exist. To obtain sufficient numbers in a trial, patients with considerable heterogeneity are often included, which again mitigates against obtaining clear answers. Selecting more homogeneous groups may be one answer. In a recent randomised trial, Kwakkel (1999) selected a more homogeneous group of patients with primary middle cerebral artery stroke. Extra treatment was targeted at either the arm or leg and some significant differences were reported in variables monitored between those in the control and the augmented groups. However, to achieve the total of around 100 patients, patients were recruited from *seven* hospitals over a 3-year period. Multi-centre trials represent a great deal of organisation and are very expensive. There is also a problem that extrapolation of results from a homogeneous population to a general population is not always justified.

Clearly this is an area where much more work needs to be done. The challenges are to develop appropriate methodologies for evaluating physiotherapy, and to try to raise the profile of physiotherapy research among potential funding bodies. This is a task for both physiotherapy clinicians and researchers, and also for physiotherapy managers.

CLINICIANS AND RESEARCHERS

There is a gap between clinicians and researchers which both need to address urgently. Clinicians certainly need to acquire the skills to be able to read the literature more critically, and to be able to decide which research results are relevant to their patients. Therapist researchers also have an obligation to write more clinician-friendly articles and to moderate their language to make it more accessible, easy to read and understandable. Learned journals have certain conventions and styles to which the aspiring researcher must conform to have a chance of publication, but other options are available. One way where there may be a meeting point is through case reports. These are often written by clinicians; they are usually highly readable and they are starting to build up a knowledge base for future investigation in a more rigorous way. Clinicians should urge their researcher colleagues to ask and investigate questions that are applicable in practice. They need to enter into dialogue with researchers and be confident enough to challenge them to clearly demonstrate the value of their research.

The idea of EBP and research is clearly a new emphasis for many physiotherapists. First, it involves a major shift in thinking. Clinical practice tends to be based on educational texts which are not always well referenced, and the advice of 'authority figures'. Clinicians, at least in the UK, update their clinical practice by attending courses, rather than by reading the literature on recent research, which presents a challenge for those providing education for undergraduate and postgraduate students as well as for practising clinicians.

Kuhn (1970) in his book on the philosophy of science discusses the growth and development of professions. Well-developed scientific disciplines such as chemistry and biology are seen as paradigmatic, where research follows a distinct agreed paradigm and there is consensus on the models used, and a common language. Getting to the stage of being a scientific discipline is a lengthy process, often taking many centuries. Physiotherapy is clearly a long way from this stage but shares common characteristics with professions said to be in the pre-paradigmatic period. This is characterised by 'frequent and deep debates over legitimate methods and solutions to problems ... though these serve rather to define schools rather than to produce agreement.' This seems to describe the current position in physiotherapy rather accurately.

Those who have followed the early innovators in neurological physiotherapy have advanced the early ideas but have often tended to be over influenced by the originators in a way that is commonly found in the history of science. It has been shown that disciples who follow originators demonstrate more rigid adherence to principles (Kuhn 1970). This can cause stagnation in that followers are clearly reluctant to lose anything of the original ideas and yet, while alive, most originators continue to refine and develop their methods and ideas. A constant process of change and development is necessary, both because we are refining the art of physiotherapy but also because new evidence and experience will constantly become available. Strict adherence to any clinical method without evidence to support it means that treatment can become stuck in a time warp. What is needed is for those who follow in the footsteps of others to use their own skills to build on the earlier work and take their ideas forward. These ideas need to be written down and updated as practice advances. It is said that we always stand on the shoulders of others to make our achievements, and this should be acknowledged. However, slavish adherence over time to the original ideas is not productive. What has to be done is to describe current practice and new developments and to submit them to clinical evaluation. It is no longer legitimate to maintain that something works without supporting evidence.

Therapists often feel strongly that they owe all patients a duty of care which should be reflected in terms of similar treatment time for all. However, unless programmes are tailored to individual patient needs and to likely outcomes of treatment, they are unlikely to produce optimum results. Very lengthy treatment programmes which produce little effect may be demoralising for the patient. A stroke patient who stays in hospital for 3 months and still cannot walk when discharged will have become institutionalised and may find resettlement back home more difficult than an earlier discharge with full social support.

Hospitals and countries vary widely in the amount and type of treatment they offer for different conditions. For example, the amount of time spent in hospital following a stroke can vary from weeks to months and therapists are often the ones to make the decision to keep patients in longer. However, to date, there is little evidence beyond the anecdotal to suggest that keeping patients in hospital for months only for rehabilitation achieves better results than earlier discharge home with continuing treatment when necessary.

A more flexible system could be where patients are consulted and their wishes taken into account and a type of triage principle operated. At one end of the spectrum early transfer of patients with mild disabilities to health clubs and gymnasia would not only help to maintain fitness but would do so in a normal atmosphere, weaning the patient, particularly younger ones, from hospital at the earliest opportunity. At the other end of the spectrum there should be a recognition that for some patients with severe disabilities long hospital stays are unlikely to be successful, and the emphasis may have to be on prevention of secondary disabilities with full social support. Concentrating on those patients in the middle range, where success has been shown to be more likely (Kalra et al 1994) might be a better allocation of resources. We need to have clear criteria for deciding on allocation of patients to the different streams, with the opportunity to change streams should later recovery occur. Another option is for therapists to focus more specifically on educating the nurses and other ward staff in working with patients with neurological conditions in a more formal way (Holmqvist & Wrethagen 1986).

The challenge is considerable but the future looks bright if both clinicians and researchers can come together to address the important issues and be prepared to think in innovative ways, and perhaps abandon some of the shibboleths that have ruled for so long. Many of the changes now being forced on physiotherapy practice are long overdue, such as clearly demonstrating what does and what does not achieve good results and being able to predict the likely outcome of different treatment programmes. If the pro-fession can grasp the opportunities now and hone their problem-solving skills both in the clinical situation and in the wider world of service provision, in the future, improved treat-ment and management can be offered to neuro-logical patients.

REFERENCES

Affolter F 1980 Perceptual processes as prerequisites for complex human behaviour. International Rehabilitation Medicine 3: 3–9

Bithell C 2000 Evidence based physiotherapy. Physiotherapy 86: 58–60

Bobath B 1970 Adult hemiplegia evaluation and treatment. Heinemann Medical Books, Oxford

Bobath B 1990 Adult hemiplegia evaluation and treatment. Heinemann Medical Books, Oxford

Brocklehurst J C, Andrews A, Richards B, Laycock P 1978 How much physical therapy for patients with stroke? British Medical Journal 1: 1307–1310

Brosseau L, Tousignant M, Budd J et al 1997 Inter and intra tester reliability of the balance performance monitor in a non patient population. Physiotherapy Research International 2: 150–167

Brunström S 1970 Movement therapy in hemiplegia, a neurophysiological approach. Harper and Row, Hagerstown, New Jersey

Carr J H, Shepherd R B 1982 A motor relearning programme for stroke. Heinemann Medical Books, Oxford

Chomsky N 1969 The acquisition of syntax in children 5–10. MIT Press, Cambridge

Grimley Evans J 1995 Evidence based and evidence biased medicine. Age and Ageing 24: 461–463

Haas B, Whitmarsh T 1998 Inter and intra tester reliability of the balance performance monitor in a non patient population. Physiotherapy Research International 3: 135–148

Hadorn D C 1996 Rating quality of evidence for clinical practice guidelines. Journal of Clinical Epidemiology 49: 749–754

Harms Ringdahl K 1998 What is physiotherapy? Editorial. Physiotherapy Research International 3: iv–v

Holmqvist L W, Wrethagen N 1986 Educational programmes for those involved in the total care of stroke patients. In: Banks M (ed) Stroke. Longman, Singapore

International Classification of Impairments, Disabilities and Handicaps (ICIDH) 1980 World Health Organisation, Geneva, Switzerland

International Classification of Functioning and Disability (ICIDH-2) 1999 World Health Organisation, Geneva, Switzerland

Kalra L, Smith D H, Crome P 1994 Stroke in patients over 75 years: outcome and prediction. Postgraduate Medical Journal 69: 33–36

Kuhn T 1970 The structure of scientific revolutions. University of Chicago Press, Chicago

Kwakkel G 1999 Intensity of leg and arm training after primary middle cerebral artery stroke: a randomised trial. Lancet 354: 191–196

Langhorne P, Wagenaar R, Partridge C J 1996 Physiotherapy after stroke: more is better? Physiotherapy Research International 1: 75–88

Lloyd G E R 1996 On ancient medicine. In: Polarity and analogy. Cambridge University Press, Cambridge, p 6

Logigian M K, Samuels M A, Falconer J, Zagar R 1983 Clinical exercise trial for stroke patients. Archives of Physical Medicine Rehabilitation 64: 364–367

Luria A R 1963 The role of speech in the regulation of normal and abnormal behaviour. Pergamon Press, Oxford

Magnus R 1926 Some results of studies of the physiology of posture. Lancet ii: 585–588

Magoun H W, Rhines H 1948 Spasticity, the stretch reflex and the extrapyramidal system. C C Thomas, Springfield, Illinois

Munson R 1981 Why medicine cannot be a science. Journal of Medical Philosophy 6: 183–208

Partridge C J, De Weerdt W 1995 Different approaches to physiotherapy in stroke. Reviews in Clinical Gerontology 5: 199–209

Piaget J 1936 Origins of intelligence in children (reprinted 1952). International Universities Press, New York

Riddock G, Buzzard E F 1921 Reflex movements and postural reactions in quadriplegia and hemiplegia with special reference to those of the upper limb. Brain 44: 397–489

Rosner B S 1970 Brain functions. Annual Reviews in Psychology 21: 555–594

Sackett D L Rosenberg W M, Gray J A, Haynes R B, Richardson W S 1996 Evidence based medicine: what it is and what it isn't. British Medical Journal 312: 71–72

Sherrington C S 1931 Reflex inhibition as a factor in the coordination of movements and postures. Quarterly Journal of Experimental Physiology 6: 251–259

Stephenson R, Edwards S, Freeman J 1998 Associated reactions: their value in clinical practice. Physiotherapy Research International 3: 69–76

Tonelli M R 1990 In defense of expert opinion. Academic Medicine 74: 1187–1192

USA Office of Technology Assessment of the Congress of the United States 1995 The impact of RCTs on health policy and medical practice. US Government Printing Office, Washington DC, 1983

Index